GUIDE TO

Nursing Management and Leadership

GUIDE TO

FIFTH EDITION

Nursing Management and Leadership

Ann Marriner-Tomey, R.N., Ph.D., FAAN

Dean and Professor
Indiana State University School of Nursing
Nursing Management Consultant
Terre Haute, Indiana

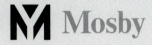

St. Louis Baltimore Boston Carlsbad Chicago Naples New York Philadelphia Portland
London Madrid Mexico City Singapore Sydney Tokyo Toronto Wiesbaden

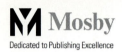

Mosby

Dedicated to Publishing Excellence

A Times Mirror Company

Publisher   Nancy L. Coon
Executive Editor   N. Darlene Como
Developmental Editor   Dana Knighten
Project Manager   Peggy Fagen
Editing and Production   Graphic World Publishing Services
Designer   Jeanne Wolfgeher

FIFTH EDITION

Copyright © 1996 by Mosby–Year Book, Inc.

Previous editions copyrighted 1980, 1984, 1988, 1992

Printed in the United States of America
Composition by Graphic World, Inc.
Printing/binding by R.R. Donnelley & Sons Company

Mosby–Year Book, Inc.
11830 Westline Industrial Drive
St. Louis, MO 63146

Library of Congress Cataloging-in-Publication Data

Marriner-Tomey, Ann, 1943-
     Guide to nursing management/Ann Marriner-Tomey.—5th ed.
       p.   cm.
     Includes bibliographical references and index.
     ISBN 0-8151-6401-7
     1. Nursing services—Administration.   I. Title.
     [DNLM: 1. Nursing, Supervisory.   WY 105 M359g 1995]
     RT89.M39   1995
     362.1'73'068—dc20
     DNLM/DLC
     for Library of Congress   173573   95–18304
                                                        CIP

96 97 98 99 00 / 9 8 7 6 5 4 3 2 1

To David and Natasha

Preface

Management skills are as important to nurse administrators as their clinical knowledge and skills. Unfortunately, beginning in the early 1960s, nursing education emphasized clinical skills at the expense of managerial expertise, and nurses who were interested in leadership and management had to turn to other disciplines. The bias was reflected in the dearth of writings on management in nursing literature and has been corrected only in the last decade.

The rapid changes during the 1980s with the increase in better educated personnel and increased technology to handle management functions brought about a focus on leadership. Computers could now be used to help make policy and procedure changes, calculate budgets, design organization structures, order supplies and equipment, project staffing patterns, keep personnel records, manage patient classification systems, complete staffing schedules, and communicate with personnel, all of which saved managers considerable time from when these and other managerial functions were done by hand. It became apparent that the leadership needed to get work done through others was increasingly important. Additionally, transformational leaders who had vision and could motivate associates to work toward common goals through active participation could help organizations survive and even thrive during rapid change.

Guide to Nursing Management and Leadership is designed to teach nursing students about the management process and leadership and to supply the practicing nurse with practical information about nursing administration. The management process—plan, organize, staff, direct, and control—is the conceptual framework. Leadership content is integrated. I have drawn on hundreds of articles on such topics as staffing and quality assurance that have appeared in the nursing literature, synthesizing and organizing the content to make it readily retrievable and more meaningful. In addition, I have incorporated the contributions of other disciplines' sources—notably business and the social sciences—that are not readily available to most nurses. This type of approach is long overdue in nursing and should help prepare middle and top managers to deal with the tasks before them. Portions of this book have appeared as articles in the *American Journal of Nursing, Journal of Nursing Administration, Nursing Leadership, Nursing Management,* and *Supervisor Nurse.* Articles are identified at the end of each chapter, related books at the end of each section, and general books in the General Bibliography.

I want to express appreciation to Sherri Beaver and Chian-Huei Ling for doing computer searches and to Jan Arnett, Frederic Arnold, Fran Drake, Kandi Dunn, Betsy Frank, Debbi Perkins, and Marina Wolf for consultation regarding content. I also want to thank my loving husband for enriching my private life while supporting my professional activities and helping me maintain balance.

ANN MARRINER-TOMEY

Contents

Part Four   Direct   265

Chapter 16 Theories of Leadership,   267

Chapter 17 Development of Management Thought,   280

Introduction: The Management Process

The management process is universal. It is used in one's personal life as well as one's professional life. One applies it to management of oneself, a patient, a group of patients, or a group of workers. Although management process, principles, and tools can be used in a variety of situations, this presentation will focus on the process in nursing administration and the management of an agency and workers.

The management process is composed of five major functions: (1) planning, (2) organizing, (3) staffing, (4) directing, and (5) controlling (see Figure I-1). Planning is the first function, and all other functions are dependent on it. Conceptual thinking and problem solving are crucial. Data are gathered and analyzed so that alternatives can be identified and evaluated in the decision-making process. The manager must forecast what is needed for the future, set objectives for the desired results, and develop strategies for how to achieve the goals. Priorities must be set, and the strategies need to be sequenced in a time frame to accomplish the goals. Policies and procedures are developed in the planning phase. Policies are standing decisions about recurring matters, and procedures standardize methods. Budgets are used as planning and controlling tools to allocate resources. Planning is the basis for time management, which will in turn facilitate the implementation of the plans.

Organizing is the second managerial function. Having planned, the manager now organizes so that personnel can implement the plans with efficiency and effectiveness. An organizational structure is established and shown on an organizational chart. Relationships are delineated, depicted on the organizational chart, and described in position descriptions that define the scope of responsibilities, relationships, and authority. Job analysis, evaluation, and design help define qualifications for persons in each position on the organizational chart.

Staffing includes recruiting, selecting, orienting, and developing personnel to accomplish the goals of the organization. It also involves determining assignment systems, such as case method, functional, team, modular, primary nursing, case management and/or managed care, and selecting staffing schedules to meet the needs of clients, personnel, and institution. There are many variables to be considered, and the more accurately they are assessed, the higher the probability of containing costs while providing high-quality care.

After managers have planned, organized, and staffed, they must direct personnel and activities to accomplish the goals of the organization. Knowledge of one's leadership style, managerial philosophy, sources of power and authority, and political strategies is important. To get work done by others, the leader must resolve conflicts and motivate and discipline staff. People are led by envisioning the preferred future, modeling desirable behavior, encouraging accomplishments, and enabling others. All these tasks require good communication skills and assertive behavior.

Controlling is the last step in the management process. It ensures progress toward objectives according to plan and involves setting standards, measuring performance against those standards, reporting the results, taking corrective actions, and rewarding performance as appropriate. Controls should be designed for specific situations and should reveal potential or actual deviations promptly enough for corrective action to be effective.

Leadership is integrated throughout the book. The difference between leadership and management is the difference between effectiveness and efficiency (see Table I-1). Effectiveness is related to leadership, vision, and judgment. Efficiency is related to management and mastering routines. It is best when an administrator is both a leader and a manager. Things are managed. People are led. Bennis and Nanus (1985) have indicated that managers do things right and leaders do the right thing. Both leadership and management are important in administration.

During the late 1980s, there was great emphasis on restructuring the workplace toward professional nursing practice and self-governance to retain nurses. This lent itself to an egalitarian philosophy. In keeping with this philosophy, the term *supervisor*

Table I-1 Comparison of Leadership and Management

Concept	Leadership	Management
Motto	Do the right thing	Do things right
Challenge	Change	Continuity
Focus	Purpose	Procedures, structure
Method	Strategy	Schedules
Outcomes	Journeys	Destinations
People	Potential	Performance
Questions	Why?	Who? What? When? Where? How?
Time frame	Present to future	Past to present

was changed to *manager* and *subordinate* to *staff associate* in the fourth edition of the book. During the early 1990s, multidisciplinary teams flourished and nurses needed to work more autonomously to provide health care in the community in response to health care reform. The fifth edition reflects this shift in emphasis and the increased need for critical thinking skills that has accompanied it.

One

Plan

Nature and Purpose of Planning

Planning is the first function of management. All other management functions—organizing, staffing, directing, and controlling—depend on planning. Nurse managers need to be familiar with the decision-making process and tools so that they can identify the purpose of the institution, state the philosophy, define goals and objectives, prepare budgets to implement their plans, and effectively manage their time and that of the organization.

Chapter 1

Strategic and Operational Planning

Chapter Objectives

◆ Identify at least two differences between strategic and operational planning.

◆ Describe at least five changes in health care delivery systems that need to be taken into account in strategic planning.

◆ Identify at least five benefits of strategic planning.

◆ Explain the relationships among purpose, philosophy, goals, and objectives.

Major Concepts and Definitions

Strategic planning	long-range planning extending 3 to 5 years into the future
Operational planning	short-range planning that deals with day-to-day maintenance activities
Belief	conviction that certain things are true
Value	the worth, usefulness, or importance of something
Purpose	an aim to be accomplished; mission statement
Philosophy	statement of beliefs and values that directs behavior
Goal	the end to be accomplished
Objective	something aimed at or striven for; things done to achieve the goal

PLANNING PROCESS

There are two major types of organizational planning: long-range or strategic planning and short-range or operational planning. Strategic planning extends 3 to 5 years into the future. It begins with in-depth analysis of the internal environment's strengths and weaknesses and the external opportunities and threats so that realistic goals can be set for the preferred future. It determines the direction of the organization, allocates resources, assigns responsibilities, and determines time frames. Strategic planning goals are more generic and less specific than operational planning.

Nurse managers are more likely to be involved in the operational or short-range planning. Operational planning is done in conjunction with budgeting, usually a few months before the new fiscal year. It develops the departmental maintenance and improvement goals for the coming year.

History of Strategic Planning

Private business started using strategic planning in the mid-1950s when the demand for products began to level off and decline and substitute products became available from foreign competitors. The health care industry started during the mid-1970s when the federal government established restricted payment regulations. Third-party payers also developed restrictions, and payment shifted from the federal government to individuals and other payers. This increased price sensitivity and competition. Alternative delivery systems such as preferred provider arrangements, health maintenance organizations, self-help and wellness programs, and ambulatory services proliferated. As chief executive officers looked at job redesign to increase productivity while cutting costs, mergers, acquisitions, joint ventures, and informal networking increased.

High-cost technology responded to the competitive environment, with greater acuity of care in acute-care settings, tertiary settings, and homes. At the same time the population was aging, increasing numbers of the population were under- and uninsured. Quality of life and ethics also became important issues. Consequently, strategic planning became prevalent in health care settings and literature during the 1980s.

Purpose of Strategic Planning

Strategic planning clarifies beliefs and values: What are the organization's strengths and weaknesses? What are the potential opportunities and threats? Where is the organization going? How is it going to get there? It gives direction to the organization, improves efficiency, weeds out poor or underused programs, eliminates duplication of efforts, concentrates resources on important services, improves communications and coordination of activities, provides a mind-expanding opportunity, allows adaptation to the changing environment, sets realistic and attainable yet challenging goals, and helps ensure goal achievement.

Leaders need vision that is realistic and feasible. Development of a strategic vision involves analysis of the agency's environment, capabilities, and resources; development and articulation of a conceptual image; clarification of values; development of a mission statement; identification of goals and objectives; and identification of strategies for reaching the goals. The strategic vision should be clear, cohesive, consistent, and flexible.

Strategic Planning Process

It is important that top-level administrators are committed to strategic planning. Otherwise, such planning may just be viewed as busy work. Managers need to be taught the importance of long-range planning and the way to do it.

A situation audit or environmental assessment analyzes the past, current, and future forces that affect the organization. Expectations of outside interests such as opinion leaders, governmental officials, insurance companies, and consumers are sought. Expectations of inside interests such as doctors, staff, administrators, and patients are collected.

The management team can use a grid to visualize the situation audit (see Worksheet 1-1 at the end of this chapter). The past, present, and future are represented on the horizontal axis. Clients, competition, market share, environmental-demographic, economic, legal, political, technological, resources-facilities, financial, and human resources and other criteria are represented on the vertical axis.

A WOTS-up (weaknesses, opportunities, threats, and strengths) analysis worksheet is also helpful. Each quadrant of a paper is labeled as one of the four categories, and appropriate factors are listed in each quadrant for a bird's-eye view of the situation audit (see Worksheet 1-2 at the end of this chapter). Internal strengths or weaknesses may include management development, qualifications of staff, medical staff expertise, abundance or scarcity of staff, financial situation, cash flow position, marketing efforts, market share, facilities, location, and quality of services.

Threats may be shortage of nurses, decrease in patient satisfaction, decrease in insured patients, increase in accounts receivable, decrease in demand for services, competition, regulations, litigation, legislative changes, unionization, and loss of accreditation.

Opportunities include nurse and physician recruitment, referral patterns, new programs, new markets, diversification, population growth, improved technology, and new facilities.

After the situation audit is done, the management team writes a purpose or mission statement, identifies organizational goals and objectives, plans strategies to accomplish the objectives, identifies required resources, determines priorities, sets time frames, and determines accountability.

PURPOSE OR MISSION STATEMENT

Organizations exist for a purpose. Clarification of the purpose is the first priority for planning. Most nursing services exist to provide high-quality nursing care to clients. Some also encourage teaching and research. Each specialty area, with its own specific purposes, contributes to the overall purpose of the institution: The purpose of the in-service education department is to orient staff to the job and to provide educational programs to improve the quality of the staff work. The burn unit exists to provide good-quality nursing service to patients with burns.

Purpose influences philosophy, goals, and objectives. For example, if a progressive care unit exists to help patients adjust to their diseases, it should be staffed with professional nurses particularly skilled in teaching and counseling. If, however, the unit's purpose is to cut hospital and patient expenses, it may be a minimal care unit with reduced services given by nonprofessional workers. The relationships among the purpose, philosophy, goals, and objectives should be examined periodically for consistency. See Box 1-1 for an example of a purpose statement.

PHILOSOPHY

The philosophy articulates a vision and provides a statement of beliefs and values that direct one's practice. It should be written, included in appropriate documents, and reviewed periodically. If the philosophy is stated in vague, abstract terms that are not easily understood, it is useless. Conflicting philosophies between overlapping units cause confusion and should be avoided. Workers are most likely to interpret the

Box 1-1   **SAMPLE PURPOSE**

The purpose of General Hospital is to combine scientific knowledge with unselfish service for healing the body, mind, and spirit. Related instruction, public service programs, and research will be facilitated in the interest of high-quality health care.

Box 1-2

SAMPLE PHILOSOPHY
DEPARTMENT OF NURSING SERVICE*

Nursing has a significant role in a society that values the maintenance and improvement of health along a positive continuum for individuals and groups. Nursing functions dependently, interdependently, and independently in its relationship with other health care providers—all of whom share goals of prevention of disease and disability, care of the ill, promotion and maintenance of optimal health for individuals and groups, and achievement of a dignified death.

The worth, dignity, and autonomy of individuals (employees, patients, and others) are recognized, as is each individual's right to self-direction and responsibility for his or her own life. Although individuals vary in their ability to adapt to stressors in a dynamic environment, each possesses the ability and potential to learn to adapt more constructively. Additionally, each has basic physical, social, emotional, and spiritual needs that are expressed in the environment in which the individual lives and must be responded to on the basis of the uniqueness of that individual and his or her environment, needs, and previous experiences.

The function of the department of nursing service is to provide an organizational structure conducive to provision of high-quality nursing care, most effective use of resources, and support and participation in education and research programs. It must manage the activities for which it is directly responsible and provide for the professional growth of its employees.

In addition, the department of nursing service encourages the use of the most up-to-date knowledge available, constantly adding to that body of knowledge, teaching others to employ the knowledge constructively to improve health care and its delivery system, and providing a milieu in which these activities can take place. In fulfilling this responsibility the department of nursing service encourages knowledge expansion by providing assistance with, and participation in, the educational and research activities of the medical center. Opportunities for knowledge acquisition are provided by workshops, classes, seminars, conferences, clinical experiences, and so on, for all nursing personnel and by encouragement of personnel's continuing their own developmental and educational pursuits.

The primary emphasis of the department of nursing service is the provision of patient care; therefore, all nursing personnel (including the administrative staff) must maintain a clinical component and excellence in nursing practice.

Research and educational pursuits are directed toward the amelioration of the provision of health care to all individuals and groups in our society, the improvement of the provision of health care delivery system, and the effective use of nursing personnel (inclusive of role expansion and innovative uses of nursing personnel) based on competence, education, skill, knowledge, ability, and training.

To achieve the level of nursing care desired, the nursing care provider must develop respectful, understanding relationships and use systematic problem-solving and decision-making processes based on accurate assessments, appropriate knowledge, and sound judgment. The nursing care provider must be able to effectively interact with individuals and groups under stress and to terminate those interactions when they are no longer needed or can no longer be used by the recipient.

> The department of nursing service recognizes the need to strive toward the achievement of shared goals for nursing with the school of nursing and to provide opportunities for the involvement of the nursing service in the educational process and nursing education in the nursing care process. The department of nursing service collaborates with medical and hospital administration in the management of the hospitals, determines and manages its own practice, and works with other departments in the hospitals to improve care provision, resource use, and educational and research endeavors. Additionally, the department of nursing service shares responsibility with other major departments and divisions in the medical center aimed at excellence of care provision, effective resource use, and support of educational and research endeavors.
>
> *Adapted from Department of Nursing Service Philosophy, University of Colorado Medical Center.

philosophy from the pronouncements and actions of the leaders in the institution. Therefore, conformity of action to belief is important.

When developing or reevaluating a philosophy, the manager should consider theory, education, practice, research, and nursing's role in the total organization. Poteet (1988) identified three approaches that can be used to incorporate nursing theory into the philosophy. An eclectic approach would select ideas from various nursing theories and incorporate them into the philosophy statements: a theory might be adopted and integrated into the philosophy, or another might be referred to throughout. Attaching an explanation of the theory to the philosophy would also be useful.

Myra Levine and Dorothea Orem focus on nursing therapeutics. Dorothy Johnson and Sister Callista Roy emphasize the client. Imogene King, Margaret Newman, Ida Orlando, Josephine Patterson, Loretta Zderad, Joyce Travelbee, and Ernestine Wiedebach discuss interaction. Martha Rogers focuses on the environment and human being interactions.

It is appropriate to comment on skill levels needed, advanced preparation for certain positions, need for continuing education, provision of educational opportunities for students, and specific practice modalities. Value of applying research findings to practice, supporting research efforts, and nursing's role in the overall organization should also be clarified in the philosophy. See Box 1-2 on p. 6.

GOALS AND OBJECTIVES

Goals and objectives state actions for achieving the purpose and philosophy. In fact, if the purpose and philosophy are to be more than good intentions, they must be translated into explicit goals. The more quantitative the goal, the more likely its achievement is to receive attention and the less likely it is to be distorted. Goals are central to the whole management process—planning, organizing, staffing, directing, and controlling. Planning defines the goals. The institution is organized and staffed to accomplish the goals. Direction stimulates personnel toward accomplishment of the objectives, and control compares the results with the objectives to evaluate accomplishments.

Box 1-3   **SAMPLE GOALS AND OBJECTIVES**
DEPARTMENT OF NURSING SERVICE*

I. *Goal:* Staff development programs continue to increase in importance as a result of technological advances and increased specialization. Programs designed to meet this increased need for knowledge must be promoted, as must leadership development programs.
Objective: To increase effectiveness and efficiency of staff development programs with emphasis on clinically specialized knowledge and leadership development programs.
  A. To continue the development, implementation, and evaluation of programs for nursing service personnel.
  B. To evaluate and revise as appropriate the patient care coordinator orientation and ongoing staff development program.
  C. To develop an orientation and ongoing staff development program for staff associates.
  D. To evaluate the efficiency and effectiveness of the nursing assistant program and role and recommend appropriate alternatives.
II. *Goal:* Personnel use must be efficient and effective with responsibility and tasks performed correlated with education, knowledge, and competence.
Objective: To evaluate and increase efficiency and effectiveness of nursing service personnel.
  A. To increase the use of interunit consultation among nursing service personnel.
  B. To coordinate and evaluate the preoperative teaching program with the surgical patient care units and the preoperative patient assessment performed by operating room personnel.
  C. To evaluate the cost-effectiveness of delivery systems.
  D. To initiate the development of standards of performance for selected nursing service job classifications.
  E. To evaluate various staffing methodologies by considering flexibility in addition to efficiency and effectiveness.
III. *Goal:* Health care costs continue to raise significant concern as increasing external controls are implemented. All nursing service positions must be justifiable with specific, validated tools.
Objective: To evaluate and justify staffing patterns in each patient care area.
  A. To complete the implementation of the patient classification tool in all inpatient clinical areas.
  B. To identify a tool to measure patient complexity in the ambulatory care setting and test the validity of the tool.
  C. To use data comparing hours of patient care provided with hours of patient care needed to adjust staffing patterns.
IV. *Goal:* Accountability of the health care provider and regulation of health care quality continue to receive increased emphasis by external agencies; therefore, concurrent and retrospective audit of nursing care must be ongoing, with data collected used for quality of care improvements and maintenance.

Objective: To establish and implement a concurrent audit system while continuing retrospective audits for the purpose of quality of care improvements.

A. To complete one new retrospective audit in each clinical area.
B. To continue combined medical and nursing audits in each clinical area.
C. To reaudit all diagnoses that required corrective actions to determine the effectiveness of the actions.
D. To delineate the type of concurrent audit system to be used and initiate its implementation.

*Adapted from Department of Nursing Service Goals, University of Colorado Medical Center.

Goals and objectives may address services rendered, economics, use of resources—people, funds, and facilities—innovations, and social responsibilities. Objectives are selective rather than global, are multiple, and cover a wide range of activities. The immediate, short-term, and long-term goals need to be balanced, interdependent, and ranked in order of importance. It is common to have more short-term than long-term goals.

Classic theory contends that the board of directors and top administration should determine institutional goals. Behavioral scientists are interested in having workers involved in setting goals and identifying real versus stated goals. The real goals can be identified by observing the day-by-day decisions and actions. Service interest, profit motives, governmental regulations, union representation, and personal goals all influence decision making.

It is appropriate for the board of directors and top administrators to set institutional goals and objectives; for the vice president for nursing, directors of nurses, and patient care coordinators to set the goals and objectives for the nursing service; for the staff associates to determine the unit goals and objectives; and for the nurses to determine their goals and objectives with their immediate manager. The overlap created by the vice president and director's working on institutional and nursing service goals and the patient care coordinator's contributing to nursing service and his or her unit's goals help facilitate continuity and compatibility of goals. Participation in the determination of goals and objectives increases commitment, transforming them from stated to real goals. Because goals are dynamic, they change over time. They should be reviewed periodically so that they can be changed in an evolutionary rather than a radical manner. Goals should be specific rather than vague and challenging yet reachable. Necessary support elements should be available. See Box 1-3.

The planning process is a critical element of management. It must be learned by nurse administrators, because it will not happen by accident. Planning is largely conceptual, but its results are clearly visible. The statement of the purpose or mission, philosophy, goals, and objectives are all consequences of planning. They set the stage for smooth operations.

BIBLIOGRAPHY

Bryant L, Dobal M, Johnson E: Strategic planning: collaboration and empowerment, *Nurs Connections* 3:31-36, Fall 1990.
Buchana A: Strategic planning for tomorrow's success, *Caring* 11:52-57, November 1992.

Carroll AB: Three types of management planning: making organizations work, *Management Quarterly* 34:32-36, Spring 1993.

Duncan H: Strategic planning theory today, *Optimum* 20:633-674, Winter 1989/1990.

El-Namaki MSS: Creating a corporate vision, *Long Range Plann* 25:25-29, December 1992.

Eubanks P: Tallahassee Memorial: focusing the culture on customer service, *Hospitals* 66:40-42, August 5, 1992.

Howard LS, Mabon SA, Piland NF: Nursing department strategy, planning, and performance in rural hospitals, *JONA* 23:23-34, April 1993.

Lantz J, Fullerton JT, Dowling W: A community strategic planning for elder services, *JONA* 23:47-52, October 1993.

Matejka K, Kurt L, Gregory B: Mission impossible? Designing a great mission statement to ignite your plans, *Management Decision* 31:34-37, 1993.

Muller-Smith P: Beyond the basics: enhancing management skills, *J Post Anesthesia Nursing* 8:410-412, Dec 1993.

Peters J: On vision and values, *Management Decision* 31:14-17, 1993.

Peters J: On objectives, *Management Decision* 31(6):28-30, 1993.

Poteet GW, Hill AS: Identifying the components of a nursing philosophy, *J Nurs Adm* 18:29-33, 1988.

Smeltzer CH, Hinshaw AS: Integrating research in a strategic plan, *Nurs Manage* 24:42-44, February 1993.

Smith HL, Mabon SA, Piland NF: Nursing department strategy, planning, and performance in rural hospitals, *JONA* 23:23-34, April 1993.

Thomas AM: Strategic planning: a practical approach, *Nurs Manage* 24:34-38, February 1993.

Wilson I: Realizing the power of strategic vision, *Long Range Plann* 25:18-28, October 1992.

Zabriskie NB, Huellmantel AB: Developing strategic thinking in senior management, *Long Range Plann* 24:25-32, December 1991.

CASE STUDY

Lake View Hospital is a 98-bed general hospital. Its organizational chart is shown in the Appendix. It is one of two hospitals serving an industrial community with a population of about 90,000. Patients are being discharged earlier so there is an increasing vacancy rate on the medical-surgical units. At the same time there is an increasing demand for geriatric services and ambulatory care. Demands for home health have also increased.

CRITICAL THINKING AND LEARNING ACTIVITIES

Using the case study above, complete the following tasks:

1. Consider current trends and do a situation audit using Worksheet 1-1. Hypothesize about the information not provided in the case study based on what is happening in your community.

2. Do a WOTS-up analysis using Worksheet 1-2.

3. Write the purpose of Lake View Hospital.

4. Write the philosophy for Lake View Hospital.

5. Develop the goals and objectives for one of the units.

✍ Worksheet 1-1

Situation Audit			
Criteria	Past	Present	Future
Clients			
Competition			
Market share			
Environment			
Demographics			
Economics			
Laws			
Politics			
Technology			
Facilities			
Finances			
Human resources			

✍ **Worksheet 1-2**

WOTS-Up Analysis

Weaknesses	Strengths

Threats	Opportunities

Chapter
2

Decision-Making Process

Chapter Objectives

◆ List five steps in the decision-making process.

◆ Identify at least six techniques to increase creativity.

◆ Describe at least two ethical positions that can be used to consider moral dilemmas.

Major Concepts and Definitions	
Decision-making process	the process of selecting one course of action from alternatives
Critical thinking	the ability to question philosophically and exercise careful judgment when evaluating a situation
Creativity	intellectual inventiveness
Consultation	an interactive, helping relationship between two parties
Ethics	a moral philosophy that examines how means are related to ends and how to control means to serve human ends

DECISION-MAKING PROCESS

Decision-making, the process of selecting one course of action from alternatives, is a continuing responsibility of nurse managers. They are confronted by a variety of situations. Hospital or agency policies provide guidelines for dealing with routine situations. Exceptional instances can make decisions more difficult and may require a mature sense of judgment. Problem solving is a skill that can be learned, and because staff nurses can learn by observing their leaders, good decision making by the leader may do more than solve immediate problems; more important for the long term, it can foster good decision making by staff nurses.

Decision making relies on the scientific problem-solving process: identifying the problem, analyzing the situation, exploring alternatives and considering their consequences, choosing the most desirable alternative, implementing the decision, and evaluating the results. See Box 2-1.

Identify the Problem and Analyze the Situation

The first step in the decision-making process is defining the problem. What is wrong? Where is improvement needed? Sometimes the problem seems obvious and can be

Box 2-1   **DECISION-MAKING PROCESS**

1. Identify the problem and analyze the situation

2. Explore the alternatives

3. Choose the most desirable alternative

4. Implement the decision

5. Evaluate the results

dealt with routinely. If the employee repeatedly reports late to work or abuses the privilege of sick leave, the manager can respond in accordance with agency policies. However, when managers are concerned only with the infraction, they may be dealing with the effect rather than the cause of the problem. Consequently, similar situations may continue. It is important to define the factors that are causing the problem. For instance, two staff nurses may each complain about the intrusion of the other into his or her work. Initially the problem may appear to be a personality clash or a political power struggle. However, the cause may be the manager's failure to define the job responsibilities of each nurse. As long as the manager concentrates on the symptom instead of the problem, the difficulties will arise. It is only when the real problem has been identified that effective decision making can be initiated.

Nurse managers can identify the problem by analyzing the situation. All too frequently, decisions are made and implemented before all the facts have been gathered. To prevent this the manager should have a questioning attitude. What is the desirable situation? What are the presenting symptoms? What are the discrepancies? Who is involved? When? Where? How? With answers to these questions managers can develop tentative hypotheses and test them against what they know. Progressive elimination of hypotheses that fail to conform to the facts reduces the number of causes to be considered. Feasible hypotheses should be further tested for causal validity. When managers believe they have identified the cause or causes of the problem by analyzing available information, they should begin exploring possible solutions.

Explore the Alternatives

There are usually a number of ways to solve a problem. Some may be quick and economical but less effective than their alternatives. Others may be more effective but less economical. If various alternatives are not explored, the course of action is limited.

When solving a problem, managers should determine first whether the situation is covered by policy. If it is not, they must draw on their education and experience for facts and concepts that will help them determine alternatives. Using one's experience is probably the most common approach to solving problems, but it may be inadequate. The more experience the manager has had, the more alternatives may be suggested to solve a variety of problems. However, health care changes rapidly, and solutions to yesterday's problems may not work today. Consequently, managers should look beyond their own experiences and learn how others are solving similar problems. This can be done through continuing education, professional meetings, review of the literature, correspondence, and brainstorming with staff. Inductive and deductive reasoning are both appropriate.

Choose the Most Desirable Alternative

The number and quality of alternatives depend largely on the creativity and productivity of managers and their staff. Leadership that prevents immediate acceptance of an apparently obvious solution and facilitates group exploration of decision-making opportunities (such as problems to solve) usually increases the number of alternatives and the quality of problem solving.

Eagerness to reach a decision may lead to premature solutions; on the other hand, considering only a few alternatives in haste blocks good decisions. Avoidance of the real problem, lack of clear problem definition, insufficient data, early statement of attitude by a status figure, mixing of idea generation and idea evaluation, lack of staff commitment because the superior who makes the decision does not implement it, and decisions made by large groups also interfere with reaching effective solutions.

One alternative is not always clearly superior to all others. The manager must try to balance such factors as patient safety, staff acceptance, morale, public acceptance, cost, and risk of failure. Criteria for calculating the value of decisions are useful. The following questions may be asked: Will this decision accomplish the stated objectives? If it does not, it should not be enforced and another option should be used. Does it maximize effectiveness and efficiency? One should use available resources before seeking outside assistance. Finally, can the decision be implemented? If not, it obviously will not solve the problem.

Implement the Decision

After a decision has been made, it must be implemented. A decision that is not put into action is useless. The manager will need to communicate the decision to appropriate staff associates in a manner that does not arouse antagonism. The decision and procedures for its implementation can be explained in an effort to win the cooperation of those responsible for its implementation. The manager will need to select the staff associate to implement the decision and provide the direction to initiate action. Managers may need to control the environment so staff associates can function as planned. Once the decision has been implemented, it should be evaluated.

Evaluate the Results

The final step of decision making is evaluation of the results of the implementation of the chosen alternative. Evaluative criteria may have to be developed. Audits, checklists, ratings, and rankings can be used to review and analyze the results. Because solutions to old problems sometimes create new problems, additional decisions may need to be made and evaluated.

CRITICAL THINKING

Elements of reasoning are essential dimensions that provide general logic to reason. They include purpose or goal; central problem or question at issue; point of view or frame of reference; empirical dimension; conceptual dimension; assumptions, implications, and consequences; and inference and conclusion. See Box 2-2.

Purpose or goal.   All reasoning has purpose and needs clarity, significance, achievability, and consistency of purpose.

Central problem or question at issue.   All reasoning is an attempt to solve a problem, figure something out, or answer a question. To answer a question or solve a problem one must understand what it requires. There needs to be clarity and significance of the question, and the question needs to be relevant and answerable.

Box 2-2   **ELEMENTS OF CRITICAL THINKING AND REASONING**

Purpose or goal
Central problem or question at issue
Point of view or frame of reference
Empirical dimension
Conceptual dimension
Assumptions
Implications and consequences
Inference and conclusions

Outlined from Paul R: *Critical thinking,* Santa Rosa, CA, 1993, Foundation of Critical Thinking.

Point of view or frame of reference. All reasoning is done from a point of view. Reasoning is improved when multiple, relevant points of view are sought and when those points of view are articulated clearly, empathized with logically and fairly, and applied consistently and dispassionately.

Empirical dimension. Reasoning is only as sound as the evidence it is based on. The evidence should be clear, relevant, accurate, adequate, fairly gathered and reported, and consistently applied.

Conceptual dimension. Reasoning is only as relevant, clear, and deep as the concepts that form it. Concepts should be clear, deep, neutral, and relevant.

Assumptions. All reasoning is based on assumptions. Reasoning can only be as sound as the assumptions on which it is based. Assumptions should be clear, consistent, and justifiable.

Implications and consequences. All reasoning has implications, consequences, and direction. Understanding the implications and consequences is important to reason through a decision or issue. One must consider the clarity, completeness, precision, reality, and significance of articulated implications.

Inference and conclusions. All reasoning has inferences by which one draws conclusions and gives meaning to the data. Reasoning is only as sound as the inferences it makes and the conclusions it come to. Inferences should be clear and justifiable. Conclusions should be consistent, profound, and reasonable.

CREATIVE DECISION MAKING

The Creative Process

The creative process has steps similar to those of the problem-solving process, but the emphasis is different. Decision making stresses choice of a solution, whereas the creative process emphasizes the uniqueness of the solution. Creativity is a latent quality, activated when a person becomes motivated by the need for self-expression or by the stimulation of a problem. Thus the first phase of the creative process is a felt need. Similarly, when decision makers are confronted with a problem, they start seeking a solution.

The second phase of creative problem solving is a work stage known as preparation, from which creative ideas emerge. Innovation is partially dependent on the number of options considered. By exploring relationships among potential solutions, one may identify additional solutions. Many decisions are made after slight preparation and therefore result in commonplace solutions. Superficial analysis of obvious information does not facilitate creative answers. Extensive use of libraries for data collection is useful; the creative person may take notes on readings, develop them into files with other clippings and ideas, review these materials, and combine the most appropriate aspects of old solutions into new answers.

Incubation, the third phase, is a period for pondering the situation. Repetition of the same thoughts, with no new ideas or interpretations, is a sign of fatigue and indicates that it is a good time to start the incubation period. Switching one's attention provides a necessary respite, and yet the unconscious mind continues to deal with the problem. A time should be set to reexamine the situation and review the data collected during the preparation phase.

Illumination is the discovery of a solution. It may come to mind in the middle of the night or during the performance of another task. It is recommended that the idea be written down so the details can be preserved. Having paper and pencil readily available at all times (including in the bedside stand) is helpful.

It is rare for an illumination to be ready for adoption. Verification, the fifth and final phase of creative decision making, is the period of experimentation when the idea is improved through modification and refinement. The advantages and disadvantages of each alternative must be weighed; resources and constraints, such as personnel, finances, facilities, and equipment, have to be evaluated, and potential technical and human problems should be considered. Some decisions have failed at implementation because potential problems were not anticipated and dealt with. It would be unfortunate for an otherwise useful alternative to be rejected for a disadvantage that could be easily overcome. By comparing the advantages and disadvantages of the options, the manager can choose the most desirable alternative.

Encouraging Creativity

The thinking mechanism of the human brain has been conceptualized as having two sides. The right side is intuitive and conceptual and is used for uninhibited creative thinking. The left side is analytical and sequential. If we use the analogy of driving a car, the right side of the brain is a green light that keeps us going until we have generated a multiplicity of ideas. The left side is a red light that says stop and question whether this is worthwhile. The judicial left side of the brain analyzes and evaluates the creative ideas generated by the right side of the brain. We need to use both sides. We are usually socialized to use the left side more than the right side, but the right side can be stimulated. Box 2-3 lists some creative thinking techniques.

Box 2-3   **CREATIVE THINKING TECHNIQUES**

Brainstorming
Brainwriting
Collective notebook technique
Convergent thinking
Delphi technique
Divergent thinking
Drawing
Forecasting alternative future scenarios
Lists
Meditation
Modeling
Reverse brainstorming
Stepladder technique
Synetics
Visualization

Convergent thinking.   The problem is divided into smaller and smaller pieces to find a more manageable perspective.

Divergent thinking.   One's view of the problem is expanded. The problem is considered in different ways.

Brainstorming.   Under favorable circumstances a group working together can identify more ideas than an individual or that group of individuals working separately. Brainstorming is a technique leaders can use to create a free flow of ideas. They should encourage the members to contribute a large number of freewheeling ideas without fear of criticism or ridicule. This can improve the quality of ideas offered and result in new combinations through rearrangement, reversal, substitution, and other modifications.

Brainstorming seems to work best for simple and specific problems. Complex problems can be divided into parts and handled separately. If the problem is too complex, the discussion may lack focus and be very time-consuming. Brainstorming may be most useful when group members understand at least part of the problem. Although the session may not produce a viable solution, its stimulation may continue beyond the meeting and cause employees to take another look at their routinized activities.

Creativity is probably fostered best in permissive atmosphere in which mutual respect prevails and people are encouraged to express their views and ideas even if they are at variance with current policies and practices. A free interchange of ideas with considerable borrowing and adaptation fosters the production of creative ideas. This is a divergent way of thinking that apparently generates the largest number of creative ideas when people look for what can be used from "wild" ideas rather than criticizing them because they won't work.

Reverse brainstorming.   This encourages convergent thinking to break down ideas into smaller parts; analyze and focus on a particular problem or part of a problem. It is done verbally and works best for auditory or verbally oriented people.

Brainwriting.   Brainwriting encourages free association and recording of ideas without verbal interaction. A problem is identified. Participants are given a blank piece of paper and told to write at least four ideas, suggestions, solutions, and so forth. The paper is then passed to someone else. Reading others' ideas is intended to stimulate more ideas, which are then written on the page. The process continues until no one can think of anything else to write.

Collective notebook technique.   A problem is identified and participants are instructed to record thoughts and ideas about the problem for a specified period. Each participant gives his or her notebook to another person, who reads it, looks for patterns, and synthesizes the content. The participants then meet, analyze the results, and make recommendations to solve the problem.

Stepladder technique.   This technique structures the entry of group members into the group to ensure that each member contributes to the decision-making process. Initially, two group members try to solve a problem. Then a third member joins the core group and presents a preliminary solution to the problem. The entering person's presentation is discussed by all three persons. The process is repeated as group members are added.

   Each member is given the group's task and time to think about it before presenting to the group. The entering person presents preliminary solutions before the group comes to a final decision. There is a discussion after each entering person presents. The final decision is delayed until all members of the group have presented and are available to participate in the final decision.

The Delphi technique.   The Delphi technique allows members who are dispersed over a geographic area to participate in decision making without meeting face to face. A problem is identified, and members are asked to suggest potential solutions through the use of a questionnaire. Members anonymously return the first questionnaire, and the results are centrally compiled. Each member is sent a copy of the results; after viewing them, members are asked for their suggestions again. Review of the results of the first questionnaire typically triggers new solutions or stimulates changes in original positions. This process continues until consensus is reached. Little change usually occurs after the second round.

   The Delphi technique insulates group members from one another's influence and does not require physical presence, so it is particularly appropriate for scattered groups. Unfortunately, it is time-consuming and may not develop as many alternatives as the other techniques.

Lists.   The checklist method is used to assemble criteria on a checklist, sort it, prioritize it, eliminate items, and add others. An attribute list records characteristics. They are then rearranged in possible combinations of ideas. The scamper technique lists verbs that are idea-generating. *Scamper* is an acronym for substitute, combine, adapt, modify, put to other uses, eliminate, and reverse.

Drawing. Drawings can be used to evoke and record creative insight because intuitive consciousness communicates more readily in symbols and impressions than in words.

Synetics. Synetics is the joining together of apparently irrelevant elements. A problem is identified and a brief analysis given. The problem is then simplified to clarify it and reinterpreted in analogy or metaphor. The group then plays with the analogy. The analogy or metaphor chosen to represent the problem is considered in depth. The problem is thus redefined in a new light.

Visualization. Free association can be used to create a big dream approach. First, desired outcomes are visualized and then visually run backward to identify a new approach. Imagine what you would like: a phone that tells you who is calling before you answer it, that shows who is talking to you, that you do not have to touch to answer, that rings wherever you are (office, home, car, beach). Once you have imagined what you want, you can begin dreaming about how to make your dream a reality. This technique allows you to pretend that you already have what you want and facilitates concentration on the outcomes.

Forecasting alternative future scenarios. The future is often more a matter of choice than of chance. The choice is enhanced by forecasting potential scenarios—status quo, least preferred, most preferred, and not likely—and selecting the most desired. The process includes assessing the present situation, identifying its strengths and weaknesses, recognizing the driving forces in the environment, constructing possible alternative future scenarios, identifying the preferred future, developing a plan of action, implementing the plan, and evaluating the implementation.

Modeling. Look at how others are doing what you wish to do. However, be cautious: what works for someone else, somewhere else, may not work for you here and now. Similarly, what worked for you somewhere else or at some other time may not work now. Seek out what can be used or adapted, given the current situation and the preferred future.

Meditation. The optimal state for peak performance of athletes is relaxed concentration, or "playing loose." Meditation can generate a more focused state of relaxed attention.

Developing Creative Thinking Attitudes

People need to be open-minded about new ideas and the ideas of others. Inquiring minds are never satisfied. Creative people are not unduly concerned about the opinions of others, because many great ideas are first ridiculed and later accepted. People need to put aside critical, analytical, and judicial thinking while working creatively and move beyond their personal habits and attitudes. After numerous ideas have been generated, they can be judged and the best selected. Trust, acceptance, and good humor help create an environment conducive to creative problem solving. Creative people have an inner motivation, mental ability, objectivity, tolerance for complexity, enjoyment of risk taking, and ability to find problems.

Blocks to Creativity

Negative attitudes, self-censorship, lack of confidence, lack of effort, habits, conformity, and reliance on authority all block creativity.

CONSULTATION

Consultation is a helping relationship. It is a process of interaction between the consultant, who has the specialized knowledge and skills, and the consultee, who asks for assistance with problem solving. It has a beginning and an end and is a temporary, voluntary, educational relationship. The consultee identifies a problem and seeks help from an expert. Because the consultant is usually not a part of the hierarchical structure of the organization, the consultant is an outsider who advises. Implementation of the recommendations depends on the consultee, thus giving the process a take-it-or-leave-it quality. The consultation process usually involves problem solving, but the consultant may play several roles: helping identify problems, educating staff about related issues, identifying obstacles to problem solving, offering advice about how to solve problems, acting as a change agent, developing interpersonal relationships, mediating conflicts, or performing tasks that organizational members do not have the skill to perform. The consultant typically collects and analyzes data, recommends or intervenes, and then terminates the relationship.

Consultants become known by doing something and telling others about it, volunteering to present workshops and speeches, publishing books and articles, being active in professional organizations, circulating flyers and announcements, and being included in lists of consultants.

An internal consultant knows the system, history, political realities, norms, and language better than an outside consultant and will probably devote more time to the problem. Internal consultants are viewed as less costly because they are usually not compensated extra for consultative services. Unfortunately, there are disadvantages to hiring internal consultants. They may be part of the problem; lack perspective to see the whole; have no independence of movement; have no adequate power base; encounter resistance because of their relationship with the hierarchy, vested interest, or organizational politics; or have a limited background.

An external consultant has a more diverse background, brings new ideas and a different perspective to the situation, is independent of the power structure, and is consequently high powered. Unfortunately, the external consultant does not know the history and politics of the institution and may not care about them.

Once it has been determined that there is a need for consultation, what the purpose is, and who the consultant should be, a contractual agreement is necessary. The agreement may be verbal or written, but it should determine the fee, hours of the consultant's time, expected outcome, and criteria for termination. The fee may be negotiated as a flat fee, a fee based on hours spent at the agency that includes travel and preparation time, or an hourly rate for all the time the consultant spends on the project, including research and report writing. The hours are largely controlled by the compensation structure. The consultant may have a regular schedule or be "on call." In most cases the outcome is accepted whether it is judged acceptable or not. Common outcomes are a written analysis with recommendations, decisions reached, systems devised or revised, and projects completed. Usually the termination occurs at a natural closure point such as the resolution of the problem or completion of the project. However, contingency plans should be made in case there are personality conflicts or the project takes too long and exceeds the budget.

ETHICAL ASPECTS OF DECISION MAKING

Ethics is a moral philosophy, a science of judging the relationship of means to ends, and the art of controlling means so they will serve human ends. It involves conflict, choice, and conscience. When there is a conflict, there is a choice between conflicting alternatives. The choice is influenced by values. Values are learned first from important adults and are modified by association with people of different values. Value modification and reinforcement are lifelong processes. A value is consciously prized and cherished, freely chosen from alternatives, and acted on in a variety of ways. Ethical choices must also consider wants, needs, and rights: people may want what they do not need. Someone may want a dessert but not need it; in fact, it may be harmful. People often need what others also need. One who needs food to prevent starvation may have a right to receive food from people who have plenty, but not from someone who would starve without it. That would infringe on the other person's rights, and duty and right are correlated: it is one's duty to protect rights. A legal obligation is legislated, but it may not be ethical. A moral dilemma occurs when a decision has equally unsatisfactory alternatives.

There are several ethical positions that do not solve dilemmas. However, they do provide ways to structure and clarify them. *Utilitarianism* is a community-oriented position that focuses on the consequences and prefers the greatest amount of good and happiness for the most people, or the least amount of harm. In contrast, *egoism* seeks solutions that are best for oneself without regard for others. One's own pleasure is the concern. *Formalism* considers the nature of the act and the related principles without thought to personal position or consequences of the actions: be honest; remember the golden rule. *Rule* ethics expects obedience to laws, rules, professional codes, and authority. *Fairness* considers distribution of benefits and liabilities from the viewpoint of the least advantaged. Benefit to the least advantaged is the norm in this type of decision making.

There are also models for ethical relationships. In the *priestly model,* the manager is paternalistic and makes decisions without considering others' values or seeking others' input. Although nurses may have expertise that qualifies them to make some decisions, they have no right to make moral decisions affecting other people. Autocratic leadership may use the priestly model. The *engineering model* suggests that one person presents facts to another and sets aside her own code of ethics to do what the other wants; staff working for line authority may provide an example of this model. The *contractual model* provides a contract that identifies general obligations and benefits for two or more people. It deals with the morals of both parties and is appropriate for superior-subordinate relationships. In the *collegial model,* individuals share mutual goals and reach decisions through discussion and consensus. When there are shared values, this model helps build teams and minimize conflict.*

---

* Robert Veatch's models for ethical medicine are discussed in Aroskar MA: Ethics of nurse-patient relationships, *Nurse Educ* 5:18, 1980.

To make an ethical decision, one must first consider what is intended to be a means and an end and then determine what good or evil is found in the means and the end. If a major evil is intended either as a means or an end, it is an unethical decision.

If the ramifications of the decision are probable, but not willed as a means or an end, there are several factors to consider. The good or evil of each alternative should be evaluated: a necessary good outweighs a useful good; paying workers wages outweighs paying for profit sharing. Urgency increases the necessity; therefore, physical needs must be met before self-actualizing needs. An agency should provide adequate wages for food and shelter before providing continuing education. The probability of an outcome should be considered: a possible negative outcome is outweighed by a probable good; one will work to earn a living even though there is a slight risk of back strain. The intensity of one's influence is considered because one's impact on someone else may have undesirable consequences; for instance, if an employee is fired for incompetence, it may cause a hardship for the employee's family. If the manager did not tell the employee what was expected or how to do the job, the manager would have been a considerable factor in that employee's poor job performance. Firing the employee would seem evil. If, however, the staff associate is frequently tardy or absent through no fault of the manager, the consequences of firing the worker seem justified. If there is no proportionate reason for permitting an evil, the act is unethical. If there is an alternative that provides more good and less risk of evil, it should be chosen; if there is not, there is proportionate reason for risking an evil.

MORAL REASONING

Levels of moral development have been identified as (1) premoral or preconventional when behavior is motivated by social or biological impulses with no sense of obligation to rules; (2) conventional when the person accepts standards of the group with little critical reflection, uses literal obedience to the rules, and feels obligation; and (3) autonomous when the person thinks and judges for himself, considers the purpose and consequences of the rules, and does not accept the group standards without reflection.

Moral choice involves selecting one of two or more values that conflict. Ten universal moral values are distributive justice, law, liberty, life, property, punishment, roles and concerns of affection, roles and concerns of authority, sex, and truth.

The level of moral development determines what a person finds valuable, how she defines the value, and why she finds it valuable. First, a person considers the power of the person involved. Second, she looks at satisfying her own needs. Third, the individual considers relationships with others and then sees life as inherently worthwhile aside from other considerations. Moral judgment is necessary but not sufficient for mature moral action. People may do wrong even when they know better.

ETHICS COMMITTEES

Complex ethical issues regarding patient care and policymaking must be addressed. Institutional ethics committees deal with ethical questions that often require painful choices for patients, particularly for infants and those elderly adults who are unable to make their own decisions.

The following issues must be addressed within the institution's philosophy, both when forming an institutional ethics committee and through ongoing study and evaluation of the existing committee: responsibility, accountability, economic costs, efficacy, role of the committee in patient care decisions, privacy for the patients and families, and committee composition, structure, meetings, and access. Nursing should be represented on the committee.

BIBLIOGRAPHY

Alvino J: Future problem solving in the year 2000—challenges and opportunities for business, *Business Horizons* 36:16-22, November-December 1993.

Anonymous: Ideas, *American Salesman* 35:29-30, March 1990.

Burk ME: *Library Management* 14:4-8, 1993.

Busby A, Raub JR: Implementing an ethics committee in rural institutions, *JONA* 21:18-25, December 1991.

Czerwinski BS: An autopsy of an ethical dilemma, *JONA* 20:25-29, June 1990.

Donley R: Ethics in the age of health care reform, *Nurs Econ* 11:19-24, January-February 1993.

Drummond H: Another fine mess: time for quality in decision-making, *J General Management* 18:1-14, Autumn 1992.

Hamburger D: The project manager: risk taker and contingency planner, *Project Management J* 21:43-48, June 1990.

Johnson LJ: The influence of assumptions on effective decision-making, *JONA* 20:35-39, April 1990.

Johnson V: Intuition in decision-making, *Successful Meetings* 42:148-153, February 1993.

Kessler FA: How to avoid common pitfalls of consensus decision making, *Oil & Gas Journal* 91:34-36, September 27, 1993.

Marriner A: The decision-making process, *Supervisor Nurse* 8:58-67, February 1977.

Martin K, Leak G, Aden C: The Omaha System: a research-based model for decision making, *JONA* 22:47-52, November 1992.

Miller S: An ethical nursing practice model, *JONA* 23:22-25, March 1993.

Rogelberg SG, Barnes-Farrell JL, Lowe CA: The stepladder technique: an alternative group structure facilitating effective group decision making, *J Appl Psychol* 77:730-737, 1992.

Schlick JD: Critical thinking skills, *Quality* 31:15-18, August 1992.

Schwartz RH: Nurse decision-making influence: a discrepancy between the nursing and hospital literatures, *JONA* 20:35-39, June 1990.

Silver WS, Mitchell TR: The status quo tendency in decision making, *Organ Dyn* 18:34-46, Spring 1990.

Williams I: Business decisions: a spiritual approach? *Management Services* 34:14-16, December 1990.

CASE STUDY

Your organization has limited funds for personnel raises. You represent your unit on the agency budget committee. Should you give everyone the same dollar amount raise, thus giving a lower percentage raise to personnel with larger salaries? Should you give the same percentage raise across the board, thus giving people with higher salaries more money? Should the raises be stratified, giving different categories of people different dollar or percentage raises? What are other options?

CRITICAL THINKING AND LEARNING ACTIVITIES

1. Using Worksheet 2-1, problem solve the situation in the case study.

2. Using Worksheet 2-2, determine what your decision in the case study might be given different ethical viewpoints.

3. Identify a problem or try to generate a list of uses for a pencil. Divide the class in half. Half the class uses brainstorming to solve the problem or generate a list of uses for a pencil. The other half uses brainwriting for the same assignment. Compare the results. Discuss your feelings about using the techniques.

4. Do some self-assessing and determine your own level of moral development—premoral, conventional, or autonomous.

✍ Worksheet 2-1

Problem-Solving Tool

Define the problem:

Explore alternatives and expected results from each alternative. Consider the time to implement, cost of implementation, and probability of acceptance of the implementation.

What is the most desirable alternative?

Ethical Decisions

Given a problem, what would your decision be using the following ethical philosophies?

Utilitarianism—greatest amount of good and happiness for the most people or least amount of harm

Egoism—best for oneself without regard for others

Formalism—golden rule

Rule ethics—obedience to laws, rules, professional codes, and authority

Fairness—benefit to the least advantaged

Chapter

3

Decision-Making Tools

Chapter Objectives

- ◆ List at least five decision-making tools.
- ◆ Identify at least three models.
- ◆ Describe how to use a Gantt chart.
- ◆ Describe how computers can be applied in nursing.

Major Concepts and Definitions	
Tool	an instrument used to accomplish an end
Model	an abstraction or representation of something more complex
Probability	the likelihood of an event's occurrence
Simulation	an imitation of an event or process
Game theory	a simulation of system operations
Gantt chart	a tool used to visualize multiple tasks that need to be done
Decision tree	graphic tool to visualize alternatives available, chance events, and probable consequences
PERT	*program evaluation and review technique*
CPM	*critical path method* to calculate time estimate for activities
Queuing theory	a mathematical technique used to determine efficiency of intermittent services
Linear programming	matrix algebra or linear mathematical equations used to determine the best way to use limited resources for maximal results
Computer	an electronic machine that performs rapid calculations or compiles, correlates, and selects data by means of stored instructions and information
Vroom and Yetton Model	a tool used to identify autocratic, consultative, and group decision processes

DECISION-MAKING TOOLS

Most decisions involve varying degrees of uncertainty. Leaders and managers use research of various kinds to minimize the uncertainty of their decisions.

Probability Theory

Probability theory can be applied when risk or uncertainty is present in a decision. It operates on the assumption that factors occur in accordance with a predictable pattern. For example, if a person tosses a coin 200 times, we can predict that it will show heads 100 times and tails 100 times. Deviations can be set within a predictable margin. Inferences based on statistical analysis of existing data can be used to predict results.

Sometimes a sample of the population may be analyzed. Measures of probable error become increasingly important when one is dealing with a sample because the smaller the probable error, the greater the amount of confidence that can be put in the findings. One must consider the reliability of sampling and the additional time and expense involved in collecting more information. Probability can become a substitute for otherwise unknown information: when probabilities can be substituted for unknowns, the margin of error for the solution may be limited but not completely removed.

There are three criteria that assume that previous experience is necessary to work with probability. In the "maximax" criterion managers maximize the maximum possible gain. Managers are optimistic about the factors influencing their decision and select the option from which they can achieve the best results. This is a dangerous criterion in that it does not consider possible complications. When applying the "maximin" criterion, managers are pessimistic and expect the worst possible results. They select the option that allows them to maximize the least favorable results. They consider what complications can occur for each option, assume that everything that can go wrong will go wrong, and select the alternative that offers the best results when everything possible goes wrong. The "minimax" criterion can be applied when managers have made a decision they regret. Something unexpected prevented them from achieving the most favorable results; managers then subtract the complication from the most favorable results and try to minimize their regrets.

Uncertainty arises when the manager has to make a decision for which there is no historical data on which to calculate probabilities. Under uncertain conditions there is no best criterion to apply. The manager considers objective and subjective options according to his or her own optimistic or pessimistic philosophy and guesses which alternative will render the most desirable results.

Simulation, Models, and Games

Simulation is a way of using models and games to simplify problems by identifying the basic components and using trial and error to determine a solution. Through simulation, the manager may compare alternatives and their consequences. The computer may be used to help solve simulations. These methods may be used to study organizational changes, scheduling, assembly line management, and time sequences.

A model represents something else, most commonly objects, events, processes, or systems. It is a technique of abstraction and simplification for studying something under varying conditions. Manipulation is used to test the impact of proposed changes on the system without disturbing the subject of the model. Almost all quantitative methods used to guide decision making are models. They are particularly useful because of their convenience and low cost compared with manipulating real occurrences. Although models vary considerably in the accuracy with which they represent real situations, they increase predictive capabilities over such methods as guesswork and intuition.

Models are developed to describe, explain, and predict phenomena. The critical element of model building is conceptualization. Consequently, models can provide abstractions that facilitate communication. Models vary in the degree of abstraction used: a life-size mannequin is a realistic model that nursing students use to learn to make occupied beds; a model of a building or a piece of equipment built to scale is quite concrete, whereas blueprints or photographs, organizational charts, and mathematical models are abstract.

The more variables added to the model, the more realistic but cumbersome it becomes. The objective of modeling is to provide a simplified, abstract version of reality. Managers must strive for the appropriate level of abstractness. They may base their decision on an oversimplified model if they do not attempt to expand their knowledge of the situation. Simplified models may be useful for quantitative analysis and prediction, but one must be cautious, because a person with the least knowledge of a situation may be the most certain about how to solve the problem. If description and understanding are important, more comprehensive models should be developed. Continuing to research a problem may contribute to a more realistic model, but it may also delay the decision too long. The cost of gathering additional information may be prohibitive; therefore, the cost of model refinement needs to be balanced against the benefits obtained.

Game theory is a simulation of system operations. The player tries to develop a strategy that will maximize gains and minimize losses, regardless of what the competitor does. War games are commonly used to train personnel and to test plans and equipment under field conditions. Management games are used primarily to train personnel rather than to solve competitive problems. They are particularly useful for training in decision making by simulating real-life operations in a laboratory setting.

Gantt Chart

Gantt charts, named for their developer, Henry L. Gantt, are highly developed schedules that allow one to visualize multiple tasks that have to be done. A Gantt chart is a grid with columns labeled *Tasks, Assigned Responsibility,* and *Time Frame,* which may be minutes, hours, days, weeks, months, years, or decades, depending on the longevity of the project. A line is drawn through the time frame while a task is in process. An X is put at the point where that task is completed. One typically works backward from due dates.

A person is told on Monday that a report is due Friday at 4 PM. The person needs to collect information, type the report on the computer, revise the report, and submit it. The person will use 3 days to collect the information and 1 day to type or word process it, incubate the ideas overnight, do any revision needed Friday morning, and submit the report Friday afternoon. See Figure 3-1.

Task	Responsible	Mon	Tue	Wed	Th	Fr
Collect information	ME	— — — — — — — — ·				
Type report	ME				X	
Revise report	ME					X
Submit report	ME					X

Figure 3-1 Gantt chart.

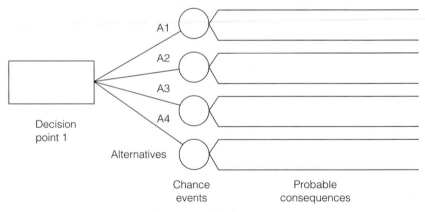

Figure 3-2 Decision tree.

Decision Trees

A decision tree is a graphic method that can help managers visualize the alternatives available, outcomes, risks, and information needs for a specific problem over a period. It helps them to see the possible directions that actions may take from each decision point and to evaluate the consequences of a series of decisions. The process begins with a primary decision having at least two alternatives. Then the predicted outcome for each decision is considered, and the need for further decisions is contemplated. The matrix resembles a tree as the decision points are diagrammed (Figure 3-2).

The results diagrammed on the tree are founded on the manager's experience and judgment but may be supported by computational data. For complex problems, probability statistics may be used to explore further factors that favor or oppose expected events. Although the decision tree does not depict an obviously correct decision, it allows managers to base their decision on a consideration of various alternatives and probable consequences. It helps them realize that subsequent decisions may depend on future events. Decision trees are useful for short- and medium-range planning as well as for decision making. Unfortunately, decision trees for more than 2 or 3 years become cumbersome and speculative.

In Figure 3-3 the nursing staff decides to have a ward picnic for the psychiatric patients. The alternatives are to hold the picnic indoors or outdoors, and the chance events are rain or no rain. If the picnic is scheduled indoors and it rains, the patients may be crowded but dry; there will be no bugs; and the staff will be proud of their decision. If the picnic is scheduled indoors and it does not rain, the patients may feel crowded; the room may seem stuffy; the party will lack a picnic atmosphere; and the staff may regret not scheduling it outside. On the other hand, if the picnic is scheduled outdoors and it rains, the participants will get wet; the food will be ruined; and spirits will be dampened. If the picnic is scheduled outdoors and it does not rain, it will be a pleasant experience.

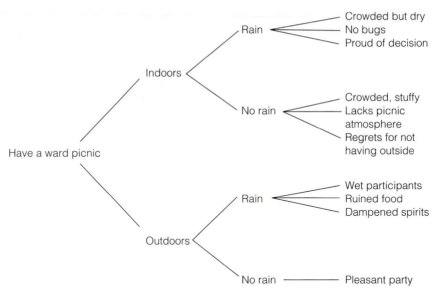

Figure 3-3   Decision tree for psychiatric ward picnic.

Program Evaluation and Review Technique (PERT)

PERT is a network system model for planning and control under uncertain conditions. It involves identifying the key activities in a project, sequencing the activities in a flow diagram, and assigning the duration of each phase of the work. It is particularly appropriate for one-of-a-kind projects that involve extensive research and development.

PERT recognizes that certain tasks must be completed before the total project can be completed and, furthermore, that subtasks must be completed before others can be started. The key events are identified, numbered, labeled, or numbered and labeled on the flow chart. The activities that cause the progress from one event to another are indicated by arrows, with the direction of the arrow showing the direction of the work flow.

PERT also deals with the problem of uncertainty with respect to time by estimating the time variances associated with the expected time of completion of the subtasks. Three projected times are determined: (1) the optimistic time (t_0), which estimates the completion time without complications; (2) the most likely time (t_m), which estimates the completion time with normal problems; and (3) the pessimistic time (t_p), which estimates the completion time given numerous problems. Thus the shortest, average, and longest times needed to complete an activity are calculated. The expected time (t_e) is calculated from these figures by the following formula:

$$t_e = \frac{t_0 + 4(t_m) + t_p}{6}$$

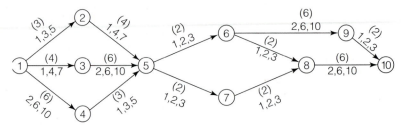

Figure 3-4 PERT model. This PERT model indicates that subtask 1 must be completed before 2, 3, and 4 can be done; 2, 3, and 4 before 5; 5 before 6 and 7; 6 before 9; 6 and 7 before 8; 8 and 9 before 10. A coding system can be used to determine what the numbers mean. For example, 1 = program planned, 2 = staff informed. Arrows show direction of work flow. Optimistic, most likely, pessimistic, and expected times are recorded for each activity.

If the optimistic time is 2 weeks, the most likely time 4 weeks, and the pessimistic time 6 weeks, the expected time is

$$t_e = \frac{2 \text{ weeks} + 4(4 \text{ weeks}) + 6 \text{ weeks}}{6} = \frac{24 \text{ weeks}}{6} = 4 \text{ weeks}$$

The PERT model helps the manager determine priorities (Figure 3-4). Use of resources can be considered when setting priorities. Assignments may be changed temporarily, overtime may be allowed, or temporary help hired to facilitate the activity flow and to manipulate the time required to move from one event to another.

Critical Path Method (CPM)

CPM, closely related to PERT, calculates a single time estimate for each activity, the longest possible time. A cost estimate is figured for both normal and crash operating conditions. Normal means the least-cost method, and crash refers to conditions in less than normal time. Simple sequences can be worked out manually and more complex ones by computer. CPM is particularly useful where cost is a significant factor and experience provides a basis for estimating time and cost. Managers can observe the critical path and compare the progress to the projected dates.

Network analysis techniques facilitate planning and result in objective plans by making it possible to identify the critical path and show interrelationships between parts, thus facilitating improvements in structure and communications. They are particularly useful for task force or project forms of organization and for projects.

Queuing Theory

Queuing theory deals with waiting lines or intermittent servicing problems. It is a mathematical technique for determining the most efficient balance of factors related to intermittent service. It is particularly applicable when units to receive service arrive in a random fashion but the time required for service is predictable. It balances the cost of waiting versus the prevention of waiting by increasing service, by acknowledging that although delays are costly, eliminating them may be even more costly. Decreasing or eliminating the waiting line to reduce waiting line costs causes an increase in cost of labor and physical facilities. The time of arrival is an important factor in determining the optimal size of facilities and staffing. Sometimes actual observations may be made and tallies kept of how many units or clients require service each hour of the workday or during certain seasons. For example, through observation one may determine that many junior and senior high school students attend sexually transmitted disease (STD) or family planning clinics during after-school hours. The STD or family planning clinics in a small college community may have fewer demands for service during holiday seasons and summer vacation because many students have returned to their hometown communities. The manager may adjust staffing accordingly. In the hospital setting, the manager may choose to use part-time people or split shifts to help compensate for an increased workload during the morning when most patients are bathed and once-a-day treatments are given, and again during late afternoon or early evening when most patients are admitted.

When observations cannot be made for an extended period to determine a stable pattern of workload, the Monte Carlo technique may be applied. It provides a large sample of random numbers that may be generated by a computer to determine rather precise predictions of servicing load per hour.

Linear Programming

Linear programming uses matrix algebra or linear mathematical equations to determine the best way to use limited resources to achieve maximal results. The technique is based on the assumption that a linear relationship exists between the variables and that the limits of the variations can be calculated. Three conditions are necessary for linear programming: (1) Either a maximal or minimal value is sought to optimize the objective. The value may be expressed as cost, time, or quantity. The manager may wish to minimize time and expense while maximizing quantity and quality of production. She may wish to reduce the time lost through inefficient allocation of resources or minimize the number of people required to do a job. (2) The variables affecting the goal must have a linear relationship; the ratio of change in one variable to the change in another variable must be constant. If it takes 3 minutes to do a task, it should take 15 minutes to do the task 5 times. (3) Constraints or obstacles to the relationships of the variables exist. Linear programming would not be needed if there were no restrictions.

Simple allocations can often be made by observation and experience, but in large operations the problems may be complex and involve thousands of possible choices. Linear programming is a sophisticated shortcut technique in which a computer can be used to determine solutions. It may be used to determine a minimal-cost diet for meeting certain nutritional standards or for assigning community health nurses to territories. A school of nursing might use this technique to determine class sizes, class hours, and instructors by feeding into a computer equation containing such variables as student's desire or requirement to enroll in particular classes, number of students, number of professors qualified to teach the course, and the hours available to conduct the course. Because linear programming depends on linear relationships and many decisions do not involve them, the manager may need to apply nonlinear programming.

ADVANTAGES AND LIMITATIONS OF QUANTITATIVE TOOLS FOR DECISION MAKING

Quantitative tools lend themselves to a rational, systematic approach to problem solving for decisions that can be expressed mathematically. They encourage disciplined thinking. They are not limited to the six or seven variables the human mind can consider at one time, and they may evaluate thousands of interrelationships simultaneously. Decisions made with the use of quantitative tools are likely to be superior to those that rely heavily on judgment. Unfortunately, many managerial problems involve intangible, nonmeasurable factors that reduce the effectiveness of the tools. The mathematical expressions are based on assumptions; if those assumptions are not true for a given situation, the tool becomes useless.

COMPUTERS

Computers provide several advantages over paper-based record systems. Information can be stored in smaller areas, search and analytical tasks can be performed, and information can be obtained faster and more efficiently. Unfortunately, if used improperly, computers can magnify weaknesses in an organization.

Computers can be applied in nursing in three major categories: (1) clinical systems, (2) management information systems, and (3) educational systems. In clinical systems, computers help with patient histories, medical records, and patient monitoring. Computerized record systems can improve the usability of patient information because data from the chart can be rearranged to be useful to various health care professionals. Physicians can enter their diagnoses, protocols, and notes directly into the computer, saving nurses transcribing time. The instructions can be printed out at the appropriate auxiliary department. Nurses can also record their notes directly into the computer and spend less time and energy accumulating and summarizing data to develop care plans. Standard screens with standard choices increase efficiency for recording observations and doing care plans. Nurses are made aware of changes that require their intervention quickly because information from ancillary departments can be sent automatically to the nursing station terminal. The computer can sort and analyze data and facilitate communication about the patients among health care providers.

Patient monitoring systems record patient responses and can alert nurses to changes. Computers can record the patient's progress on paper or on the monitor, sound an alarm, and often transmit information from the patient's bedside to monitors at the nursing station. In addition to monitoring patients continuously and detecting changes, computers can analyze and interpret the data. Through computer monitoring, nurses can respond quickly to changes in patients' conditions.

Computers have many applications in management information systems. They can be used for patient classification systems, supplies and material management, staff scheduling, policy and procedure changes and announcements, patient charges, budget information and management, personnel records, statistical reports, administrative reports, and memos.

Box 3-1

VROOM AND YETTON NORMATIVE MODEL

Vroom and Yetton address decision making as a social process and emphasize how managers do rather than should behave in their normative model. They identify the following alternative decision processes: A = autocratic, c = consultative, G = group, I = first variant, and II = second variant.

Types of Management Decision Styles*

AI   You solve the problem or make the decision yourself, using information available to you at that time.

AII   You obtain the necessary information from your subordinate(s), then decide on the solution to the problem yourself. You may or may not tell your subordinates what the problem is in getting the information from them. The role played by your subordinates in making the decision is clearly one of providing the necessary information to you, rather than generating or evaluating alternative solutions.

CI   You share the problem with relevant subordinates individually, getting their ideas and suggestions without bringing them together as a group. Then you make the decision that may or may not reflect your subordinates' influence.

CII   You share the problem with your subordinates as a group, collectively obtaining their ideas and suggestions. Then you make the decision that may or may not reflect your subordinates' influence.

GII   You share a problem with your subordinates as a group. Together you generate and evaluate alternatives and attempt to reach agreement (consensus) on a solution. Your role is much like that of chairman. You do not try to influence the group to adopt "your" solution and you are willing to accept and implement any solution that has the support of the entire group.

(GI is omitted because it applies only to more comprehensive models outside the scope of the article.)

DECISION RULES

Vroom identifies seven rules that do most of the work of the model. Three rules protect decision quality and four protect acceptance.*

1. *The Information Rule.*   If the quality of the decision is important and if the leader does not possess enough information or expertise to solve the problem by himself, AI is eliminated from the feasible set. (Its use risks a low-quality decision.)

2. *The Goal Congruence Rule.*   If the quality of the decision is important and if the subordinates do not share the organizational goals to be obtained in solving the problem, GII is eliminated from the feasible set. (Alternatives that eliminate the leader's final control over the decision reached may jeopardize the quality of the decision.)

3. *The Unstructured Problem Rule.*   In decisions in which the quality of the decision is important, if the leader lacks the necessary information or expertise to solve the problem by himself, and if the problem is unstructured, i.e., he does not know ex-

actly what information is needed and where it is located, the method used must provide not only for him to collect the information but to do so in an efficient and effective manner. Methods that involve interaction among all subordinates with full knowledge of the problem are likely to be both more efficient and more likely to generate a high-quality solution to the problem. Under these conditions, AI, AII, and CI are eliminated from the feasible set. (AI does not provide for him to collect the necessary information, and AII and CI represent more cumbersome, less effective, and less efficient means of bringing the necessary information to bear on the solution of the problem than methods that do permit those with the necessary information to interact.)

4. *The Acceptance Rule.* If the acceptance of the decision by subordinates is critical to effective implementation, and if it is not certain that an autocratic decision made by the leader would receive that acceptance, AI and AII are eliminated from the feasible set. (Neither provides an opportunity for subordinates to participate in the decision, and both risk the necessary acceptance.)

5. *The Conflict Rule.* If the acceptance of the decision is critical, and an autocratic decision is not certain to be accepted, and subordinates are likely to be in conflict or disagreement over the appropriate solution, AI, AII, and CI are eliminated from the feasible set. (The method used in solving the problem should enable those in disagreement to resolve their differences with full knowledge of the problem. Accordingly, under these conditions, AI, AII, and CI, which involve no interaction or only "one-on-one" relationships and therefore provide no opportunity for those in conflict to resolve their differences, are eliminated from the feasible set. Their use runs the risk of leaving some of the subordinates with less than the necessary commitment to the final decision.)

6. *The Fairness Rule.* If the quality of decision is unimportant and if acceptance is critical and not certain to result from an autocratic decision, AI, AII, CI, and CII are eliminated from the feasible set. (The method used should maximize the probability of acceptance as this is the only relevant consideration in determining the effectiveness of the decision. Under these circumstances, AI, AII, CI, and CII, which create less acceptance or commitment than GII, are eliminated from the feasible set. To use them is to run the risk of getting less than the needed acceptance of the decision.)

7. *The Acceptance Priority Rule.* If acceptance is critical, not assured by an autocratic decision, and if subordinates can be trusted, AI, AII, CI, and CII are eliminated from the feasible set. (Methods that provide equal partnership in the decision-making process can provide greater acceptance without risking decision quality. Use of any method other than GII results in an unnecessary risk that the decision will not be fully accepted or receive the necessary commitment on the part of subordinates.)

As one asks the diagnostic questions and applies the rules to specific situations, one may eliminate all but one decision style from the feasibility set. However, it is more likely that several decision styles could be used and still protect both the decision quality and acceptance requirements. Then the time factor is used to determine which of the feasible options will require the least time.

Vroom and Yetton focus on three classes of outcomes that influence the ultimate effectiveness of decisions: (1) the quality of the decision, (2) acceptance of the decision by the subordinates, and (3) available time needed to make the decision. The authors found that managers can diagnose a situation quickly and accurately by answering seven questions.*

Problem Attributes	Diagnostic Questions
A. The importance of the quality of the decision.	Is there a quality requirement such that one solution is likely to be more rational than another?
B. The extent to which the leader possesses sufficient information/ expertise to make a high-quality decision by himself.	Do I have sufficient information to make a high-quality decision?
C. The extent to which the problem is structured.	Is the problem structured?
D. The extent to which acceptance or commitment on the part of subordinates is critical to the effective implementation of the decision.	Is acceptance of decision by subordinates critical to effective implementation?
E. The prior probability that the leader's autocratic decision will receive acceptance by subordinates.	If you were to make the decision by yourself, is it reasonably certain that it would be accepted by your subordinates?
F. The extent to which subordinates are motivated to attain the organizational goals as represented in the objectives explicit in the statement of the problem.	Do subordinates share the organizational goals to be obtained in solving this problem?
G. The extent to which subordinates are likely to be in conflict over preferred solutions.	Is conflict among subordinates likely in preferred solutions?

*Reprinted by permission of the publisher: Vroom V: A new look at managerial decision making, *Organizational Dynamics* 1(4):69, 1973. Copyright © 1971 by AMACOM, a division of American Management Associations.

In educational systems, computer-assisted instruction allows students to proceed at their own speed, provides immediate feedback, and allows dissemination of information to remote areas.

When using computers as decision-making tools, nurses should take advantage of good commercial software that is available and should investigate the possibility of using existing systems. Securing the confidentiality of patient and personnel records by carefully locking up diskettes or by constructing a passwords system is very important.

The Vroom and Jago model (1988) is a computer-friendly revision of the Vroom and Yetton model (1973) (see Box 3-1). It provides an additional number of problem attributes, deletes the decision rules, changes dichotomous variables to continuous variables, and provides mathematical formulas to determine decisions.

BIBLIOGRAPHY

Arbel A: Approximate articulation of preference and priority derivation, *Eur J Operat Res* 43:317-326, December 18, 1989.

Barry CT: Information systems technology: barriers and challenges to implementations, *JONA* 20:40-43, February 1990.

Marriner A: The decision making process, *Supervisor Nurse* 8:58-67, February 1977.

Porter M, Miller TR: Uses and abuses of financial modeling, *Topics in Health Care Financing* 19:34-45, Fall 1992.

Sainfort FC et al: Decision support systems effectiveness: conceptual framework and empirical evaluation, *Organizational Behavior & Human Decision Processes* 45:232-252, April 1990.

CASE STUDY

You are the nurse manager of a home health care agency. Because of your computer management programs you know how many supplies have been used in specific time frames and can anticipate how much of what will be needed in the future. Using the Vroom and Yetton normative model in Box 3-1, analyze the problem attributes and determine if you should use an autocratic, consultative, or group decision process to make a fast, economical, quality, and acceptable decision regarding ordering supplies for the unit.

CRITICAL THINKING AND LEARNING ACTIVITIES

1. Develop a Gantt chart to do an assignment, prepare for a test, do your housework, or perform a similar task. Write the steps that must be accomplished down the left side of the page. Put a time frame across the top of the page. Put a line through the grid when the step is in process and an *X* where it is completed.

2. Draw a PERT chart for the activities involved with a new addition to a health care facility. Consider completion of the building; ordering equipment and supplies; recruitment, selection, and orientation of staff; development of goals; development of budget; and admission of the first patients.

3. Use a decision tree to decide when and where to have a unit holiday party. Consider your alternatives, such as having the party in the afternoon or evening; having it at the health care agency, a private residence, or a public place; including only those employed at the agencies or including their families as well. Estimate the probable consequences. See Figures 3-2 and 3-3 on pp. 34-35 as examples.

Chapter

4

Behavioral Aspects of Decision Making

Chapter Objectives

◆ Describe the interrelationship of values, attitudes, perceptions, personality, and roles.

◆ Identify and define at least six group roles.

◆ Compare advantages and disadvantages of group participation in decision making.

◆ Identify five stages of group process and the major activity in each stage.

Major Concepts and Definitions

Values	basic convictions or principles
Attitudes	mental states of readiness
Perceptions	consciousness, awareness
Personality	a relatively stable set of characteristics and temperaments
Roles	expected behaviors in given situations
Myers-Briggs Type Indicator	a method of self-examination of one's strengths and weaknesses and how one differs from others
Group process	how the group functions

INDIVIDUALS AS DECISION MAKERS

Three major behavioral characteristics influence decision making: (1) perception of the problem, (2) a personal value system, and (3) the ability to process data. Perception is a psychological process that makes sense out of what one sees, hears, smells, tastes, or feels. It is affected by one's previous experiences and personal value system; thus, people may perceive the same situation differently. There are also differences in ability to process data, to remember facts, and to explore alternatives.

Values

Values represent basic convictions about what is right, good, or desirable; as a result, they help an individual decide which mode of conduct is preferable to others. Value systems list an individual's values in order of their relative importance and provide the foundation of attitudes, perceptions, personality, and roles. These values cloud objectivity and rationality by containing interpretations of what is right and wrong and implications that certain behaviors or outcomes are preferred over others. They are relatively stable and enduring and generally influence decisions and behaviors.

Attitudes

Attitudes are mental states of readiness that are organized through experience and exert specific influences on a person's response to the people, objects, and situations to which they are related. Attitudes, like values, are learned from parents, teachers, and peers, but attitudes are less stable than values. They influence decisions and behavior and are close to the core of personality.

In the late 1950s, Leon Festinger proposed the theory of cognitive dissonance to explain the linkage between attitudes and behavior. *Cognitive dissonance* means a perceived inconsistency or incompatibility between attitudes and behavior. Festinger maintained that this inconsistency is uncomfortable and that people will try to reduce the dissonance and consequently the discomfort. People seek a stable state with a minimum of dissonance. For example, if someone thinks he is being paid more than he is worth, he is likely to work harder, but if he thinks he is underpaid, he may slow down and do less.

Perceptions

Perception involves receiving, organizing, and interpreting stimuli. The perceptions then influence behavior and form attitudes. People select various cues that influence their perceptions and consequently often misperceive another person, group, or object.

- *Selective perception* means that people select information that supports their viewpoints. Knowing oneself increases the accuracy of perception of others. People tend to identify their own characteristics in others. Consequently, people who accept themselves are more likely to view others favorably.

- A *stereotype* is a judgment made about people on the basis of their gender or ethnic background that can contribute to selective perception.

- A *self-fulfilling prophecy* occurs when people expect certain behavior, use selective perception to see it, and treat others as if it were so. For example, if a nurse manager thinks certain ethnic groups are lazy and irresponsible, he or she may not assign them challenging tasks. That could lead to boredom and demotivation, which reinforce the stereotype, creating a self-fulfilling prophecy.

Personality

Personality is a relatively stable set of characteristics, temperaments, and tendencies that are significantly formed by inheritance and by social, cultural, and environmental factors.

Roles

Role theory is a collection of concepts, definitions, and hypotheses that predict how actors will perform in certain roles and under what circumstances given behaviors can be expected. *Roles* are acts or behaviors expected of a person who occupies a given social position. *Positions* are locations in social systems, such as nurse or teacher. People who occupy positions collectively share common behaviors. Specific behaviors associated with positions constitute roles. Positions and roles have counterparts or counterroles such as nurse-client, teacher-student, or leader-follower.

Positions may be *ascribed* or *achieved*. A person has little or no control over ascribed positions such as age, sex, or birth order in the family. Some degree of control is possible for achieved positions such as marital status, occupation, and social status.

Role structure involves individuals, behaviors, and positions. The *individual,* or actor, ego, referent, or self, has a set of attributes that can be described from a variety of viewpoints. An interactionist would look at the interaction of roles, the psychiatrist at personality, and the structuralist at position tasks. *Behaviors* are actions taken by the role enactor. These acts are learned and influenced by norms. They are often voluntary and goal-directed. *Prescription* refers to what should be done by a person in a certain position. *Positions* often require specific skills, intelligence, or temperament and may be held based on one's age, sex, and education. Positions often imply titles such as nurse or teacher. People in positions are exchangeable, but the positions are not.

Role socialization is a process of acquiring specific roles and involves role expectations, role learning, and role enactment. *Role expectations* are beliefs held by others about the specific behaviors inherent in specific positions; they may be general or specific, formal or informal, extensive or narrow in scope. Some expectations are very clear, whereas others are not. General expectations allow more latitude in the implementation of the role than do specific ones. For example, nurses should be kind and gentle in general. More specifically, nurses use two-way communications skills. Some formal expectations are written, such as codes of ethics and behavioral objectives, whereas informal expectations are communicated indirectly. Expectations for age and sex are extensive in scope in that they transcend other roles. Expectations that apply in only a few positions are narrow in scope. Thus, only nurses working in cardiac intensive care units are expected to read and interpret electrocardiograms, and only nurse managers are expected to write a budget.

Role learning involves locating oneself accurately in the social structure. It begins at infancy and early childhood as one prepares to assume adult responsibilities. It involves the development of basic skills such as language, interpersonal competence, and role taking. *Role taking* is the ability of the person to act out perceptions of how she and others would behave in certain positions. Playing nurse is an example of learning role taking.

Role enactment refers to behaviors and is related to the number of positions held, the intensity of involvement in those positions, and the preemptiveness of them. People hold multiple positions at any one time, a situation that sometimes causes conflict and difficulty with role enactment. One may not have enough time to implement each role effectively, and there can be conflicts among various role expectations. A professional nurse who takes a course will have less time for child care. Intensity of involvement is the degree of effort exerted to enact a role. It may vary from noninvolvement to engrossing involvement. For example, a nurse may merely pay for membership in an organization or may become an officer and serve on several committees. Preemptiveness is the amount of time a person spends enacting one role as compared with others.

Role stress or role dissonance is the difference between role enactment and role expectations. The greater the difference, the greater the stress. *Role ambiguity* results from a lack of clear role expectations. *Role shock* arises from discrepancies between anticipated and encountered roles. *Role conflict* is a consequence of contradictory or mutually exclusive roles.

MYERS-BRIGGS TYPE INDICATOR

The Myers-Briggs Type Indicator is a useful method for performing self-examinations to understand one's strengths and weaknesses and how one differs from others. Myers and Briggs identified four dimensions of psychological type: attitude toward life, perception function, judgment function, and orientation to the outer world. Each of

Table 4-1   Myers-Briggs Type Indicator

Dimensions	Contrasting	Categories
Attitude toward life	Introversion	Extroversion
Perception	Sensing	Intuiting
Judgment	Thinking	Feeling
Orientation to outer world	Judging	Perceiving

the four dimensions has two categories, thus forming sixteen different types, as shown in Table 4-1.

Introverts like to work alone, think before they act, do not like interruptions, like quiet for concentration, may work on a project for a long time, are interested in ideas, are careful with details, may have difficulty remembering names and faces, and may have trouble communicating.

Extroverts like to be around people, communicate freely, may act without thinking, like variety and action, and may become impatient with slow jobs.

Sensing types tend to be good at detail work, are not usually inspired, rarely make errors of fact, are patient with routine details, enjoy using skills they know, like established ways of doing things, and work steadily step by step to the end.

Intuitive types like solving new problems, enjoy learning new skills, follow their inspirations, and work in bursts of energy to reach conclusion quickly.

Thinking types value logic, organize ideas into logical sequences, tend to be brief and businesslike, and may seem impersonal.

Feeling types value sentiment, tend to be friendly and agreeable, may undervalue thinking, and are likely to ramble. They are usually stronger in social skills than in executive ability.

Judging types like to plan their work and follow the plan, make decisions quickly, and get things done.

Perceiving types are curious, may start too many projects, and may have trouble finishing them or coming to a conclusion.

Leaders should know their own styles and those of people with whom they work. When leaders are aware of their own limitations, they can consult opposite types to compensate. By knowing their associates' strengths and weaknesses, they can maximize the strengths, minimize the weaknesses, and develop strong teams.

GROUP PROCESS

Group process is critical for group development. How the group functions, communicates, and sets and achieves objectives are all related to group dynamics. Both

**Box
4-1**   **GROUP PROCESS ROLES**

GROUP TASK ROLES	GROUP MAINTENANCE ROLES	DYSFUNCTIONAL ROLES
Initiator-contributor	Gatekeeper	Aggressor
Information seeker	Encourager	Dominator
Opinion seeker	Harmonizer	Recognition-seeker
Information giver	Compromiser	Special-interest pleader
Opinion giver	Follower	Blocker
Elaborator	Group observer	Self-confessor
Coordinator	Standard setter	Help seeker
Orienter		Playboy
Critic		
Energizer		
Procedural technician		
Recorder		

task-oriented behavior and maintenance-oriented behavior are necessary for adequate group development.

People who assume group-task roles coordinate and facilitate the group's efforts to identify the problem, explore alternative options, identify the ramifications of the options, choose the most viable option, and implement and evaluate the plan. There are numerous group-task roles , and any member of the group may fulfill a number of these roles in successive participation (see Box 4-1).

Initiator-contributors propose new ideas or different ways of approaching a problem. Their task is to identify the problem, clarify the objectives, offer solutions, suggest agenda items, and set time limits. The *information seeker* searches for factual information about the problem, whereas the *opinion seeker* clarifies values pertinent to the problem and its solutions. Unlike the information seeker, the *information giver* identifies facts, shares experiences, and makes generalizations. *Opinion givers* state their beliefs and what they think the group should value. Their focus is on values rather than on facts. The *elaborator* develops suggestions, illustrates points, and predicts outcomes. Relationships are clarified by the *coordinator*. The *orienter* summarizes the discussion, activities, and points of departure to provide perspective on the group's progress toward its goal. Evaluation of the problem, content, and process is done by the *critic,* who may measure the group's achievement against a set of standards. The *energizer* stimulates the group to increase the quantity and quality of their work. The *procedural technician* facilitates group action by arranging the room for the meeting, distributing the materials, working the audiovisual equipment, and generally functioning as the "go-for"—the person who goes for what is needed. An account of the discussion, suggestions, and decisions is kept by the *recorder.*

The roles of group building and group maintenance focus on how people treat each other while accomplishing a task. The *gatekeeper* regulates communication and takes actions to ensure everyone an opportunity to be heard. *Encouragers* radiate warmth and approval. They offer commendation and praise and indicate acceptance and understanding of others' ideas and values. *Harmonizers* create and maintain group cohesion, relieving tension through their sense of humor and helping others reconcile their disagreements. *Compromisers* promote group process by yielding status, admitting mistakes, modifying their ideas for the sake of group cohesiveness, maintaining self-control for group harmony, or by generally making compromises to keep the group action oriented. The *follower,* acting as a passive audience, goes along with the group. The *group observer* keeps records of the group process and gives interpretations for evaluation of the proceedings. The quality of the group process is compared with standards by the *standard setter.*

Some members of the group may try to satisfy their individual needs irrespective of the group tasks or maintenance roles. For example, *aggressors* meet their needs at the expense of others by disapproving of others and deflating their status. The *dominator* asserts authority or superiority through flattery, interrupting others, and by giving directions authoritatively. *Recognition-seekers* call attention to themselves by boasting and acting in unusual ways. The *special interest pleader* speaks for an interest group and addresses issues that best meet that need. The *blocker* is negative, resistant, and disagreeable without apparent reason and brings issues back to the floor after the group has rejected them. The *self-confessor* uses the group to express personal feelings, whereas the *help-seeker* expresses depreciation, insecurity, and personal confusion that elicit sympathetic responses. The *playboy* has a lack of involvement in the group process and appears nonchalant. A high incidence of individual roles in a group requires self-diagnosis to suggest what group-training efforts are needed. Having a trained observer record who is fulfilling what roles during a meeting can be revealing. On a form similar to the one shown in Worksheet 4-1 at the end of this chapter, an observer records each time a participant plays a certain role.

GROUP FACTORS IN DECISION MAKING

A group comprises two or more people who perceive themselves as sharing common interests and who come together to accomplish an activity through face-to-face interaction. People join groups to satisfy security, fulfill social and esteem needs, enhance their personal status and careers, sustain friendships, and accomplish goals. In organizations, formal groups are deliberately created to perform specific tasks. These may be command groups formed of a manager and staff associates or temporary task groups composed of people who do not necessarily report to the same manager. The informal group evolves naturally.

Within an agency it is unusual for individuals to complete the decision-making process alone. Even if an individual makes the decision, others will probably be involved in the implementation. Commitment to the decision is important to its implementation and may be increased by participation in the decision-making process. One should be aware, however, that there are disadvantages as well as advantages to group participation in decision making.

Advantages of Group Participation in Decision Making

Because of their broader experiences, groups have a wider range of knowledge to draw on than does the individual. Participation allows nurses to express their views and attempt to persuade others, thereby increasing self-expression, innovation, and development. People are more apt to be committed to implementation if they have had the opportunity to share in the decision-making process. Group decisions, however, are time-consuming and expensive. Still, because of the members' diverse backgrounds, it may be less time-consuming for a group to make a decision than for an individual to gather information and analyze it. In the end this may be no more expensive than having a higher-paid manager make the decision.

Disadvantages of Group Participation in Decision Making

Group decisions may result from social pressures. Staff associates may be influenced by their desire for group acceptance or by an attempt to appease her manager. Hierarchical pressures can reduce the staff associate's participation to acquiescence to the manager's desires. Formal status is likely to inhibit interaction when the manager has less expertise than the staff. A competent manager is more likely to possess self-confidence and allow interaction. It is not always easy to determine another's competence, and one cannot expect the level of expertise to match the degree of participation.

Group participants change and so do the problems. A minority may rule if an individual or a few people dominate the group. Members may become more interested in winning an argument than in determining the best alternative. Choosing the most acceptable solution may produce consensus, which is not necessarily the optimal alternative and may simply foster the status quo.

Groupthink

When a group becomes too cohesive and demands too much conformity, the group is likely to develop patterns of behavior that interfere with good decision making. Symptoms of groupthink include high cohesiveness of the group, the illusion of invulnerability, collective rationalization, a tendency to moralize, self-righteousness, a feeling of unanimity, stereotyping of other groups, pressure to conform, and self-censorship to keep quiet. Opposing ideas are discouraged and dismissed.

Group norms form gradually and informally in a variety of ways. People bring expectations with them from past situations. The first pattern that emerges in a group often sets group expectations, and important incidents establish precedents. Explicit statements by group members and conscious decisions by the group also help determine norms. Norms apply to behavior, not to thoughts and feelings. They are generally developed only for behavior that is considered important by most group members and usually allow for a range of acceptable behaviors. Group norms are enforced because they make predictable what behavior is expected of group members, reinforce specific roles, and help avoid embarrassing interpersonal problems. They probably reflect the preferences of powerful group members and help ensure group success.

Group cohesiveness occurs when members of the group like each other and want to be members of the group. A charismatic leader, good reputation of the group, shared goals, similarity of attitudes and values, and small enough size to allow interaction increase group cohesiveness. There is a direct correlation between cohesiveness and conformity to group norms. However, group norms may not be consistent with those of the organization.

There are several steps a manager can take to discourage groupthink. When assigning a policy-planning mission to a group, the leader should be impartial instead of stating preferences and expectations. At least one member of the committee can be assigned the role of devil's advocate. One or more outside consultants or qualified internal colleagues who are not core members of the group can be invited to each meeting on a staggered basis to challenge the views of the core members. Members of the core group can discuss the group's deliberations with trusted colleagues periodically and report their reactions back to the group. The group may be divided into subgroups to meet separately under different leadership, report back to the larger group, and discuss differences. Two or more independent groups may be assigned to explore the same policy question. Results can then be compared. The leader should encourage each committee member to be a critical evaluator and to air objections and doubts diplomatically. This can be reinforced by the leader's acceptance of criticism of his or her own suggestions.

COMMITTEE ASPECTS OF DECISION MAKING

A committee is a group of people chosen to deal with a particular topic or problem. The authority delegated to committees varies widely. A staff committee serves merely in an advisory capacity. A line committee is a plural executive responsible for making decisions affecting affiliates. Formal committees are part of the organizational structure and have specific duties and authority. Informal committees have not been delegated authority and are often primarily for discussion. Formal committees tend to be permanent; informal committees are more likely to be temporary. Committees are usually most useful when appointed for a specific purpose. A committee appointed to collect data, analyze findings, and make recommendations is an ad hoc committee. There are advantages and disadvantages to decision making by committees.

Advantages of Committee Decision Making

Although the ultimate responsibility for a decision is the top administrator's, that burden can be shared through the use of committees. Group deliberation and judgment can be advantageous for decision making. Complex problems may be more manageable when department heads and specialists participate. Sharing in the decision-making process increases the department head's understanding of the situation and commitment to the decision. Most decisions based on consensus after deliberation are widely satisfactory. The unanimity of committee decisions helps increase the support and confidence of subordinates.

Disadvantages of Committee Decision Making

Although the top administrator's burden for decision making can be shared by committees, it requires more leadership ability to conduct business in that manner. Committee decisions may make managers appear to be a figurehead and decrease their prestige in the community. Weak administrators may in fact be controlled by their staff instead of being in control themselves. They may use committees to avoid responsibilities or to delay decisions. A committee may have a fixed responsibility, but it is the group rather than the individual that is held accountable because it is difficult to identify who is responsible for a poor decision. A committee decision is a slow, ponderous process that is consequently expensive. Pressures for unanimity may discourage input from more aggressive and creative members. Consensus through compromise may decrease the quality of the decision. Indecisiveness can result in adjournment without action taken and contribute to a minority tyranny of the strongest members.

Committee Functioning

Despite the obvious disadvantages and misuses of committees, there is an increasing emphasis on group participation. Committee decisions are particularly useful for policy formulation and planning. Consequently, the manager should consider how to maximize the use of committees.

There are several kinds of committees, including (1) interdepartmental committees involving nursing with nonnursing departments, (2) committees based on organizational position and job function, (3) standing committees, and (4) task forces. Interdepartmental committees help coordinate goals and activities among departments and help solve interdepartmental problems. The situational problems between departments can best be solved by people with firsthand experience, rather than by committees. Consequently, alternatives to committee meetings should be considered for problem solving. Dual leadership is sometimes used to give equal consideration to each department. That tends to result in a lack of leadership. Alternating chairpersons may serve the same purpose as having co-chairpersons.

Committees based on organizational position and job function provide a vehicle for group cohesion and power. Standing committees represent focal points of action in the institution. In hospitals, standing committees may be formed to make recommendations about patient care evaluation, continuity of care, patient education, and staff development. Schools of nursing often have standing committees for bylaws, curricula, admissions, progression, and graduation. A task force is a time-limited committee that assesses a situation, makes recommendations, and is dissolved. People with the most knowledge and skills related to the problem should serve on the task force.

Defining the scope and authority of the committee helps members know what their responsibilities are. Members should know whether they are simply to discuss an issue, provide the manager with ideas, make recommendations, or be responsible for the decision. With their job clearly defined, there is less chance that committee members will waste their time dealing with issues beyond the scope of their responsibility. An awareness of the limits placed on them also allows committee members to evaluate their work better. It may be advisable to review committees periodically to dissolve those no longer needed, consolidate those duplicating responsibilities, and create new ones.

The size of the committee is important. It should be large enough to facilitate deliberation and have a membership with a breadth of knowledge and expertise. If it is too large, it encourages indecision and inefficiency, because the larger the group, the more time it takes to allow each member to participate and for the group to reach a consensus. Effective committee size may range from five to fifteen. Five is considered an ideal size if the five members have adequate knowledge and skills. Appropriate membership is critical for effective committee functioning. Members need the necessary knowledge and skills, should possess authority, must be suitably representative, and should be able to work well within a group.

Feedback to and from nonmembers and administration enhances committee effectiveness. Developing input channels helps foster group acceptance for committee recommendations. For example, staff nurses may give input to the patient care coordinator who represents them at administrative team meetings. Periodic status reports to administration and nonmembers are not only a means of communication, they help committee members focus on goals and evaluate progress.

Good leadership can increase the effectiveness of a committee. The chairperson can facilitate committee work by preparing agendas, circulating reports before meetings, making research results available to members, collecting necessary facts before the meeting, defining the proposal for action, and conducting the meeting efficiently. Agendas circulated to members well in advance of meetings allow committee members to know what to expect and to come to the meeting prepared to deal with the subject. The circulation of reports and other information before the meeting helps prevent the waste of meeting time while members review studies or think aloud. It reduces the chances of a decision being railroaded, a report being meekly accepted, or postponement of a decision until after members have more opportunity to study the proposal.

Stages of Group Development

Committees go through stages of group development. They typically form, organize, solve problems, implement solutions, and disband. During the forming stage, individuals are likely to feel anxious, fearful, doubtful, and self-protective. The leader concentrates on putting the members at ease, explaining the purpose, developing a workable climate, and exerting leadership. Tension tends to be high, suspiciousness is common, and disagreement emerges with the power struggles that occur during the organizing phase. The leader needs to clarify goals, policies and procedures, code of conduct, and communication patterns. Loyalty, trust, confidence, dignity, and pride develop during problem solving. The leader seeks to approve recommendations by consensus through a systematic and logical approach. Self-interest, excitement, recognition, and rewards are common during implementation. The leader tends to the plan of action, the acceptance of decisions, and the generation of feedback. Members may have positive or negative feelings about disbanding. The leader should express appreciation and give positive reinforcement.

Role of Chairperson

The committee chairperson needs to handle members who create various problems during the meeting, such as the overly talkative, the inarticulate, and the ramblers. In general, the chairperson lets the group take care of the overly talkative as much as possible. Embarrassing or sarcastic remarks are not appropriate. The overly talkative may be slowed down with some difficult questions or interrupted with a comment like "That's an interesting point. Let's see what the group thinks of it." Input can be invited from all committee members, starting with the others first. The rambler is likely to talk about everything except the subject. When the member stops for a breath, the chairperson thanks the member, refocuses attention by restating the relevant points, and moves on. Some members may come up with comments that are obviously incorrect. The chairperson can say something like "That's one way of looking at it," or "I see your point, but can we reconcile that with (the true situation)?" Side conversations can be distracting. The chairperson tries not to embarrass the people involved. One can be called by name and asked an easy question, or the last opinion can be restated and one asked his or her opinion of it. When two or more members clash or the committee is divided into factions, the chairperson should emphasize points of agreement, minimize points of disagreement if possible, and draw attention to objectives. The inarticulate may lack the ability to put thoughts into proper words; the silent person may feel timid, insecure, bored, indifferent, or superior. Interest can be aroused by asking people for their opinions. That technique can also be used to encourage people to talk. The action of the chairperson depends on what is motivating the committee member.

The chairperson should keep the discussion on the subject and help integrate committee deliberation. Thus, rather than resorting to compromise, members may develop a point of view that differs from the preconceived notions that they brought to the meeting. The chairperson should not force members to take a position until after the subject has been fully considered. Members who take a premature stand may feel the need to defend that position for the sake of winning an argument rather than for the quality of the decision. The chairperson can encourage each member to be a critical evaluator and to consider the consequences of an action. Outside experts may be invited in, or task forces can be selected to study issues and report back to the committee. It may be useful to have a follow-up meeting after a consensus has been reached to allow for, and to deal with, second thoughts.

Committees permit simultaneous participation, and yet people may still leave the meeting with varying interpretations of what happened. Consequently, it is advisable to have a secretary take minutes and for the chairperson to circulate the draft for modification before having the minutes approved by the committee. Chairpersons should also follow up on the decisions made and report their findings to the committee. Was the recommendation implemented? If so, what were the results? If not, why not?

Continuum of Participation

Participation in decision making is based on the principle that all members of a group or organization should be encouraged to contribute to decisions. The extent of participation allowed depends on such factors as organizational philosophy, mana-

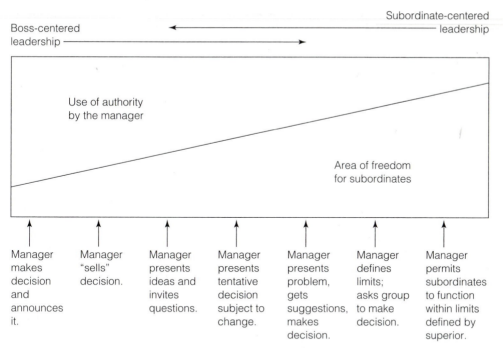

Boss-centered
leadership ———

Subordinate-centered
leadership

Use of authority
by the manager

Area of freedom
for subordinates

| Manager makes decision and announces it. | Manager "sells" decision. | Manager presents ideas and invites questions. | Manager presents tentative decision subject to change. | Manager presents problem, gets suggestions, makes decision. | Manager defines limits; asks group to make decision. | Manager permits subordinates to function within limits defined by superior. |

Figure 4-1   Continuum of leadership behavior and participation. (From Tannenbaum R and Schmidt WH: How to choose a leadership pattern. *Harvard Business Review* 51:164, May-June, 1973).

gerial style, and organizational climate. Agencies that discourage participation have an authoritarian climate. Directions and control are located at the top of the hierarchy, where decisions primarily are made by top management. They are communicated down to staff, and unquestioned obedience is expected. Agencies that allow greater participation at lower echelons are democratic in nature. Tannenbaum and Schmidt developed the continuum of leadership behavior and participation related to the degree of authority used by the leader and the amount of freedom granted subordinates in reaching decisions (see Figure 4-1). The actions on the extreme left characterize the manager who maintains a high degree of control, whereas the actions on the right characterize the leader who releases a high degree of control. Neither extreme is without limitations.

Manager makes decision and announces it.   In this situation managers identify the problem, explore alternative solutions, choose one of them, and then report their decision. They provide no opportunity for others to participate, may or may not give consideration to others' thoughts and feelings, and may or may not imply coercion.

Manager "sells" decision.   Here managers identify the problem and make a decision. However, instead of merely announcing the decision, they try to persuade subordinates to accept it. This procedure recognizes the possibility of some resistance and seeks to reduce it by such acts as explaining to employees what they gain from the decision.

Manager presents ideas and invites questions.   Now managers who have made a decision and have tried to persuade staff associates to accept it, provide an opportunity for others to ask questions to get a fuller explanation of their thinking and intentions. This discussion allows exploration of the implications of the decision.

Manager presents tentative decision subject to change.   In this situation managers present their tentative decision for reaction by the people who will be affected by it. They reserve the power to make the final decision but takes others' thoughts and feelings into account when making the decision.

Manager presents problem, gets suggestions, makes decision.   Now managers identify the problem but get suggestions from staff associates before making a decision. This approach uses the knowledge and experiences of others. Managers select what they consider the best solution from the expanded list of alternatives developed by themselves and others.

Manager defines limits, requests group to make decision.   Managers identify the problem, set the boundaries within which the decision must be made, and give the group, including themselves, the power to make the decision.

Manager permits group to make decisions within prescribed limits.   This represents the extreme degree of group freedom where the group identifies the problem, explores alternatives, and makes the decision. The only limits imposed on the group's decision are from top-level administration. Managers commit themselves in advance of the decision making to help implement the decision of the group. They may or may not be a part of the group decision making. If so, they act with no more authority than any other member of the group.

Whether the manager chooses a more autocratic or democratic approach depends on several factors. The following questions should be asked: How important is the quality of the decision? Does the manager have sufficient information to make a good decision? If not, others should be involved in the decision. If so, have prior autocratic decisions been accepted by the staff associates? If not, others should be involved. Is acceptance of the decision critical for its implementation? If so, the implementers should be involved with the decision making. Staff associates should be included in decision making if they share organizational goals and are not in conflict with preferred solutions.

TEAM DEVELOPMENT

The group factors in decision making, committee aspects of decision making, and stages of group development all apply to team development. Organizational cultures that are people oriented, goal directed, and quality driven are conducive to team development (see Box 4-2).

The role of the manager in the development of self-managing teams is as follows:

- Show a willingness to help establish teams
- Set goals and expectations

Box 4-2 CHARACTERISTICS OF CULTURES THAT SUPPORT TEAMS

Value employees' interpersonal requirements
Promote cooperative rather than competitive relationships
Encourage individual accountability and responsibility
Recognize individual contributions
Have positive visions of the future
Have short- and long-term goals
Have quality standards
Believe in their products and services
Are people oriented
Support the community

From Hicks RF, Bone D: *Self-managing teams,* Menlo Park, Calif, 1990, Crisp Publications.

Box 4-3 BENEFITS OF SELF-MANAGED TEAMS

Increased productivity
Commitment to the organization
Commitment to the job
Common commitment to goals and values
Increased effort toward stated goals
Shared ownership and responsibility for tasks
Proactive approach to problems
Faster response to change
Increased employee development
Flexible work practices
Motivation through peer pressure rather than management mandates
Less need for management interventions
Increased employee satisfaction
Better work climate
Synergy

Adapted from Harrington-Mackin D: *The team building tool kit,* New York, 1994, American Management Association; and Hicks RF, Bone D: *Self-managing teams,* Menlo Park, Calif, 1990, Crisp Publications.

- Give the team feedback to help it self-correct as it proceeds
- Acquire needed resources, such as education, consultation, supplies, and equipment
- Allow processing time
- Protect the team from the political obstacles and road blocks that may occur when people in the hierarchy feel threatened because they believe they are losing decision-making power

The manager can help ensure the team's success through its infancy by selecting members who work well together, are mature problem solvers, have positive attitudes, are future oriented, are willing to take risks, and are interested in working in a self-managing team. Building a successful experience is also important. Documenting and communicating success make it easier to take the next steps. Verbal feedback to the organization about the successes of the team is very powerful. The manager should make sure that the commitment, time, and resources are available for success. Encourage the team to go slowly enough to do it right and consequently move faster in the long run. Employees should then start feeling autonomy, responsibility, accomplishment, and belongingness that contribute to job satisfaction and synergy (Hicks and Bone, 1990). Box 4-3 lists some of the benefits of self-managed teams.

BIBLIOGRAPHY

Anonymous: To succeed, listen, *Industry Week* 241:36-40, November 16, 1992.

D'Aquila NW, Habegger D, Willwerth EJ: Converting a QA program to CQI, *Nurs Manage* 25:68-71, October 1994.

Fritz R: A systematic approach to problem solving and decision making, *Supervisory Management* 38:1045-263X, March 1993.

Johnson V: The groupthink trap, *Successful Meetings* 41:145-146, September 1992.

Kirkpatrick DL: The power of empowerment: how much is too much or not enough? *Training & Development* 46:29-31, September 1992.

Marriner A: Behavioral aspects of decision making, *Supervisor Nurse* 8:40-47, May 1977.

Nickols FW: How to figure out what to do, *Training* 28:31-39, August 1991.

Schwartz AE, Levin J: Making the best decision: steps to take, methods to avoid, *Nonprofit World* 8:28-30, November-December 1990.

Sims RR: Linking groupthink to unethical behavior in organizations, *J Business Ethics* 11:651-662, September 1992.

CASE STUDY

There is a popular workshop coming to town. Because of the census you can manage to allow only two staff members to attend even though you think most would like to attend the workshop. Using the Vroom and Yetton normative model (Chapter 3, Box 3-1), you have assessed that the quality of the decision is not very important but the acceptability of it is. Consequently, you are going to involve the group in the decision.

Will you (1) present ideas and invite questions, (2) present the problem, get suggestions, and make the decision, or (3) define limits and ask the group to make the decision.

Identify advantages and disadvantages of group participation in this decision making.

CRITICAL THINKING AND LEARNING ACTIVITIES

1. Using Worksheet 4-1, Group Roles Grid, identify the number of times members of a group play various roles during a class activity or group meeting.

2. Identify the stage of development of a group to which you belong.

3. Observe the activities and behaviors of the chairperson of a committee meeting that you attend.

Group Roles Grid

Names

Roles

Initiator-contributor								
Information seeker								
Opinion seeker								
Information giver								
Opinion giver								
Elaborator								
Coordinator								
Orienter								
Critic								
Energizer								
Procedural technician								
Recorder								
Gatekeeper								
Encourager								
Harmonizer								
Compromiser								
Follower								
Group observer								
Standard setter								
Aggressor								
Dominator								
Recognition seeker								
Special interest pleader								
Blocker								
Self-confessor								
Help seeker								
Playboy								

Chapter 5

Time Management

Chapter Objectives

◆ Describe how planning relates to time management.

◆ Identify at least five ways to streamline paperwork.

◆ Identify at least five ways to make telephone communication efficient.

◆ Describe at least five ways managers can help meetings be effective and efficient.

◆ Discuss responsibility, authority, and accountability as they relate to delegation.

Major Concepts and Definitions	
Delegation	to entrust a task to another person who serves as one's representative
Responsibility	obligation; what must be done to complete the task
Authority	power to make final decisions and give commands
Accountability	liability for satisfactory completion of work
Planning	preparing a scheme for doing
Time management	controlling use of time for maximum productivity

TIME MANAGEMENT

If productivity were only a function of time, one would expect all to produce equally. And yet, although everyone has the same number of hours in a day and the same number of days per week, some people accomplish more than others. Granted, some people work longer and harder than others to accomplish more, but some just make better use of their time. Because nurses work long hours, they should work smarter—not harder—to get more done in less time.

MAXIMIZE MANAGERIAL TIME

Inventory Activities

Nurse managers may start a plan for maximizing use of their time by conducting an inventory of their activities. After recording what they did every 15 minutes for a typical week, they assess how they spent their time. How much time was spent in which activities? Was the way the time was spent determined by conscious decisions, habit, work demands, default, or spontaneity? What do they like to do? What activities do they want to increase? What do they want to decrease? How can they reduce the time wasters? (See Box 5-1.)

Set Goals

Next, nurses determine their short-, medium-, and long-range goals. What do they want to accomplish? What do they want to do soon? Which goals must be completed before others? Which will take the longest to achieve? Setting priorities helps resolve goal conflicts and directs how they will spend their time.

Plan Strategies

Once they have determined and ranked their goals, they plan strategies for how to accomplish them. What activities must they do? What are low-priority activities that can be eliminated? Next the nurse manager schedules activities. A tickler box with divider cards for months and weeks can be used by filing task cards behind the

Box 5-1   TIME WASTERS

Poor planning	Telephone interruptions
Failure to establish goals	Unorganized office visits
Failure to set objectives	Poorly planned meetings
Failure to plan strategies to accomplish	Lack of delegation
goals	Lack of information
Unwillingness to say no	Poor communication
Ineffective use of transition times	Lack of feedback
Cumbersome paperwork	Procrastination
Poor filing system	Indecisiveness
Poor reading skills	Haste
Poor listening and memory techniques	Management by crises

appropriate month and week card. As they look at their major responsibilities for a whole year, they may have some flexibility in determining when certain jobs are done and can use those to help balance the workload around tasks that have to be done at certain times, such as preparing the budget. Various calendar systems can also be used: one may do major project planning on a year-at-a-glance calendar; desk ink blotters that depict a month at a time can help regulate that month's work; a week-at-a-glance or a day-at-a-glance calendar is convenient for carrying in one's purse. Daily work sheets depicting what work should be done during which hour may also be useful. Computer scheduling is increasingly popular.

Plan Schedule

Nurse managers need to assess their peak and low times to plan a detailed schedule more effectively. Are they most alert and creative in the early morning or late at night? Are they slow starters in the morning? Do they reach a low energy point in the middle of the afternoon? The nurse's prime internal time—the most creative time for working alone—is a good time to schedule work that should not be interrupted. When is their prime external time, their best time to work with others? If they reach a low point in the afternoon, that may be a good time to schedule office visits. They may offer their guests a cup of coffee or tea, which tends to facilitate communication, sip on their own drinks, and listen.

Time should be set aside for certain activities each day. Scheduled activities are recorded. Scheduled and unscheduled times are noted, and contact and thinking times are identified. The secretary may be given available hours for scheduling office visits.

A few minutes at the beginning of each day should be allowed for planning. A running list of what needs to be done in order of importance can be made each morning to plan what will be done that day. Desk-organizing files—which are merely folders with such labels as *urgent, return calls, dictate, read, file,* and *low priority*—can help determine what to do each day. Scheduled free time can be used to deal with these activities. A few minutes at the end of the day are used to evaluate what happened.

Say No

Learning how to say no graciously saves time. It is advisable for nurse managers to acknowledge the request, state and explain their position, check back for understanding with the other person, and avoid defensiveness. For example, when asked to speak at a meeting they might respond, "I would love to discuss our institutional goals with your committee. However, I have another commitment at that time. Barbara Jones and Sue Smith are both very familiar with the institutional goals. Perhaps you could ask one of them to speak. Does that sound agreeable to you?"

Use Transition Times

Managers can accomplish much during transition times. Incoming mail may be read while one is on "hold" when returning phone calls. Reports can be read while commuting to and from work or audiotapes can be listened to while driving. Isometric exercises can be done at almost any time. Lunch and coffee breaks may be used for personal business. Because many people are watching their weight, lunch breaks may be better used for exercise, such as walking and jogging, or for meditation than for eating a large lunch.

Streamline Paperwork

Much time can be saved by streamlining paperwork. Scheduling a block of time to answer mail prevents interruptions. If the situation warrants, a standard reply can be used. Some responses can be made on the query memo if no file copy is needed, and typing carbon responses to letters onto the back of the query letter saves filing time and space. Color coding is useful, and recording of destruction dates on files reduces the need to review the materials later. Dictation usually takes less time than writing by hand, and calls can be used when a record is not necessary. Computerization and electronic mail also save time. Selective reading by scanning tables of contents and reading summaries at the end of long responses and reports saves time. Managers should not concentrate on details unless necessary, as they are quickly forgotten. Scanning for major points is often adequate.

Improve Reading

Learning speed-reading techniques such as tapping, L pattern, S swirl, area reading, and reading for meaning can help overcome common reading problems of single-word fixation, involuntary regression by rereading, subvocalization of words as one reads, and inability to concentrate.

Improve Memory

Listening and memory techniques also save time. When listening for understanding, one should assume value in what the speaker is saying by being attentive, delaying judgment, maintaining eye contact, and using attentive body language. One then needs to assess the content of the information by focusing on central ideas, looking for

**Box
5-2**   **MEMORY TECHNIQUES**

VERBAL TECHNIQUES	PHYSICAL TECHNIQUES	MENTAL TECHNIQUES
Repeating	Note taking	Focusing
Clarifying	Filing	Imaging
Summarizing	Follow-up memos	Linking
		Locating
		Chunking

relationships between ideas, and selecting an organizing structure such as main and supporting ideas, advantages and disadvantages, or putting information into chronological order. One should analyze the information by listening to what is being said, identifying how it is being said by inferring emotions from body language and tone of voice, and considering the speaker's motivation for saying it. Distractions may have to be reduced so the listener can concentrate.

Verbal, physical, and mental techniques can be used to stimulate memory (see Box 5-2). Repeating, clarifying, and summarizing are effective verbal techniques. Physical techniques for stimulating memory are note taking, filing, and follow-up memos. Focusing, imaging, linking, locating, and chunking are mental techniques:

- *Focusing* by putting attention on one thing at a time helps block out distractions.

- *Imaging* creates a vivid mental image that helps one remember something. When introduced to Leona Dean, the nurse might picture her leaning on a dean of a specific school to help remember her name.

- *Linking* makes associations between things that make them easier to remember later. Associations may be cause and effect, parts of a whole, or things that are near each other, logically go together, contrast with each other, or happen concurrently. Creating an association that leads from point one to point two to point three and creating an image of those associations will help one remember a speech.

- *Locating* is a memory technique that uses a known structure, often one's home, to arrange and remember information by putting it in specific locations. One might progress through an orientation program by visualizing the hallway in the office and thinking of who is in each office as one walks through the hall and what service that person provides new staff.

- *Chunking* helps one remember by dividing large amounts of information into smaller, more manageable pieces. One could chunk information needed into separate sections of a report, or the nurse could locate what items are needed in specific, separate offices.

Use Telephone Calls

Telephone calls instead of office visits or correspondence save time. Secretaries can screen calls so that other activities are not interrupted and, in fact, may be able to handle much of the business. A call-back system can be used to complete the business the secretary cannot handle. If late morning and late afternoon are chosen for returning calls, calls are likely to be kept short, because people are eager to eat lunch or to go home.

Paging and beeping systems, call forwarding, call back, call waiting, speed dialing, three-way calling, and conference calls make telephoning more efficient. A long cord or cordless phone allows one to move around and work while using the telephone. Car phones can be used during transition times.

Forms for telephone messages are less likely to get lost than scraps of paper. It is helpful for phone messages to be collected in one place. One should keep a list of commonly called phone numbers handy. If major topics for conversation are outlined before making a call, it is less likely that one will forget something and need to call back. One can set the tone of the call. A businesslike call started by "What can I do for you?" will accomplish more in less time than a friendly call started with "How are you?" Conference calls also save time by focusing more on business than socializing. The purpose for the conversation helps determine whether a meeting or a conference call is necessary.

Schedule Office Visits

Secretaries may also screen office visits. Again, they may be able to handle much of the business themselves. When managers schedule reception hours, secretaries can schedule appointments for the appropriate length of time and inform managers of the purpose of the meeting so that they can be adequately prepared. One may need to close the office door to complete a task without interruptions. Sitting with one's back to the door may decrease interruptions because people will notice that the manager is busy.

Control Visit Time

The length of a meeting can be better controlled if it is not in the manager's office. Managers may go to the staff associates' work area or meet visitors in a reception area, where they are free to leave whenever they desire. By standing up when someone drops into the office, managers prevent the visitor from sitting down, thus controlling the situation. They can assess the priority, make an appointment for another time, keep the visit short, or invite the visitor to sit down for a longer discussion. Many drop-in visits can be prevented by scheduling lunch with staff associates on a regular basis. This allows the manager opportunity to keep informed, discuss matters of common interest, and eat lunch at the same time. Staff can be informed through memos and routing slips.

Use Meetings Effectively

Managers spend considerable time in meetings, much of which is wasted. Meetings are used for participative problem solving, decision making, coordination, information sharing, and morale building. Managers first consider the purpose of the meeting; if it is not necessary, they do not conduct it. Key participants are identified, and if they cannot attend, the meeting is not held. People who do not need to attend are not invited. Managers should consider alternatives to a meeting, such as a memo, telephone call, or conference. Staff associates can represent the manager at some meetings both to save managerial time and to develop the staff associates. Managers may limit their time in meetings by attending only that segment when they are to make a contribution. Scheduling meetings before lunch and quitting time facilitates ending meetings on time. A centrally located meeting place saves travel time. The purpose of the meeting should be clearly defined, and an agenda should be circulated before the meeting.

Meetings should start on time, because time is expensive. Starting a meeting 15 minutes late for twenty people who earn $10 an hour costs $50 in downtime. Stating the purpose of the meeting and following the agenda are the manager's responsibilities. The manager should start with high-priority items so that only low-priority items will be left over. The manager should control interruptions, restate conclusions, make assignments and deadlines clear, and end the meeting on time. If the business is completed early, the manager dismisses the meeting. Minutes are circulated preferably within a day after the meeting; this allows people to be informed without having to attend the meeting unless their input is specifically needed. Minutes also remind participants of their assigned tasks.

Delegation

The manager needs to evaluate the risk involved in delegating by assessing the criticality of the expected results and the confidence in resources. The planning strategy ascertains specifications, including the expected results, rationale, requirements, and constraints. The delegated authority should be specified, and support needed should be anticipated. When communicating the delegated assignment, the manager should ensure understanding, give and receive feedback, and address concerns. To monitor the delegated assignment, the manager should set up a milestone-tracking system, review scheduled status reports, and give feedback on the interim reports. Support is provided by responding to the delegatee's needs, acknowledging the status reports, and being available for guidance and problem solving. The manager should intervene only when the action seems warranted and, even then, by avoiding interference and explaining one's actions. Reverse delegation can be avoided by clarifying specifications, transferring authority, and expressing confidence in the delegatee. The results should be evaluated by examining the specifications, evaluating the monitoring results, and giving feedback on the final results.

Reasons for delegating.   Delegation saves time and can help develop others. Delegation maximizes the use of the talents of staff associates. It uses latent abilities in personnel that contribute to their growth and development. Staff members learn by doing. Their involvement tends to increase their motivation and commitment to accomplish goals while freeing the manager to manage. This also reduces managerial costs.

Conditions that facilitate delegation.   Several conditions facilitate delegation. First, managers need to understand the concept of delegation and have a generally positive attitude toward people. They need to overcome feelings of loss of prestige through delegation and develop a positive atmosphere for their staff. They should help achieve results through effective communication instead of by doing the job themselves. Thus, they concentrate on the accomplishment of overall goals and objectives rather than the day-to-day details.

Top management clarifies policies, goals, and objectives, and these are further developed by each succeeding lower level. For example, top management sets the overall budget, but each department then works with its own budget. Specifying goals and objectives directs personnel and determines priorities and the use of resources. Management by objectives promotes this.

Job descriptions provide a definition of the responsibility and authority involved with each position. Everything that must be done for the organization to meet its goals is part of someone's job. Consequently, job descriptions are based on the functional needs of the agency and clarify the responsibility of the individual's position and the objectives of the work.

Before writing job descriptions, management decides which assignments to delegate. To do so, managers should be aware of the capabilities and characteristics of their staff associates. Testing of employees to learn what they can and cannot do and providing the necessary training helps overcome many personnel failures. Staff members are often asked to perform skills for which they are not qualified or in which they are not interested. People tend to put off tasks they find unpleasant and then do them poorly. It is not necessary to delegate equally. By knowing individual capabilities, the manager can delegate according to the associate's interests and abilities.

Job descriptions are not always advantageous in small or rapidly changing organizations, because those staffs often assume different roles at different times. Generalization is more common than the specialization required in larger, more stable organizations. Some employees outperform the requirements of their job descriptions, whereas others are not able to do some of the duties described. Job descriptions can be redefined according to the person's capability and organizational needs. If employees are unable to handle the required duties, they may be transferred to another area, given further training, supplied with an assistant to supplement their weak areas, or fired.

Controls based on goals, rather than means, are important. The manager checks on how well the delegated responsibilities are being performed, and the staff know whether they are meeting their responsibilities. Performance standards clarify how the manager measures achievement. These standards cover the quantity and quality of work expected and the time allowed for its accomplishment. The standards should be broad enough to allow individuality. If the standards are perceived as reasonable and fair by both manager and staff associate, they will both be happier with their jobs. Staff associates like their work to be noticed and appreciated. The manager meets their need for recognition and appreciation by having a general knowledge of what is happening, using an open door policy, expressing willingness to give assistance and support, and taking a personal interest in their problems. A "snoopervisor," however, is not appreciated.

It is the manager's responsibility to assess the results of delegation. One of the most satisfactory ways of being aware of what is happening is by being among the staff associates. Formal and informal meetings, systems of reporting, quality control, and

> **Box 5-3**   ASPECTS OF DELEGATION
>
> Responsibility
> Authority
> Accountability

statistical sampling are other means. Although inspection is perceived as unpleasant, most staff associates accept it as necessary. However, they do object to unnecessary inspections that disturb routines.

Even though people may receive satisfaction by knowing that they are doing a good job, having those efforts recognized by others is appreciated. Managers err if they do not give praise for work well done. People should also be rewarded for their continued contributions to the agency through raises and promotions. If staff associates err, they should be corrected—the sooner the better. But when staff associates participate in goal setting, when the emphasis is on the goal rather than individual personalities, and when training is a continuous process, corrections that otherwise would have been made by the manager may be unnecessary. The system encourages self-correction.

Learning to live with differences may be difficult for managers, especially if they once performed their staff associate's tasks and now find that they are being done differently. It is even more threatening when the staff associate does a better job than the manager once did. It has to be recognized that there will be differences in quantity and quality of work accomplished and methods used between the manager and staff associate or among staff associates.

Responsibility, authority, and accountability.   Assignment of responsibility, delegation of authority, and creation of accountability are the three concepts most often mentioned in relation to the delegation process (see Box 5-3). *Responsibility* denotes obligation. It refers to what must be done to complete a task and the obligation created by the assignment. The manager and the staff associate must understand what activities the staff associate is responsible for, what results are expected, and how performance is to be evaluated. Managers need a clear idea of what they want done before they can communicate that to others. To clarify them for themselves, the managers may put their ideas in writing. By so doing, they are then less likely to give incomplete directions. The assignment of responsibility is not complete, however, until the staff associate decides to accept the obligation.

Authority is the power to make final decisions and give commands. People to whom responsibility has been assigned need the authority to direct the performance of delegated duties. They need authority of sufficient scope to include all related activities without frequent consultation with their manager. The granting of too little authority is a common problem, because organizational policies and procedures are often limiting, and sometimes the person may have little control over the actions of others.

People with delegated authority perform for the manager. Although authority is delegated so that the staff associates can fulfill their responsibilities, the manager maintains control over the delegated authority and may recall it. Delegation of authority involves the staff associate's knowledge, abilities, skills, and potential contribution and the manager's guidance. During the initial phase of delegating authority, staff associates present their ideas and plans. The manager raises questions, explores alternatives, and helps identify potential problems and ways to prevent them. Then mutual agreement is reached. The manager offers continuing support by providing staff, resources, and information needed by the staff associate for the completion of the delegated responsibility. Good communications, sharing of information, and feedback are important.

Accountability refers to liability. Staff associates incur an obligation to complete work satisfactorily and to use authority appropriately when they accept delegated responsibility. They are accountable to their manager. Managers are accountable for the performance of the task, the selection of the person to complete it, and both the staff associate's and their own performance. Head nurses are responsible for delegation to team leaders, who are accountable for delegation to team members. Each remains accountable for the work delegated.

Reasons for underdelegating. There are numerous reasons for underdelegating. Managers may think they can do the job quicker themselves, resent interruptions to answer questions, or not want to take the time to check what has been done. They may get cooperation from other departments more easily than staff associates or be unwilling to take risks for fear of being blamed for others' mistakes.

Some managers do not have confidence in their staff associates and are afraid that their staff associates will not keep them adequately informed. Or they may not trust their staff associates and complain that they lack training and sufficient experience. They may argue that their staff associates have little understanding of the organizational objectives and are specialists without the general knowledge needed for problem solving. In some cases, they may even be afraid that their staff associates will outperform them.

Therefore, managers may like to do the work themselves and feel that they can do it better. They receive personal recognition for and satisfaction from the work and prefer to do the real things instead of just plan with others. Such people often expect perfection, consider themselves indispensable, and desire to dominate. They are afraid of losing power and prestige and are aware that their poor operating procedures and practices may be exposed.

Reasons for not accepting delegation. Staff associates have their reasons for not accepting delegation. Some are dependent on their manager and find it easier to ask the boss. Others lack self-confidence and fear failure and criticism. This fear is often related to how mistakes have been handled. Emphasis on the mistake itself is more threatening than using the situation as a learning experience.

Lack of guidelines, standards, and control are additional problems. Duties are not always clearly defined, authority not specified, or necessary information and resources not readily available. Some staff associates are already overworked. The incentives are

Box 5-4 **REASONS FOR PROCRASTINATION**

EMOTIONAL REASONS	NONEMOTIONAL REASONS
To escape an overwhelming task	Lack of goals
To escape an unpleasant task	Goals without deadlines
To excuse poor work	Unrealistic time estimates
To gain sympathy	Insufficient information
To get someone else to do the job	Inadequate follow-up
	Interruptions
	Overcommitment

inadequate, and they do not want to perform work if their manager receives the credit.*

PROCRASTINATION

Reasons for Procrastination

Reasons for procrastination may be divided into two basic categories: emotional reasons and nonemotional reasons. Box 5-4 lists some of the most common reasons in each category.

Emotional reasons.   There are several emotional causes of procrastination. People may fill present moments with trivia to escape an overwhelming task or choose a pleasant task to escape an unpleasant one. Procrastination can be used as an excuse for poor work with comments such as "I just couldn't get to it until the last minute." Some play victims of circumstances to gain sympathy. Although it is preferable to delegate than to play "poor me," there are those who try to get someone else to do the job through procrastination.

Nonemotional reasons.   Lack of goals, goals without deadlines, and unrealistic time estimates are some reasons for procrastination. Some people have insufficient information to do a job, do inadequate follow-up, or have so many interruptions they can't get a job done. Others are just so overcommitted that they don't have time to do everything they have agreed to do.

Techniques to Stop Procrastination

Dividing and conquering, or breaking a large job down into smaller, more manageable tasks, is a good way to overcome procrastination. Doing a start-up task to get in the

---

* Delegation is discussed more fully in *Executive delegation: achieving results through people*, Stamford, Conn, 1985, Learning International.

Box 5-5   **TECHNIQUES TO STOP PROCRASTINATION**

Break a large job into smaller tasks	Ask yourself, "What's the best use of my
Do a start-up task	time now?"
Take advantage of your moods	Set goals
Consider the consequences of not doing	Set realistic time schedules
the task	Gather necessary information
Consider hiring someone to do the task	Avoid overcommitment
Consider switching jobs with someone	Give yourself rewards
Make a commitment to someone or a	
wager with someone	

mood and taking advantage of moods help. Considering the consequences of not doing the job can motivate some people into action.

Consider using the money you earn by doing things you like to do to hire someone to do what you don't like to do. Consider switching jobs with someone or divide up the job so you do what you like to do, such as the review of the literature, while someone else does what he or she likes to do, such as the statistical analysis of the data. Make a commitment to someone to help overcome procrastination.

It's appropriate to ask yourself, "What's the best use of my time now?" Then set goals, plan realistic time schedules, and gather the necessary information to do the job. Avoid overcommitment and give yourself rewards for jobs well done. Box 5-5 summarizes techniques to help stop procrastination.

MAXIMIZE ORGANIZATION TIME

Plan

Much time can be saved through appropriate organizational planning. The purpose for the existence of the agency should be determined, and the goals and objectives should be defined and ranked in order of importance. Nurse managers determine who is responsible for coordinating activities, who makes what decisions, and who needs to be informed about certain decisions. They also determine what decisions need to be made before others, what action needs to be taken first, and what deadlines must be set. The determining and ranking of goals focus activities and prevent people from spending time doing inappropriate or unimportant tasks. People who are adequately informed of what is expected of them do not waste time wondering what they are supposed to do. Making time estimates and setting time limits help regulate work flow. Through appropriate planning, problems can be prevented. The decreased amount of time spent in crisis management increases the time available for creative work.

Organize

The manager structures the agency to accomplish the tasks necessary to meet the agency's goals. Organizational charts help clarify who is responsible to whom and for what. Job descriptions further clarify these matters. Multiple bosses, confusion over who is responsible and who has authority for what, and duplication of tasks can be prevented with planning. Autonomy and independence reduce the amount of time otherwise spent in conflict management. Policies and procedures help clarify expectations.

Staff

Selection of well-qualified staff is critical for time saving, because they require less supervisory time for development and corrective action. Staff development further reduces time lost by better preparing staff to do their jobs. Appropriate use of personnel through assessment of work to be done, careful planning of the number and mix of personnel, and matching staff members' interests and abilities to the job further reduce waste. When nurses' interests are matched to the organizational goals and they feel appreciated, they are likely to have increased job satisfaction. Consequently there is little absenteeism and less turnover. Nurse managers should watch for chronic absenteeism, try to determine the reason, and correct it. They also expect punctuality, because tardiness is a loss of time. If nurse managers find that employees' personal problems are affecting their work, they should refer personnel for appropriate assistance so that they will have more energy to do their jobs.

Direct

It is nurse managers' responsibility to delegate what a less qualified, lower-paid person can handle. They identify the task to be delegated, determine the best person to do the job, and communicate the assignment clearly. They allow the staff associate to help determine how the task will be accomplished and keep authority commensurate with responsibility. They set controls, monitor results, and provide support as needed. It is essential that managers teach others how to do the work instead of doing it themselves. They can save considerable time by streamlining communication systems and by not holding any more meetings than necessary. The nurse manager should also facilitate open communications and assertive behavior and handle conflict immediately before it drains time and energy.

Control

Nurse managers set standards, monitor results, and give feedback. They adjust closeness of supervision to the needs of the employee, take disciplinary action as soon as it is justified, and fire personnel who are not meeting minimum standards. Good management conserves time and energy. Lack of it leads to management by crisis.

CAREER PLANNING

Choosing a Field of Nursing

There are many opportunities in nursing. From the 1930s until the 1990s about 70% of nursing was done in hospitals. Hospital nurses can do medical, surgical, obstetrical, pediatric, and psychiatric nursing or subspecialties such as intensive cardiac care.

Community health nursing, home care, hospice care, industrial nursing, school nursing, working in a physician's office or clinic, rehabilitation nursing, long-term care, and health promotion are other opportunities. The federal government offers additional options, such as a career in the army, navy, or air force, and working for the nursing service of the Veterans' Administration or the Indian Health Services. Teaching, consulting, conducting research, serving as a staff member of a professional organization, and being an independent nurse practitioner are possibilities.

To set short-term and long-range goals one considers the importance of salary, fringe benefits, retirement plans, work hours, and opportunities for advancement. Desirable climate and geographic location are also considerations. Short-term goals help position one for long-range goals. It is advisable to get some clinical experience before applying for teaching or consultation positions. Trends should be taken into consideration for long-term goals. The population is growing older and acquiring chronic diseases, health care reform is focusing on access to quality economical care, care is moving from the hospital to the community, ambulatory care and home care are increasing, and health promotion is being encouraged.

Locating Job Openings

After deciding what type of nursing one wants to do and the geographic area where one wants to practice, the nurse needs to locate job openings. Professional journals advertise positions, and college placement services and employment agencies maintain job listings. Recruiters are often at professional meetings. One can ask friends, acquaintances, and relatives if they know of openings. Employers can be contacted directly.

Résumé

A résumé is a summary of information about one's education, employment, and professional and personal history. It is typically a prerequisite for an interview, because the employer uses the résumé to determine who will be interviewed. Consequently, the résumé should be carefully developed and updated periodically.

Résumés should be printed on high-quality 8½ inch by 11 inch typing paper with a laser printer—they should never be handwritten. The contents should be well arranged, with major and minor headings to facilitate reading. The content should be concise yet complete, but not crowded. Résumés should contain the following information:

Identification. Full name, address, and telephone number should appear at the beginning of the résumé.

Job objective. Including or excluding a job objective is controversial. Some say it limits one's scope of employment, whereas others argue that the personnel manager should know what position the nurse is seeking. Separate résumés for each job, customizing the job objective, and accenting the characteristics that qualify the nurse for a particular job are appropriate.

Education.   In reverse chronological order, one should list the names and locations of schools attended, dates of attendance, and diploma or degrees conferred. Continuing education, such as workshops, in-service education, and home study courses, indicates an interest in self-improvement and is appropriate to list. If the grade point average is high it is appropriate to cite it.

Work experience.   Previous employment should be listed in reverse chronological order by identifying the name and location of each agency, dates of employment, position title, and responsibilities. New graduates can list their student clinical experiences. It is appropriate to give a reason for leaving the position.

Military service.   If the applicant has served in the armed forces, a summary of the military record should be included. Branch of service, years in the service, rank achieved, awards and distinctions, special assignments, skills, and knowledge acquired are some of the items appropriate to include.

Affiliations.   Memberships, offices, committee activities in professional organizations, learned societies, and civic and social groups may be listed. Religious and political affiliations should be used with discretion.

Honors and awards.   Scholarships, honors, and awards may be cited by stating the honor, the organization that conferred it, the location, and the date.

References.   If references are available, it should be stated that they will be provided upon request. One should always check the willingness of people who might serve as references. One may also compile a letters of reference file by asking teachers, supervisors, or peers to write letters of reference "to whom it may concern" at the time of termination. This is an opportune moment to make such a request because the nurse's performance is vivid in the reviewer's mind. It may prevent the reviewer from having to write more than one letter when copies are acceptable, and the applicant does not have to be concerned about locating the person later. Compiling one's own letter file allows the nurse to send the most informative and appropriate letters of reference. The nurse keeps the original letters and sends the appropriate photocopies with the résumé. Multiple copies with the original signature can be made, to save time.

Cover letter.   The résumé should be accompanied by a cover letter stating the applicant's interest in working for the specific agency, the special qualifications and interests the applicant brings, the applicant's availability, and how the applicant can be reached.

Interview.   An interview allows the employer to determine if the applicant meets the requirements for the position being sought, and it allows the applicant to obtain information about the agency. First impressions are important. The interviewer will quickly assess the applicant's manners and appearance. The applicant may be questioned about dependability, responsibility, and ability to work with others. The compatibility of the applicant's goals with available opportunities may be explored.

Job procurement.   A nurse is likely to apply for more than one job at a time. Once a position has been accepted, the other agencies should be informed of the decision in a friendly and professional way because the nurse may apply to that agency again in the future.

BIBLIOGRAPHY

Anonymous: Skills: using time effectively; types of management activity; delegation, *International Journal of Bank Marketing* 10:17-23, 1992.

Barter M, Furmidge ML: Unlicensed assistive personnel: issues relating to delegation and supervision, *JONA* 24:36-40, April 1994.

Brunsman R: Time control—a waste of time, *Life Association News* 88:114-117, November 1993.

Chaleff I: Overload can be overcome, *Industry Week* 242:44-48, June 7, 1993.

Hasten RI: Delegation: learning when and how to let go, *Nur 91* 21:126, 1991.

Hasten R, Washburn M: Delegation: how to deliver care through others, *AJN* 92:87-89, March 1992.

Hasten R, Washburn M: How to plan what to delegate, *AJN* 92:71, April 1992.

Hasten R, Washburn M: What do you say when you delegate work to others? *AJN* 92:48, July 1992.

Ladouceur ME: Four dimensions, *Executive Excellence* 11:11, January 1994.

Marriner A: Time management, *JONA* 9:16-18, October 1979.

Meade J: On-screen sidekick can help to organize your work, *HR Magazine* 39:36-42, January 1994.

Singhvi SS: Time management can boost white-collar productivity, *National Productivity Review* 12:463-469, Autumn 1993.

CASE STUDY

You are the charge nurse on the 3-to-11 shift. When you return from your dinner break, the ward clerk reports the following:

1. Mrs. Jones' IV has infiltrated.
2. The operating room staff are on their way to take Mr. Anderson to surgery. He has not received his preoperative medication yet.
3. A parent has asked if her daughter, who is a new surgical patient, should have bright red blood on her dressing.
4. Two patients haven't received their meal trays yet.
5. Someone spilled a bouquet of flowers in a patient's room.

   The other RN is busy with his own patients. You have yourself, a ward clerk, and an IV-certified LPN you can delegate to. Decide who should do what and in what priority. Using Worksheet 5-1 on page 78, justify your decisions.

CRITICAL THINKING AND LEARNING ACTIVITIES

1. To practice time management, record what you do every 15 minutes for a typical week and assess how you spent your time. Identify time wasters.

2. Set a goal and plan strategies to accomplish it.

3. Assess your peak and low times and plan your schedule.

4. Prepare a daily "to do" list.

✍ **Worksheet 5-1**

Effective Delegation Tool

1. Identify the task to be accomplished:

2. Identify the skill or educational level needed to complete the job:

3. Identify the person best able to complete the job in terms of capability and time available:

4. Write a clear description of what you want the employee to do:

5. Identify the outcome you expect and by when:

6. Describe the degree of responsibility and authority that the employee will have:

After presenting the necessary information to the employee, have him or her repeat what has been delegated.

Chapter

6

Financial Management

Chapter Objectives

◆ Identify at least three prerequisites to budgeting.

◆ Name and describe at least five types of budgets.

◆ Describe advantages and disadvantages of budgeting.

◆ Describe at least five strategies for cost containment.

◆ Describe at least three environmental factors that stimulated the development of a prospective payment system.

◆ List at least three of the most common methods for costing out nursing service costs.

Major Concepts and Definitions	
Accounting	a system that accumulates bookkeeping entries into summaries of the financial situation of the agency
Budget	a plan for the allocation of resources and a control for ensuring that results comply with the plans
Cost containment	to hold back costs within fixed limits
Economics	production, distribution, and consumption of wealth
Costing out	calculating the cost of specific items

BUDGETS

A budget is a plan for the allocation of resources and a control for ensuring that results comply with the plans. Results are expressed in quantitative terms. Although budgets are usually associated with financial statements, such as revenues and expenses, they also may be nonfinancial statements covering output, materials, and equipment. Budgets help coordinate the efforts of the agency by determining what resources will be used by whom, when, and for what purpose. They are frequently prepared for each organizational unit and for each function within the unit.

Planning is done for a specific time period, usually a fiscal year, but may be subdivided into monthly, quarterly, or semiannual periods. The budgeting period is determined by the desired frequency of checks and should complete a normal cycle of activity. Budget periods that coincide with other control devices—such as managerial reports, balance sheets, and profit-and-loss statements—are helpful.

The extent to which accurate forecasts can be made must be considered. If the budget forecasts too far in advance, its usefulness is diminished. On the other hand, factors such as seasonal fluctuations make it impossible to predict long-range needs from short-budget periods. Managers, therefore, necessarily revise budgets as more information becomes available. Top management and the board of directors also may prepare long-term budgets of 3, 5, or more years, but these are not used as direct operating budgets.

PREREQUISITES TO BUDGETING

Some conditions are necessary for the development and implementation of a budgetary program. First there is need for a sound organizational structure with clear lines of authority and responsibility. All employees know their responsibilities and the person to whom they are responsible; they have the authority to do what they are responsible for and are held accountable for their actions. Organization charts and job descriptions are available, and goals and objectives are set for areas of responsibilities. Budgets are then developed to conform to the pattern of authority and responsibility.

Nonmonetary statistical data—such as number of admissions, average length of stay, percentage of occupancy, and number of patient days—are used for planning and control of the budgetary process. Someone must be responsible for collecting and reporting statistical data.

Charts of accounts are designed to be consistent with the organizational plan. Revenues and expenses are reported by responsibility areas, thus providing historical data that are valuable for planning and providing budgetary control for evaluation as performance can be compared to plans. Nurse managers focus their attention on the principle of management by exception by noting what is not going as planned so they can take necessary action.

Managerial support is essential for a budgetary program. Although budgeting is done at the departmental level, it must be valued by top administration. Managers must be willing to devote their time and energy to the budgeting process. They are most likely to do that when they are familiar with the principles of budgeting and its usefulness for planning and controlling, through budget education.

Formal budgeting policies and procedures should be available in a budget manual, in which objectives of the budgetary program are defined, authority and responsibility for budgeting are clarified, and instructions for budget development are discussed in detail. Samples of standardized forms are available. A calendar of the budgeting activities with the schedule for each stage of the program is presented. Procedures for review, revision, and approval of budgets are discussed in detail.

APPLIED ECONOMICS

Economic goods are goods or services purchased by consumers from suppliers to provide a benefit to the consumer. Goods and services are acquired through exchange, generally of money. *Wealth* is the value of the consumer's resources. *Income* is additional resources gained over time. Consumers do not have the wealth to buy everything they want, so they must make choices about what to purchase.

Utility is the benefit consumers get from the purchase of goods and services. It helps determine how much the consumer is willing to pay. *Marginal utility* is the additional utility gained by consuming one more unit. Marginal utility is not the same for all consumers or for additional units. The person who likes chocolate is more willing to pay for a chocolate candy bar than a person who does not like chocolate but may not be as willing to buy a second or third chocolate bar. People try to maximize their total utility. To do that, a mix of goods should be consumed so that the last unit has the same marginal utility per dollar spent.

Supply and demand influence costs. *Supply* is the amount of goods or service that suppliers are willing to provide at a given price. *Demand* is the amount of goods or service the consumers are willing to buy at that price. For an equilibrium price, the quantity offered and the quantity demanded are the same. As supply goes up and demand goes down, the price is likely to go down. As the supply goes down and the demand goes up, the price is likely to go up.

Elasticity of demand is the degree to which the demand for a good or service decreases in response to a price increase and increases in response to a price decrease. The demand for health care is generally inelastic.

Economies of scale indicate that the cost of providing goods or services falls as quantity increases and fixed costs are shared with the larger volume. Large volumes can eventually lead to decreasing returns to scale as more personnel and supplies are needed.

Incentives encourage action. Managers may use them to encourage good use of scarce resources. Health insurance deductibles are incentives to encourage desirable behavior.

Market efficiency is the optimal allocation and use of goods and services resulting from supply and demand.

Redistribution of resources may be done to improve equality.

Market failure occurs when the free market does not operate efficiently and may result from lack of information, lack of direct patient payment, monopoly, government intervention and induced inefficiency, and other externalities.*

ACCOUNTING

Accounting is a system that accumulates bookkeeping entries into summaries of the financial situation of an enterprise. The fundamental equation of accounting is

$$\text{Assets} = \text{Liabilities} + \text{Fund balance}$$

Assets are the valuable resources owned by the agency. *Liabilities* are what the agency owes. *Fund balance* is the agency's assets. The *balance sheet* is a financial statement that shows the financial position of the agency and a specific time. The *income statement,* or statement of revenues and expenses, shows the financial results of the agency's activities for a specified period. *Depreciation* is the allocation of a portion of the cost of an asset with a multiyear life over the years the asset will be used. A *journal* is a book or computer file recording the financial events of the agency in chronological order. *Ledgers* are sets of individual accounts where information from the journal is transferred or posted so that the balance in any account can be determined and reported. *Fund accounting* is an optional accounting system used by not-for-profit agencies to establish a complete, distinct set of accounting records for separate accounts of agency assets. These assets may be restricted and unrestricted funds set aside for specific purposes such as endowments, renovations, or buildings (Finkler and Kovner, 1993).

Several terms must be understood to interpret financial accounting reports. *Entity* is a definable organizational unit. The accountant considers only transactions between one entity and another. Transactions that occur within the entity or do not involve it are not considered. If each department is an entity, performance can be compared between departments. However, if the agency as a whole is the entity, the transfer of resources from one department to another is not taken into account. Accounts deal only with *transactions,* definable changes in the financial situation of an entity: income, expenditure, depreciation. *Cost valuation* values goods at their cost minus

---

* Finkler SA, Kovner CT: *Financial mangement for nurse managers and executives,* Philadelphia, 1993, WB Saunders.

any depreciation. *Double entry* compares the assets, what is owed to or owned by the entity, with the liabilities, what is owed by the entity to others. Accountants are to balance total assets with the total liabilities and net worth. The double entry makes it possible to know where the entity stands financially at any given time. *Accrual* allows one to determine the overall assets and liabilities by entering transactions on the accounting records at the time a commitment is made rather than waiting until it is billed or paid. *Matching* is the principle of matching revenues with expenses during a budget period.

There are several standard accounting practices. *Consistency* means that categories of transactions may not be changed during or between reporting periods without noting the changes and providing comparable figures. *Materiality* means that transactions can be combined for accounting purposes unless one transaction has a significant impact by itself. *Conservatism* is the act of understating revenue and overstating expenses to provide a margin of safety. *Industry practices* are specific to industries. Special fund accounts designated by donors and a separate account for charitable care provided are examples of industry practices.

TYPES OF BUDGETS

Operating, or Revenue-and-Expense, Budgets

The operating budget provides an overview of an agency's functions by projecting the planned operations, usually for the upcoming year. The operating table reveals an input-output analysis of expected revenues and expenses. Among the factors that nurse managers might include in their operating budgets are personnel salaries, employee benefits, insurance, medical-surgical supplies, office supplies, rent, heat, light, housekeeping, laundry service, drugs and pharmaceuticals, repairs and maintenance, depreciation, in-service education, travel to professional meetings, educational leaves, books, periodicals, subscriptions, dues and membership fees, legal fees, and recreation, such as Christmas parties and retirement teas.

Both controllable and noncontrollable expenses are projected. The manager determines the number of personnel needed and the level of skills required of each. Wage levels and quality of materials used are other controllable expenses. Indirect expenses, such as rent, lighting, and depreciation of equipment, are noncontrollable. The noncontrollable expenses and the probability of rises in material prices or labor costs during the budgetary period demand that an operating budget include some cushion funds to provide for changes beyond the agency's control.

The operating budget deals primarily with salaries, supplies, and contractual services. Nonfinancial factors, such as time, materials, and space, may be translated into dollar values. Work hours, nurse-patient interaction hours, units of materials, equipment hours, and floor space also can be assigned dollar values.

Capital Expenditure Budgets

Capital expenditure budgets are related to long-range planning. Capital expenditures include physical changes such as replacement or expansion of the plant, major equipment, and inventories. These items are usually major investments and reduce the flexibility in budgeting because it takes a long time to recover the costs. For instance, a patient may be charged per treatment or per day for use of equipment, but it may take many months or even years to recover the cost of the equipment.

The hospital administrator usually establishes the ceiling for capital expenses. Under this budget, the nurse manager must establish priorities if requests exceed availability of funds. When filling out request forms for capital items, it is advisable to include names of manufacturers and suppliers, trade-in credits, and estimates of purchase, delivery, installation, and maintenance costs. Written justification for each item should be given.

Inventories are helpful in budgeting. If supplies are checked routinely, use and replacement figures are available for projection of future needs. Central supply services enhance budgetary control, and storage space facilitates inventory maintenance. Stocked supply shelves on each unit with replacement service twice a day can provide a simplified recording system. Disposable equipment and supplies need careful evaluation to determine whether they are more economical than nondisposables.

Cash Budgets

Cash budgets are planned to make adequate funds available as needed and to use any extra funds profitably. They ensure that the agency has enough, but not too much, cash on hand during the budgetary period. This is necessary because income does not always coincide with expenditures. The manager must anticipate fluctuations in resource needs caused by such factors as seasonal variations. If managers have insufficient cash on hand, they will not be able to purchase needed resources. At the other extreme, if too much cash is available, interest or other earnings that money could generate is lost. Budgeting cash requirements may not significantly affect profits, but they do ensure a liquid position and are a sign of prudent management. Using a cash budget, the nurse manager estimates the amount of money to be collected from clients and other sources and allocates that cash to expenditures. If the budget is well planned, it will provide cash as needed and produce interest on excess funds.

Labor, or Personnel, Budgets

Personnel budgets estimate the cost of direct labor necessary to meet the agency's objectives. They determine the recruitment, hiring, assignment, layoff, and discharge of personnel. The nurse manager decides on the type of nursing care necessary to meet the nursing needs of the estimated patient population. How many aides, orderlies, LPNs, and RNs are needed during what shifts, what months, and in what areas? The current staffing patterns, number of unfilled positions, and last year's reports can provide a base for examination and proposals. Patient occupancy and the general complexity of cases affect staffing patterns. Seasonal fluctuations must be considered. Personnel budgets also are affected by personnel policies, such as salary related to position and number of days allowed for educational and personal leave. Overtime costs should be compared with the cost of new positions. Employee turnover, recruitment, and orientation cost must be considered.

Flexible Budgets

Some costs are fixed and do not change with the volume of business. Other costs vary proportionately with changes in volume. Some variable expenses are unpredictable and can be determined only after change has begun: thus the need for flexible budgets, to show the effects of changes in volume of business on expense items. Periodic budget reviews help managers compensate for changes. Relationships between the volume of business and variable costs may be predicted by a historical analysis of costs and development of standard costs.

Strategic Planning Budgets

Long-range budgets for long-range planning are often called the agency's strategic plan and are usually projected for 3 to 5 years.

Program budgets are part of the strategic plan that focuses on all the benefits and costs associated with a particular program.

Business plans are detailed plans for proposed services, projects, or programs. They contain information to assess the financial feasibility of the plan. The business plan states the objectives of the project and links them to the organization's strategic plan.

HISTORICAL APPROACH TO BUDGETING

The historical approach is most effective for calculating the relationship between volume of business and variable costs when a company manufactures a few products and each product contributes a relatively stable percentage to the total sales volume. Using the historical approach, the nurse manager may observe that there are more fractures during skiing season. Consequently, more casting materials are used at that time, and there is a need for increased staffing on the orthopedic ward. A supervising community health nurse in a small college town may note that there is less use of family planning services during the summer months and again during December when students leave for vacations. Consequently, there is less need for contraceptive devices and staffing during these months. There may be an increased demand for immunizations just before elementary schools open in the fall. By plotting on a graph the high and low volumes, the nurse manager can predict the expected costs for each level between the extreme volumes. This historical perspective helps determine the amount of supplies to stock and staffing patterns.

STANDARD COST

Standard cost may be developed to predict what labor and supplies should cost. Multiplying the standard cost by the volume predicts the variable cost. Supervising community health nurses can predict the standard number of clinic visits and the number of birth control pills that will be required by each family planning client who has chosen birth control pills as a method of contraception. Multiplying the number of pills needed by each client by the number of clients using birth control pills, nurse managers can predict the inventory needed and the cost. They also can predict the number of clinic visits needed and plan staffing.

ZERO-BASED BUDGETING

Many budgeting procedures allocate funds to departments on the basis of their previous year's expenditures. Then the department managers decide how the funds will be used. This procedure usually allows for enrichment and enlargement of programs but seldom for decreases in or deletion of programs. Obsolescence is seldom examined, and this leads to increased costs.

With zero-based budgeting, no program is taken for granted. Each program or service must be justified each time funds are requested. Managers decide what will be done, what will not be done, and how much of an activity will be implemented. A decision package is prepared. The package includes a list of the activities that make up a program, the total cost, a description of what level of service can be performed at various levels of funding, and the ramifications of including them in or excluding them from the budget. The manager may identify the activity, state the purpose, list related activities, outline alternative ways of performing activities, and give the cost of the resources needed.

After decision packages are developed, they are ranked in order of decreasing benefits to the agency. They can be divided into high-, medium-, and low-priority categories and reviewed in order of rank for funding. Resources are allocated based on the priority of the decision package. The cost of each package is added to the cost of approved packages until the agreed-on spending level is reached. Lower ranked packages are then excluded.

A major advantage to zero-based budgeting is that it forces managers to set priorities and justify resources. Unfortunately, the process is time-consuming.

PERIODIC BUDGETARY REVIEW

Managers should review the budget at periodic intervals, compare actual with projected performances, and make necessary changes. However, if changes are too frequent or too great, the original budget becomes useless. One way to minimize variance between the annual budget and the revised budget is to anticipate such factors as increased labor costs and the inflationary cost of materials. When discrepancies are found between actual performance and the budget, management must determine the cause of variation to make appropriate adjustments for future plans. A variance may not be reason for changing the budget. It may be a symptom that alerts management to the need for further investigation and explanation. What may demand change is not the budget but the situation.

SUPPLEMENTARY BUDGETS

Some budgetary flexibility may be obtained through a supplemental monthly budget. A basic or minimal budget is planned, usually for a year's time, to outline the framework for the agency's plans, establish department objectives, and coordinate departments. Then a monthly supplementary budget is prepared on the basis of the volume of business forecast for that month.

MOVING BUDGETS

The moving budget may be used when forecasting is difficult. The moving budget plans for a certain length of time, such as a year. At the end of each month, another month is added to replace the one just completed. Thus the budgetary period remains constant. The projections progress a month at a time but always for a fixed period, such as 1 year. It is an annual budget revised monthly. As January is completed, the January budget for the forthcoming year is added to the moving budget.

ADVANTAGES AND DISADVANTAGES

Advantages and Disadvantages of Flexible Budgets

The major advantage of flexible budgets is the study and analysis necessary to prepare one. Fixed and variable costs and their effect on the total cost are analyzed. Unfortunately, flexible budgets are very costly to prepare and very time-consuming. It is difficult to predict short-term variations in volume, and it is unlikely that the information can result in savings of variable expenses.

Advantages of Budgeting

Budgets plan for detailed program activities. They help fix accountability by assignment of responsibility and authority. They state goals for all units, offer a standard of performance, and stress the continuous nature of planning and control process. Budgets encourage managers to make a careful analysis of operations and to base decisions on careful consideration. Consequently, hasty judgments are minimized. Weaknesses in the organization can be revealed and corrective measures taken. Staffing, equipment, and supply needs can be projected and waste minimized. Financial matters can be handled in an orderly fashion, and agency activities can be coordinated and balanced.

Disadvantages of Budgeting

Budgets convert all aspects of organizational performance into monetary values for a single comparable unit of measurement. Consequently, only those aspects that are easy to measure may be considered, and equally important factors, such as organizational development and research efforts, may be ignored. Symptoms may be treated as causes. Reasons for the symptoms should be explored, because a decrease in revenue from the family planning clinic may be related to the way people are treated at the clinic, a new competitive service in the neighborhood, or other factors. The budget may become an end in itself instead of the means to an end. Budgetary goals may supersede agency goals and gain autocratic control of the organization. There is a danger of overbudgeting; the budget becomes cumbersome, meaningless, and expensive. Forecasting is required but uncertain because budgetary control is subject to human judgment, interpretation, and evaluation. Skill and experience are required for successful budgetary control. Budget planning is time-consuming and expensive.

BUDGETING PROCESS

Financial planning responsibilities need to be identified before budget preparation begins. The governing board, administrator, budget director, steering committee, and department heads are often involved in the budgetary process. The *governing board* is responsible for the general planning function. It selects the budget steering committee, determines the budgetary objectives, and reviews and approves the master budget. The *administrator* is responsible for the formulation and execution of the budget, by correlating the governing board's goals with the guidelines for budget preparation and supervising the budget preparation. The *budget director* is responsible for the budgeting procedures and reporting. He or she establishes a completion timetable, has forms prepared, and supervises data collection and budget preparation. The budget director serves as the chairperson of the *steering committee,* which approves the budget before it is submitted to the governing board. *Department heads* prepare and review goals and objectives and prepare the budgets for their departments.

The first step in the budget process is the establishment of operational goals and policies for the entire agency. The governing board should approve a long-range plan of 3 to 5 years that reflects the community's future health needs and other community health care providers' activities. Because the situation changes over time, flexibility is built into the plan. Then operational goals must be translated into quantifiable management objectives for the organizational units. The department heads use the organizational goals as a framework for the development of departmental goals. A formal plan for budget preparation and review including assignment of responsibilities and timetables must be prepared. Historical, financial, and statistical data must be collected monthly so that seasonal fluctuation can be observed. Departmental budgets need to be prepared and coordinated. During this phase, units of service, staffing patterns, salary and nonsalary expenses, and revenues are forecasted so that preliminary rate setting can be done. Next, departmental budgets are revised, and the master budget is prepared. At this point, operating, payroll, nonsalary, capital, and cash budgets can be incorporated into the master budget. Then the financial feasibility of the master budget is tested, and the final document is approved and distributed to all parties involved.

During the budget period, there should be periodic performance reporting by responsibility centers.

COST CONTAINMENT

The goal of cost containment is to keep costs within acceptable limits for volume, inflation, and other acceptable parameters. It involves cost awareness, monitoring, management, and incentives to prevent, reduce, and control costs.

Cost Awareness

Cost awareness focuses the employee's attention on costs. It increases organizational awareness of what costs are, the process available for containing them, how they can be managed, and by whom. Delegating budget planning and control to the unit level increases awareness. Managers should be provided a course about budgeting and be oriented to the agency budgeting process before being assigned the responsibility. They should have a budget manual that contains budget forms, budget calendar, and budget periods.

Cost Fairs

Cost fairs in frequented areas such as the cafeteria increase awareness by displaying frequently disappearing items that are labeled with the cost per unit and by posting lists of estimated costs of inventory losses. Staff development programs, unit conferences, and poster contests help increase awareness. Tagging supply items and posting a computer printout of unit charges for supplies and services are revealing. Reviewing a patient's itemized bill during a conference can also be effective.

Cost Monitoring

Cost monitoring focuses on how much will be spent where, when, and why. It identifies, reports, and monitors costs. Staffing costs should be identified. Recruitment, turnover, absenteeism, and sick time are analyzed, and inventories are controlled. A central supply exchange chart prevents hoarding of supplies and allows identification of lost items.

Cost Management

Cost management focuses on what can be done by whom to contain costs. Programs, plans, objectives, and strategies are important. Responsibility and accountability for the control should be established. A committee can identify long- and short-range plans and strategies. A suggestion box can be used, as can contests for the idea that saves the most money.

Money has been saved by means such as forming a staff pool to maximize flexibility in staffing for census fluctuations, cross-training personnel, closing units for cleaning or remodeling and encouraging staff vacations when census is low, balancing the workload among shifts to minimize peaks and valleys in assigned tasks, reducing shift overlap, charting by exception, tape-recording shift reports, revising forms, improving drug ordering and delivery systems, controlling central supplies, noncontrolling oral analgesics, modifying food services, allowing volunteers to discharge and transport patients, reducing the amount of time nurses spend in nonnursing functions, and using guest relations personnel, a discharge holding area, outpatient clinics, progressive care, ambulatory care, and cooperative care for obstetrical patients.

Cost Incentives

Cost incentives motivate cost containment and reward desired behavior. Contests for the best money-saving ideas, perfect attendance, and nurse of the month help recognize personnel efforts.

Cost Avoidance

Cost avoidance means not buying supplies, technology, or services. Supply and equipment costs should be carefully analyzed. Costs and effectiveness of disposable versus reusable items are compared. The receipt, storage, and delivery of disposables and labor and processing costs of reusable items are part of the analysis. The least expensive and most effective supplies, equipment, and services should be identified and expensive and less effective items avoided.

Cost Reduction

Cost reduction means spending less for goods and services. The amount of reduction depends on the size of the agency, previous efficiency, skill of managers, and cooperation of employees. Safety programs that reduce the costs of worker's compensation and absenteeism programs that reduce sick time, absenteeism, and turnover reduce costs.

Cost Control

Cost control is effective use of available resources through careful forecasting, planning, budget preparation, reporting, and monitoring. Cost-effectiveness compares costs and identifies the most beneficial outcomes to costs by specifying programs, identifying goals, analyzing alternatives, comparing costs per program unit of service and amount of service needed, assessing effect of the outcome, and determining cost outcome and cost-effectiveness.

PROSPECTIVE PAYMENT

A prospective reimbursement system encourages the implementation of cost-effective health care services. The Tax Equity Fiscal Responsibility Act of 1982 added case-mix into Medicare based on diagnostic-related groups (DRGs). A prospective payment system based on 467 DRG categories that provided pretreatment diagnosis billing categories for most U.S. hospitals reimbursed by Medicare was signed into law as H.R. 1900 (P.L. 98-21) by President Reagan. It used a prospective rather than the traditional retrospective time frame. Reimbursement is by case or costs related to treatment of specific DRG rather than per diem or total hospital costs divided by patient days. The payment unit is the diagnosis rather than patient day. Rates are determined from local, regional, and national rural and urban costs instead of the hospital's own costs. There are incentive payments when the length of stay is lower than average and disincentives when costs exceed the standard so that hospitals profit from cost containment. Previously hospitals were reimbursed for costs retrospectively and had little incentive to contain costs. The prospective payment system applies to all Medicare-participating hospitals, except long-term care, rehabilitation, children's, and psychiatric care hospitals.

The results of DRGs include a decrease in number of patients in acute care settings caused by early discharge, an increase in the acuteness of illness among hospitalized patients, an increase in the use of ambulatory and home care facilities, and a focus on cost-effectiveness.

ECONOMICS AND HEALTH CARE FINANCING

Economics deals with efficient allocation of scarce resources; it determines which alternative represents the most efficient use of resources. But social, ethical, and moral questions must be considered to determine whether the most efficient allocation is socially acceptable.

Enacted in 1946, the federal Hill-Burton program stimulated a postwar replenishment of hospital capital facilities. The Medicare and Medicaid legislation of the mid-1960s encouraged use of those facilities, as did the role of other third-party payers, such as Blue Cross, Blue Shield, and other insurance companies. Hospitals, physicians, and patients were aware that most of the bills would be paid by insurance companies rather than patients; this pattern promoted skyrocketing medical costs. Increasing prices of food, equipment, energy, labor, and minimum-wage workers have contributed to inflated cost of health care, which has exceeded the Consumer Price Index. Supply and demand for health care services have changed with increased life expectancy, as the proportion of the population over 65 and over 85 has increased dramatically. The aged population spends about three times as much on health care as others and accounts for several percent of the increase in health care costs. New technology prolongs the lives of terminally ill patients, but this success contributes to the increased health care costs.

The Health Care Financing Administration (HCFA) is the single largest payer of health care costs, financing about 30% of all personal health care spending. In 1981 the federal government, direct patient payments, and private health insurers and other private third parties each paid 29% of health care costs while state and local governments paid 13%. HCFA is one of four major operating components of the Department of Health and Human Services (DHHS), a cabinet-level department of the federal government.

The DHHS budget is the third largest in the world, after only the U.S. and Soviet Union budgets. HCFA is responsible for Medicare and Medicaid programs that pay for about one of every five persons' (nearly 49 million people's) health care services. Medicare is the federal health insurance program for the aged, the disabled, and those with end-stage renal disease (ESRD) requiring dialysis for transplantation. Medicare (Title XVIII of the Social Security Act) was created in 1965 to supplement the Social Security cash benefit provisions. It is divided into two administrative segments: Part A, Hospital Insurance, which pays primarily for inpatient services, and Part B, Supplementary Medical Insurance, which pays for physician care and other related services. About two thirds of Medicare expenses are for inpatient hospital services. Medicaid is a joint federal and state assistance program for low-income persons and their families. Medicaid and Medicare support about 50% of all nursing home spending, about 35% of all hospital spending, and about 20% of all physician spending. Therefore, they are the logical targets for health care financing reforms (Davis, 1983).

In 1969 the Special Council to the commissioner of insurance of New Jersey published the *Wharton Report;* its most important effect was to encourage policy-makers to favor case-mix-based reimbursement.

The Health Facilities Planning Act of 1971 empowered the commissioner of health and the commissioner of insurance to regulate Blue Cross charges. *Bureaucratic Malpractice,* a report published in 1974, cited the per diem methods of hospital reimbursement by third-party payers as having created an incentive for facilities to increase the length of hospital stay beyond medical justification. The report suggested that reimbursement to hospitals by case rather than by day (per diem) could increase efficiency.

The election of Brendan Byrne as governor of New Jersey in 1974 and his appointment of Joanne Finley as health commissioner led to a more aggressive approach to cost containment. Joanne Finley's first approach, Standard Hospital Accounting and Rate Evaluation (SHARE), employed the traditional per diem method of billing regulation. She introduced public accounting into hospital reimbursement, in the form of a uniform hospital accounting system imposed by the state. Costs were grouped into 34 cost centers, and inpatient costs were grouped into three categories: (1) non–physician-controllable costs, (2) physician costs (salaries and fees), and (3) other costs that were either not controllable by the hospital or not included in determining the SHARE reimbursement rate. A preliminary per diem reimbursement rate was determined for the hospital after the hospital's reasonable costs were determined. Similar institutions were classified according to their comparable attributes in order to apply fair standards, comparable to the customary practice of peer grouping used in the utilities field.

Unfortunately, hospital output is measurable by so many indices that peer review is confounded; it is far more complex than metered electicity or telephone time used. SHARE was an innovative model of prospective reimbursement and a step toward cost containment, but it did not offer sufficient inducement for cost containment. The New Jersey Hospital Association actively opposed further imposition of controls on rates because profits depended on per diem billing to cover costs. Institutional inertia and bureaucratic resistance resulted in a preference for covering costs rather than reducing them.

Case mix is a way of defining a hospital's output or product by identifying clinically homogeneous groups of patients who use similar amounts of tests, treatments, and services. It is useful for partitioning patient services and predicting resource allocation. Case mix by disease staging and case mix by diagnosis are two distinct concepts that have been studied by a variety of researchers. Case mix by disease staging is based on physician judgments of the progression of the condition through levels of severity. Feldstein demonstrated that case mix could explain variations in hospital costs and stressed that patient categories must be medically meaningful, not just administratively convenient and that patient categories must be homogeneous with respect to resources consumed in treatment. Feldstein's research shifted resource consumption measurement to patient diagnostic stage or episode rather than patient day (Shaffer, 1983).

However, because of its practical availability, length of stay was used by the Yale research team as the principal determinant for the cost of treating statistically determined DRGs. The first version of the DRG system included 383 categories, which were redefined because of the excessive number of outliers, or patients who did not fit into any category. DRGs are not without problems: some categories lack homogeneity and may be applicable only to the population originally tested; length of stay is not very applicable to actual costs; some physicians have differences in therapeutic philosophies, and may vary their treatment of the same disease; different treatments cost different amounts; and some diseases do not have common treatment regimens.

However, there are potential administrative applications of case-mix information, including resource allocation, pricing (rate setting and financial planning), cost and efficiency control (standard setting, measurement of productivity), and quality control (quality assurance).

COSTING OUT NURSING SERVICES

There are several benefits to costing out nursing services.

- Charging out nursing services makes it possible for the customer to pay for what he or she gets: the patient pays for the care rendered.

- Customers start to realize that direct care has a price value. This helps them comprehend costs of health care and, ideally, to value it.

- Hospitals can receive compensation for what they provide, to help maximize profits.

- Nursing can be viewed as a revenue-generating center rather than a cost.

- Charging a fee for services helps enhance the professionalism of nursing through the traditional pattern of reimbursement for services.

- Costing out nursing services stimulates productivity by visualizing productivity measures to enhance the use of human resources, contain costs, and maintain quality.

- The nursing department often accounts for 40% to 60% of an agency's budget. Better budget control through a cost accounting system facilitates improvement of managerial assessment and control of resources.

- Using a cost accounting system to assess and change the nursing department helps establish a reputation for innovation and leadership. Quick responsiveness to changes will help agencies survive in a rapidly changing environment (Flarey, 1990).

The most commonly used methods for determining hospital nursing service costs are per diem, or cost per day, of service; costs per diagnosis; costs per relative intensity measures (RIMs); and patient classification systems (costs per nursing workload measures).

Per Diem

Per diem methods are the oldest methods used for both rate setting and reimbursement. Average nursing care cost per patient day is calculated by dividing the total nursing costs by the number of patient days for a specific period. Nursing costs are usually considered as salary and fringe benefits for staff and administrative nursing personnel. These costs can be calculated for individual cost centers, subdivisions, or the entire nursing service. Per diem relates nursing costs directly to length of stay but does not identify patient needs, acknowledge differences in diagnosis, specify nursing services needed, justify care given, or provide information for management decisions.

Costs per Diagnosis

Information about the patient mix is often used to reduce the variability in nursing care requirements. The medical diagnosis is frequently used to identify groupings. DRGs use this method. Some people recommend using nursing diagnosis or nursing care standards for grouping patients according to their nursing care needs. It seems logical that nursing diagnosis could better predict nursing care needs than DRGs based on medical diagnosis.

Costs per RIMs

RIMs were developed in New Jersey to allocate nursing resources in such a way as to address the complaints that DRGs inadequately represent variability of nursing care requirements. A RIM is 1 minute of nursing resource use. RIMs are costed and allocated to DRG case-mix categories through three steps: (1) The cost of a RIM is calculated by dividing the total nursing costs for a hospital by the total minutes of care estimated or nursing resources used to provide care to all patients. (2) The number of minutes used by the total hospital population, including adjustments for downtime, such as sick leave and vacation time, is calculated. (3) The cost of care for each patient is determined by multiplying the RIM by the minutes of care required by the patient as estimated by an equation. The RIMs developmental studies used data from New Jersey hospitals to measure the time used by nursing personnel performing nursing and nonnursing activities during the entire hospitalization. Thirteen resource groups were identified by mathematical modeling of data, and equations were derived for predicting nursing resource use for each of the 13 clusters. Length of stay was the best predictor of nursing time required.

Costs per Nursing Workload Measures

Patient classification systems were developed to allocate nursing staffing before DRG-based reimbursement. Nursing workload data have been used by some to calculate the cost of the nursing component of room rate. Cost accounting methods allow calculations for whole-patient care units and for individual patients; consequently, it is possible to generate a separate charge for nursing services for individual patients. These methods are also used to allocate nursing costs to DRGs or cost centers. Unfortunately there is limited retrievability of data, because few hospitals record patient classification data for individual patients in the patient record or on a database, data collection and analysis are expensive, and practice may not adhere to standards.

In general, the key problems related to costing out nursing are a lack of comparability of data used, multiple definitions of costs, and neglect of variables that affect nursing care (Edwardson and Giovannetti, 1987).

There is still much work to do. We need a forum where administrators, researchers, educators, and staff can share ideas about cost-effectiveness. We need models to describe the relationships among cost, quality, and price of nursing functions. We need to continue to compare methods for costing out nursing care and to identify data sets needed to cost out nursing and relate that to the minimum data set identified by Werley and others. Levels of care, expected outcomes, and cost of care can be related to pricing of nursing care. Nurses must be concerned about maintaining cost-effective, high-quality health care (Johnson, 1989).

PERSONAL FINANCES

This discussion of personal finance will help the reader understand broader economic and financial principles by applying them to his or her personal situation.

Assess Personal Finances

To assess your personal finances, ask the following questions:

Assets. How much do you have?

Debts. How much do you owe?

Income. How much do you earn?

Expenditures. How much do you spend?

Savings. Are you saving enough?

After using Worksheets 6-1 and 6-2 at the end of this chapter to assess your assets and liabilities and cash flow, consider making changes in your personal finances by trying to find places to spend less and save more and looking for patterns of spending that could indicate trouble.

Money Makes Money

Make sure that your money is earning interest whenever possible. You also need cash on hand or assets located where they can be converted into cash. Banks, savings and loan associations, and credit unions offer a variety of accounts that pay interest and are insured by the federal government, including money-market deposit accounts, savings accounts, and interest-paying checking accounts. Interest rates vary. There may be a fee if your balance falls below a minimum level. There may also be annual fees, monthly maintenance charges, and per-check charges.

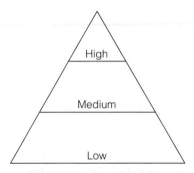

Figure 6-1 Pyramid of risk.

Financial Goals

Using Worksheet 6-3 at the end of the chapter, set and prioritize financial goals. Evaluate if your goals are realistic. Achieving your goals depends on the following factors:

- How soon you want to achieve them

- How much you can save

- How much risk you are willing to take

- What rate of return that risk will bring

There is no risk of losing your money in federally insured savings accounts within the insured limit of $100,000.00, but savings accounts pay a low interest. Money-market funds and certificates of deposit usually pay a little more than savings accounts with virtually no risk. Bonds pay more interest but have some market risk. When interest rates rise, the market value of stocks rise and the market value of bonds falls. Stocks have brought investors double-digit annual returns over time. The benefits of real estate vary over time. Your attitude toward risk will influence which investment you choose. If you cannot meet your goals in the time frame you set, you may need to (1) delay one or more goals, (2) set aside more money for savings, or (3) take more risk in the hope that your savings will grow faster.

Investment Strategies

The objectives of investment strategies are to preserve capital and to make it grow at a rate faster than inflation. To do that you need to allocate and diversify your funds. A large portion of your investments and savings should be at low risk. Fewer should be in higher-risk ventures. Spread your risk (see Figure 6-1). Box 6-1 lists some low-, medium-, and high-risk investments.

It takes discipline to save money. Savings should be treated as a fixed income, just another bill to pay each month. Payroll deductions can save your money before you get your check, and automatic bank payments can make deposits into mutual funds or savings plans. Planning for college and retirement requires big

Box 6-1   **LOW-, MEDIUM-, AND HIGH-RISK INVESTMENTS**

LOW-RISK SAVINGS AND INVESTMENTS

Certificates of deposit
Interest-paying checking accounts
Money-market funds
Savings accounts
Savings bonds
Treasury bills and bonds

MEDIUM-RISK INVESTMENTS

Growth and income mutual funds
High-quality bond mutual funds
High-quality municipal and corporate bonds
Income mutual funds
Income stocks
Long-term growth stocks
Long-term growth stock mutual funds
Rental real estate
Tax-deferred annuities
Utility stocks

HIGH-RISK INVESTMENTS

Aggressive growth stock mutual funds
Collectibles
Emerging technology company stocks
Gold and other precious metals
High-yield bonds
High-yield mutual finds
Mutual funds investing in emerging technology firms
Oil and gas partnerships
Stocks of small companies listed in the over-the-counter market

---

savings plans. Assets can be protected through insurance—health, disability, auto, home, and life.

It is important to get good financial advice. A lawyer can help with estate planning and wills. A tax adviser can help minimize taxes on various financial transactions. A stockbroker and an independent insurance agent can make valuable recommendations.*

---

* Young A: *Personal finance*, Washington, DC, 1988, Conrad and Associates, Inc.

BIBLIOGRAPHY

Cassidy SM: Medical care decisions with limited resources: can equitable decisions be made? *Benefits Quarterly* 9:94-98, First Quarter 1993.

Davis DK: The federal role in changing health care financing. 1. National programs and health financing problems, *Nurs Econ* 1:10-17, July-August 1983.

Finney RG: Budgeting: plan for the unknown, *Management Review* 82:20-23, October 1993.

Flarey DL: A methodology for costing nursing service, *Nurs Adm Q* 14:41-51, Spring 1990.

Freed DH: Cost cutting for hospitals: a heuristic approach, *Hospital Material Management Quarterly* 13:72-77, February 1992.

Fuszard B, Slocum LI, Wiggers DE: Rural nurses. 1. Surviving cost containment, *JONA* 20:7-12, April 1990.

Hesterly SC, Robinson MA: Alternative caregivers: cost-effective utilization of RNs, *Nurs Adm Q* 14:18-23, Spring 1990.

Hollander SF, Smith M, Barron J: Cost reductions part 1: an operations improvement process, *Nurs Econ* 10:325-330, September-October 1992.

Holswade SA, Jones SK, McTernan KJ: Relative costing eases clinical financial analysis, *Healthcare Financial Management* 44:94-95, January 1990.

Johnson M: Perspectives on costing nursing, *Nurs Adm Q* 14:65-71, Fall 1989.

Jones KR: Feasibility analysis of preferred provider organizations, *JONA* 20:28-33, January 1990.

Joseph AC: Ambulatory care: an objective assessment, *JONA* 20:27-33, February 1990.

Kiel JM: The importance of budgeting with nontraditional staffing patterns, *Health Care Supervisor* 11:59-69, March 1993.

Lazenby S: The psychology of budgeting, *American City & County* 107:10, June 1992.

Lentini F: Accounting for marketing success, *Journal of Accountancy* 175:44-46, March 1993.

Mailbot CB, Binger JL, Slezak LG: Managing operating room budget variances, *JONA* 20:19-26, May 1990.

Marriner A: Budgets, *Supervisor Nurse* 8:53-56, April 1977.

Marriner A: Budgetary management, *J Cont Ed Nur* 11:11-14, June 1980.

May BR: How any supervisor can control company costs, *Supervision* 51:3-5, April 1990.

Merchant KA: How challenging should profit budget targets be? *Management Accounting* 72:46-48, November 1990.

Mills ME: Operations improvement, *JONA* 20:40-44, June 1990.

Murry P: Trigger responsive budgeting, *Australian Accountant* 63:22-25, August 1993.

Nichols LM: Estimating costs of underusing advanced practice nurses. *Nurs Econ* 10:343-351, September-October 1992.

Orme CN, Parsons RJ, Baxter TD: Beating the capital budgeting blues: developing capital request evaluation criteria, *Healthcare Financial Management* 47:83-89, February 1993.

Posner BG, Brokaw L, Brown PB: Squeeze play: 40 ways to cut your losses, *Inc.* 12:68-75, July 1990.

Reis J et al: Care for the underinsured: who should pay? *JONA* 20:16-20, March 1990.

Schmidt JA: Is it time to replace traditional budgeting? *Journal of Accountancy* 174:103-107, October 1992.

Shaffer FA: DRGs: history and overview, *Nurs Health Care* 4:388-396, September 1983.

Smeltzer CH: The impact of prospective payment on the economics, ethics, and quality of nursing, *Nurs Adm Q* 14:1-10, Spring 1990.

Stout DE, Liberatore MJ, Monahan TF: Decision support software for capital budgeting, *Management Accounting* 73:50-53, July 1991.

Young DW, Pearlman LK: Managing the stages of hospital cost accounting, *Healthcare Financial Management* 47:58-80, April 1993.

CASE STUDY

Write the scenario for this case study yourself using yourself as the main character. Using Worksheets 6-1, 6-2, and 6-3, assess your financial goal priorities, assess assets and liabilities, and calculate personal cash flow.

CRITICAL THINKING AND LEARNING ACTIVITIES

1. Make a list of ways you could control costs for your personal budget.

2. Form small groups in class and brainstorm ways nurses can control hospital expenses.

3. One member of the class can get a list of costs of supplies and equipment from a local health care agency and share it with other class members.

✏ **Worksheet 6-1**

Assessment of Assets and Liabilities

Assets	Amount
Checking accounts	$ _____
Savings accounts	_____
Certificates of deposit	_____
Money-market funds	_____
Other savings	_____
Stocks	_____
Bonds	_____
Mutual funds	_____
Market value of home	_____
Other real estate	_____
Cash value of life insurance	_____
Surrender value of annuities	_____
Equity in retirement funds	_____
Equity in profit sharing plans	_____
IRAs	_____
Keoghs	_____
Collectibles	_____
Precious metals	_____
Antiques	_____
Automobiles	_____
Household furnishings	_____
Furs and jewelry	_____
Loans receivable	_____
Other assets	

Liabilities

Current bills	$ _____
Credit card balance	_____
Mortgage balance	_____
Home equity loan	_____
Auto loans	_____
Student loans	_____
Other debts	
Current net worth (assets minus liabilities)	$ _____

✍ **Worksheet 6-2**

Personal Cash Flow

Income	Monthly	Annually
Take-home pay	$ _____	$ _____
Bonuses	_____	_____
Self-employment income	_____	_____
New income from rental property	_____	_____
Interest	_____	_____
Dividends	_____	_____
Other	_____	_____
Total	$ _____	$ _____

Expenditures

	Monthly	Annually
Rent or mortgage	$ _____	$ _____
Property taxes	_____	_____
Income taxes	_____	_____
Credit card payments	_____	_____
Auto insurance	_____	_____
Homeowner's insurance	_____	_____
Food	_____	_____
Utilities	_____	_____
Furnishings	_____	_____
Transportation	_____	_____
Child care	_____	_____
Clothing and personal care	_____	_____
Medical bills	_____	_____
Dental bills	_____	_____
Educational expenses	_____	_____
Entertainment, recreation	_____	_____
Gifts	_____	_____
Contributions	_____	_____
Pocket money	_____	_____
Miscellaneous	_____	_____
Total	$ _____	$ _____
Surplus or Deficit (Income minus expenditures)	$ _____	$ _____

✍ **Worksheet 6-3**

Financial Goal Priorities

	Short Term (1 Year)	Medium Term (1 to 5 Years)	Long Term (5 to 10 Years)	Longest Term (Over 10 Years)
Buy a car				
Buy a home				
Make home improvements				
Change jobs				
Start a business				
Have children				
Pay for children's education				
Ensure adequate disability income				
Provide for survivor in event of death				
Take dream vacation				
Buy vacation home				
Reduce debt				
Increase charitable giving				
Achieve adequate retirement income				
Take early retirement				
Other				
Other				

Chapter

7

Marketing

Chapter Objectives

◆ Identify at least five factors that should be considered when making a marketing audit and ask a question to evaluate each of those factors.

◆ Describe the four *p*'s of the marketing mix.

◆ Describe the Boston consulting group's grid of potential growth and profitability possibilities for identifying marketing strategies.

◆ Identify the four stages in the life cycle of a product.

◆ Identify at least three ways to do pricing.

◆ List at least four promotion tools.

Major Concepts and Definitions	
Marketing	the analysis, planning, implementation, and control of programs for exchanges of values with target markets to achieve organizational objectives
Exchange	resource dependency
Publics	distinct groups of people or organizations that have an actual or potential interest in or impact on an organization
Market	potential arena for trading resources
Image	sum of a person's beliefs, ideas, and impressions about an object or person
Audit	identification, collection, and evaluation of information that needs to be examined to evaluate market relations
Segmentation	subsets of the total market
Marketing mix	product, price, place, and promotions
Life cycle	introduction, growth, maturity, and market decline stages of a product

MARKETING

"Marketing is the analysis, planning, implementation, and control of carefully formulated programs designed to bring about voluntary exchanges of values with target markets for the purpose of achieving organizational objectives. It relies heavily on designing the organization's offering in terms of the target markets' needs and desires and on using effective pricing, communication, and distribution to inform, motivate, and service the markets."*

Marketing Concepts

Exchange. Marketing is based on resource dependency or exchange. Organizations offer satisfactions such as goods, services, or benefits to markets that in return provide needed resources such as goods, services, time, money, or energy. Exchange involves four conditions: (1) There are at least two parties. (2) Each party offers something that the other considers valuable. (3) Each party is capable of communication and delivery. (4) Each party is free to accept or reject the offer (Kotler, 1982, p. 37).

Publics. "A public is a distinct group of people and/or organizations that has an actual or a potential interest and/or impact on an organization" (Kotler, 1982, p. 47). *Input publics* supply resources and constraints and consist of suppliers, donors, and

---

* From Kotler P: *Marketing for nonprofit organizations,* Englewood Cliffs, NJ, 1982, Prentice-Hall, p. 6.

regulatory publics. Those inputs are then managed by the organization's internal publics, such as the board of directors, management, staff, and volunteers, to accomplish the organization's mission. *Intermediary publics* are used to promote and distribute goods and services to consumers. The *consuming publics*, such as patients, clients, and students, consume the output of the organization. *Reciprocal publics* are interested in the agency, and the agency is interested in them. Patients are an example. *Sought publics* are desired by the agency but are not necessarily interested in the agency. For instance, wealthy people who are potential donors could be a sought public. *Unwelcome publics* are interested in the agency, but the agency is not interested in them. One unwelcome public consists of emergency room patients for nonemergency care. Publics are related to each other as well as to the agency, and they influence each other's attitudes and behaviors. Publics are groups that have actual or potential interests in or impact on the agency.

Market.   "A market is a potential arena for the trading of resources." It is "a distinct group of people and/or organizations that [has] resources which they want to exchange, or might conceivably be willing to exchange, for distinct benefits" (Kotler, 1982, p. 50). A market is actual or potential buyers and a place where people negotiate to transfer goods or services. The health care agency goes to the labor market to obtain employees, to the professional market to obtain physicians, and to the financial market to obtain capital.

Image.   "An image is the sum of beliefs, ideas, and impressions that a person has of an "object" (Kotler, 1982, p. 57). Publics with a positive image of an organization will be drawn to it, whereas those with a negative image will avoid or disparage it.

There are two opposite theories about image formation. *Object-determined* theory maintains that people perceive the reality of the object. They experience the object and process the sensory data in a similar way despite different backgrounds. Therefore, when people see a building in a beautiful setting they perceive it as a beautiful hospital. *Person-determined* theory maintains that people have different degrees of contact with an object; they selectively perceive different aspects of the object, and through individual ways of processing the sensory data, they experience selective distortion. In this case, some people may perceive the hospital as beautiful and others may not.

Image is a function of deeds and communications. Good deeds that others are not told about and talk without action are not enough. A strong, favorable image develops from satisfied publics who tell others their opinions.

Marketing Process

Marketing involves informing the market of services provided and fitting services to market needs. It is a complex process that generally includes the audit, market segmentation, marketing mix, implementation, and evaluation and control.

Audit.   The marketing audit involves identification, collection, and evaluation of information that needs to be examined to evaluate market relations. The *market* and *market segments* need to be identified. How large is the area to be served? Is it rural, urban, or both? How many potential customers are there? What are their ages, occupations, income levels, and interests? How many are aware of your services? Are there seasonal differences? How satisfied are the clients with the services offered now?

The *organization* should be assessed. What is the mission of the organization? What are its philosophy, goals, objectives, and priorities? What are the services provided, strengths, and weaknesses? How do your services compare with those of others? What conditions of the industry affect you? What internal and external controls affect you?

As *services* are further analyzed, note distinctive superiorities. What services are heavily used? Why? What services are underused? Why? Are there voids? If so, can they be filled? How can needed materials, supplies, and personnel be obtained? Who pays for the services?

Who are the *competitors?* How many are there? Are their numbers increasing or decreasing? Who are the principal competitors? What areas do they serve? How do their size and strength compare? How do their charges compare?

What is the profile of present and future *clients* for your services? Are client profiles different among services? What is the frequency of client usage of your services?

What are the perceptions of the *nursing market?* What are the internal perceptions of nurse recruitment? Focus groups can be formed to discuss reasons why nurses decided to work at the institution, the positive and negative aspects of the job, and ways working conditions can be improved. Interviews with directors of nursing education programs can be used to learn how the institution is perceived, where graduates of that school are going and why, and how personnel at the health care agency can influence those decisions.

What is the organization's pricing philosophy? How are *prices* determined? How are prices viewed by the staff, clients, and competitors?

In what *location* is your service provided? How accessible is it to clients? How far will clients have to travel to obtain the service? Will you travel to provide a service? If so, how far? Will you charge for travel expenses?

What is the purpose of *promotion?* Is it reaching the intended publics? Is it effective? What media are being used? What media reach whom?

Many *assessment tools* can be used to collect data for the audit. Questionnaires administered by mail, telephone, or interview, in-depth interviews, and observations are common. A consumer panel can be used to discuss relevant issues. A mediator helps keep a representative group of consumers discussing a specific topic in focus groups. Nominal groups aim at generating consensus about a particular issue. Records can be reviewed, and scientific research designs can be planned and implemented to collect data.

A *sampling plan* is important. Who will be surveyed? What will the sample size be? Large samples are more reliable than small samples. How will the sample be chosen? A random sample is the most reliable.

Statistical techniques such as frequency distributions, means, standard deviations, regression analysis, correlation analysis, factor analysis, discriminant analysis, and cluster analysis can be useful. Statistical techniques are technical; therefore, statistical consultation is often advisable.

Market segmentation.   Segmentation identifies subsets of the total market that have similar characteristics. Segmentation is based on the assumptions that consumers are different, these differences affect market behavior, and one can isolate segments within the total market. The criteria most often used to describe segments are (1) geography—rural or urban; (2) demography—age, sex, race; (3) psychography—values, habits, life-styles; (4) behavior—repeated use of services; and (5) buying process—awareness of services, benefits sought.

There are three major marketing strategies related to segments:

- Differentiated marketing aims directly and differentially at several specific segments.

- Concentrated marketing aims at a specific segment.

- Undifferentiated marketing ignores segments and deals with all as one market.

Marketing mix.   The marketing mix makes use of the audit's results related to the needs of targeted segments. It involves the four *p*'s: product, price, place, and promotions.

Product is something provided for consumption to satisfy a need or want. The inventory of services, analysis of costs, benefits, and target markets indicate which products are overused, underused, and cost-effective and which are perceived as strong or weak. This information should be used to determine the appropriate product mix.

A product line is composed of similar services that are clustered to manage process, quality, costs, and marketing more efficiently. Product line analysis is a method of analyzing products in terms of inputs and outputs and is built on total cost accounting principles. Because determination of actual cost per case is important, all costs for an admission are tracked. All hospital fixed overhead costs are allocated to patients and product lines. All costs from admission to discharge are determined and compared with the reimbursement per case. Length of stay by product line is important. When the patient's length of stay is too long, the total cost may surpass the reimbursement per case even if the daily expense is reasonable.

Product line analysis shows the relationship of inputs to outputs, gives profit and loss information for product line, attaches all costs to a product line, increases personnel's cost awareness, facilitates planning, promotes efficiency, encourages better review and control of resources, and promotes better decision making.

A Boston consulting group developed a classification system of potential growth and profitability to identify marketing strategies for products (see Figure 7-1). They created a grid with growth potential measured on the vertical axis and profitability along the horizontal axis. Low growth potential and profitability are represented at the lower left corner; the factor becomes higher toward the top and the right of the grid. Products with low profitability and low growth potential are labeled *dogs*. They drain the organization and should be divested if possible. Products in the upper left quadrant have low profitability and high growth potential. They are labeled *question marks*. Aggressive marketing to increase volume and therefore profitability is possible but risky. *Cash cows* with high profitability but low growth potential are in the lower right quadrant. That product may be maintained to use the profits to finance other

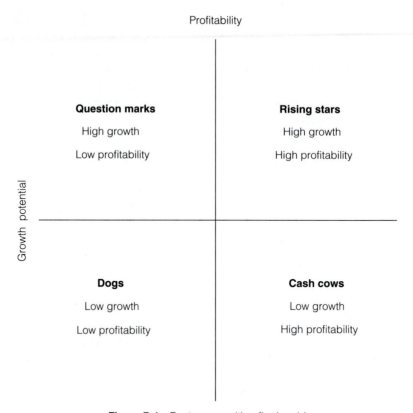

Figure 7-1   Boston consulting firm's grid.

ventures or to cover other losses. In the upper right quadrant are the *rising stars,* which have both high profitability and high growth potential. Promotional money should be put here to increase volume and profitability. After increasing growth, rising stars typically become cash cows.

Products have *life cycles*. The stages of the life cycle are as follows:

- The *introduction stage* is the beginning of a new product when the customer's response to the product and its growth potential are relatively unknown.

- The *growth stage* occurs when the number of customers and the size of the market are increased.

- The *maturity stage* is the peak market of the product. Competition enters the market to obtain a share. Marketing strategies during the maturity stage are designed to get and keep the agency's share of the market.

- The last stage is the *market decline stage,* when the market decreases because of new ideas, products, technology, or changes in customer needs.

Question marks occur during the introductory stage, when the future is risky but there is high growth potential. Rising stars form the growth stage, when profitability and growth potential are high. Cash cows are seen during the maturity stage, when there is high profitability but low growth potential. Dogs occur during the decline stage with the declining growth and profitability (Strasen, 1987).

Price is another major consideration. Because physicians rather than patients usually determine the services used and health care bills are usually paid by third-party payers, nondollar costs such as time and convenience must be considered. Minimization of nondollar costs should benefit the health care agency and the consumer.

There are several *pricing goals.*

- *Profit-maximizing pricing* tries to set the maximum price that the demand for the product or service will bear.

- *Market-share pricing* sacrifices short-term profits for long-term market domination and attempts to identify the price that maximizes the agency's share of the market.

- *Market-skimming pricing* places a high price and high profitability on a product or service when it is high demand with no competition.

- *Current-revenue pricing* tries to maximize the current revenue.

- *Target-profit pricing* attains a satisfactory profit.

- *Promotional, loss leader* pricing sets the price lower than the cost or competition to introduce customers to the new product or service. Profits are regained when the customers purchase other products.

- *Prestige pricing* sets unusually high prices to convey the image of quality or prestige.

Pricing factors include cost of product, demand for product, and competition. When considering the *cost of products* or services, one can use *mark-up pricing* by adding a certain percentage to the cost, *cost-plus pricing* by adding a fixed amount to the cost, and *target pricing* by setting the price so it yields a specific profit at a particular demand level. When considering the *demand for the product* or service, one can use *perceived-value pricing,* by setting the price according to the customer's perception of the value of the product or service, or *price-discrimination pricing,* by varying the price from one customer or place to another. There might be a sliding pay scale according to the patient's income. One hospital in a corporation might charge more or less than others because of the client's income in general or the facility's location in a rich or poor neighborhood. When considering *competition, going-rate pricing* uses the collective wisdom of the marketplace. In *sealed-bid pricing* the lowest bid gets the business (Strasen, 1987).

Place involves the physical location, appearance of the location, its accessibilty and availability, resource utilization, the expertise and courtesy of staff, referral mechanisms, and distribution. The goal is to provide the service to the consumer with efficient distribution and minimal inconvenience.

Marketing promotion informs potential consumers of the existence and availability of products and services and persuades them of the benefits to them. Tailoring services to consumer desires is important. Marketing promotion leads to awareness, understanding, interest, decision, utilization, satisfaction, reutilization, and recommendation.

Promotion tools include (1) advertising, which is any paid form of promotion; (2) personal selling, which is an oral presentation by a seller to a buyer; (3) sales promotions, which are short-term incentives for purchasing products or services; and (4) publicity, which is promotion that is not paid for by the agency. *Advertising* includes ads in newspapers, magazines, and journals, direct mail, flyers, billboard advertising, telephone directories, radio, and television. Printed materials can be used—for instance, calendars, matches, pens, telephone stickers, newsletters, and booklets about such topics as diet, exercise, poison control, and first aid. *Personal selling* includes fund-raising, lobbying, and sales calls such as presentations to community groups about health promotion, chemical dependency, weight control, exercise, birth control, and child care. *Sales promotions* include introductory offers, free samples, coupons, discounts, incentives, free lectures, and special credit cards. The best form of *publicity* is the word of mouth of satisfied customers. Other types are public service announcements, public relations campaigns, speakers bureaus, interviews, health fairs, and screening programs (Strasen, 1987).

Implementation.   Implementation can be done incrementally or as an entire package. Designing and implementing a marketing program are expensive projects and require personnel with expertise in marketing. Outside consultants can be hired when qualified people are not available within the organization. Dealing with local political conflicts, reaching communities that are out of touch with their own real demands, and sorting real demands from surface expectations are challenging tasks.

Evaluation and control.   The last phase of the marketing process is evaluation and control. It involves identifying goals and objectives, measuring planned and actual results, determining reason for variance between planned and actual results, correcting action based on causal analysis, and revising goals. Evaluation can be done more or less often—daily through weekly, monthly, yearly, or on a more extended basis to determine whether implementation is accomplishing desired results.

BIBLIOGRAPHY

Alward RR, Camunas C: Public relations: a skill for nurses, part 1, *JONA* 20:28-34, October 1990.
Barich H, Kotler P: A framework for marketing image management, *Sloan Management Review* 32:94-104, Winter 1991.
Bixler M: Maintaining your marketing consistency. *Small Business Reports* 16:27-34, January 1991.
Brown R: Making the product portfolio a basis for action, *Long Range Plann* 24:102-110, February 1991.
Brownlie DT: The marketing audit: a metrology and explanation, *Marketing Intelligence & Planning* 11:4-12, 1993.
Clift V: Plan giveaways strategically to attain specific goals, *Marketing News* 26:14, September 28, 1992.
Colangelo R, Goldrick B: Needs assessment as a marketing strategy: an experience for baccalaureate nursing students, *J Nurs Educ* 30:168-170, April 1991.
Day L: Promoting the health visiting profession, *Health Visitor,* 65:270-272, August 1992.

Del Vecchio E: Market research as a continuous process, *Journal of Services Marketing* 4:13-19, Summer 1990.

Dill PZ: Marketing the nursing practice of obstetrics, *JOGNN* 20:328-332, August 1991.

de-la-Cuesta C: Marketing: a process in health visiting, *J Adv Nurs* 19:347-353, February 1994.

Dubuque SE, Neathawk RD: Applying a marketing framework to staff recruitment and retention, *Journal of Home Health Care Practice* 5:1-8, February 1993.

Edwardson SR, Giovannetti PB: A review of cost-accounting methods for nursing services, *Nurs Econ* 5:107-117, May-June 1987.

Eppen GD, Hanson WA, Martin RK: Bundling—new products, new markets, low risk, *Sloan Management Review* 32:7-14, Summer 1991.

Fiorentiai G: Public marketing in the relationship between public administration and external environment, *Journal of Professional Services Marketing* 5:47-69, 1989.

Howard CM: Integrating public relations into the marketing mix, *Executive Speeches* 4:9-13, February 1990.

Ireson C, Weaver D: Marketing nursing beyond the walls, *JONA* 22:57-60, January 1992.

Mann N: Sharpen your marketing vision with LIMRAs marketing audit, *LIMRA's MarketFacts* 9:36-39, March-April 1990.

McCracken LJ: An attention-getting marketing strategy, *Journal of Accountancy* 170:129-132, September 1990.

Schmidt CE et al: Marketing the home healthcare agency: do nurses and physicians agree? *JONA* 20:9-17, November 1990.

Shane C: Sharing information with direct marketing, *Public Relations Journal* 47:28-29, April 1991.

Stonerock C: Maximizing market potential in home care, *JONA* 21:49-53, December 1991.

Wensley R: The voice of the consumer? Speculations on the limits to marketing analogy, *European Journal of Marketing* 24:49-60, 1990.

CASE STUDY

A school of nursing started a nurse practitioner program 1 year ago. Because of the high demand for the program twice as many students are being admitted the second year of admissions as the first year. Using Worksheet 7-1 plot the program in the life cycle and the Boston group's profitability and growth opportunity classification.

CRITICAL THINKING AND LEARNING ACTIVITIES

1. Form a small group in class and perform a brief marketing audit of your nursing program by answering the following questions: What geographic area is served? Who are the potential students? What services are provided? Who are the competitors? How do the services compare? How do the prices compare? In what location is the service provided? How accessible is it to students? How far will students travel to obtain the service? Will faculty travel to provide the service? How is the nursing program promoted?

2. Identify the market segment for your nursing program—nursing students; educational level—associate degree, baccalaureate degree, graduate degree; functional area—practice, teaching,

administering, researching, consulting; and practice area—general, medical, surgical, maternal, child, psychiatric, geriatric, community health, home care.

3. Form a small group in class and brainstorm ways you could increase the publicity for your nursing program and recruit more people into the profession.

4. Draw a grid depicting the Boston consulting firm's grid of potential growth and profitability possibilities.

5. Using Worksheet 7-1, which depicts the life cycle in one column and the Boston group's classification in the second column, identify the appropriate high or low profitability and growth opportunity for the life cycle and related Boston group's classification in the third column.

✍ Worksheet 7-1

Cycle Profitability and Growth Opportunities

Life Cycle	Boston Group Classification	High or Low Profitability; High or Low Growth Opportunity
Introduction	Question mark	
Growth	Rising stars	
Maturity	Cash cows	
Market decline	Dogs	

Bibliography
Part One

Adams JL: *Conceptual blockbusting: a guide to better ideas,* ed 3, Redwood City, Calif, 1990, Addison-Wesley.

Arndt C, Daderian Huckabay LM: *Nursing administration: theory for practice with a systems approach,* St Louis, 1980, CV Mosby.

Bagwell M, Clements S: *A political handbook for health professionals,* Boston, 1985, Little, Brown.

Bailey JT, Claus KE: *Decision making in nursing,* St Louis, 1975, CV Mosby.

Ball J, Hannah KJ: *Using computers in nursing,* Reston, Va, 1984, Reston Publishing.

Barker AM: *Transformational nursing leadership: vision for the future,* Baltimore, 1992, NLN.

Bell MJ et al: *Nursing information: where caring and technology meet,* New York, 1988, Springer-Verlag.

Belcher DW: Compensation administration, Englewood Cliffs, NJ, 1987, Prentice-Hall.

Berger MS et al, editors: *Management for nurses,* ed 2, St. Louis, 1980, CV Mosby.

Berman HJ, Weeks LE: *The financial management of hospitals,* ed 8, Ann Arbor, Mich, 1993, Health Administration Press.

Blanchard K, Peale NV: *The power of ethical management,* New York, 1989, Fawcett.

Blaney DR, Hobson CJ: *Cost-effective nursing practice: guidelines for nurse managers,* Philadelphia, 1988, JB Lippincott.

Brandt SC: *Entrepreneuring: the ten commandments for building a growth company,* New York, 1983, New American Library.

Brooten DA, Hagman LL, Naylor MD: *Leadership for change: an action guide for nurses,* Philadelphia, 1988, JB Lippincott.

Bryce HJ: *Financial and strategic management for nonprofit organizations,* Englewood Cliffs, NJ, 1987, Prentice-Hall.

Buchholz RA: *Essentials of public policy for management,* Englewood Cliffs, NJ, 1985, Prentice-Hall.

Burka JB, Yuen LM: *Procrastination: why you do it, what to do about it,* Reading, Mass, 1983, Addison-Wesley.

Byars L: *Strategic management: planning and implementation,* New York, 1987, Harper & Row.

Campbell JP, Campbell RJ: *Productivity in organizations,* San Francisco, 1988, Jossey Bass.

Charns MP, Schaefer MJ: *Health care organizations: a model for management,* Englewood Cliffs, NJ, 1983, Prentice-Hall.

Christensen W, Stearns EI: *Microcomputers in management,* ed 2, Rockville, Maryland, 1990, Aspen.

Christain WP, Hannah GT: *Effective management in human services,* Englewood Cliffs, NJ, 1983, Prentice-Hall.

Cleland VS: *The economics of nursing,* Norwalk, Conn, 1990, Appleton & Lange.

Cleverley WO: *Essentials of health care finance,* ed 3, Rockville, Md, 1992, Aspen Publications.

Cowart M, Allen RF: *Changing conceptions of health care,* Grove Road, 1981, Charles B Black.

Cox HC, Harsanyi B, Dean LC: *Computers and nursing: application to practice education and research,* Norwalk, Conn, 1987, Appleton & Lange.

Curtin L, Flaherty MJ: *Nursing ethics: theories and pragmatics,* Bowie, Md, 1982, Robert J Brady.

Dale E: *Management: theory and practice,* ed 4, New York, 1978, McGraw-Hill.

Davis AJ and Aroskar MA: *Ethical dilemmas and nursing practice,* ed 3, New York, 1991, Appleton & Lange.

Deal TE, Kennedy AA: *Corporate cultures: the rites and rituals of corporate life,* Reading, Mass, 1982, Addison-Wesley.

England GW, Negaudhi AR, Wilpert B: *The functioning of complex organizations,* Cambridge, Mass, 1981, Oelgeschlager, Gunn, & Hain.

Feldstein PJ: *Health care economics,* ed 4, New York, 1993 Delmar.

Finkler SA, Graf CM: *Budgeting concepts for nurse managers,* ed 2, Philadelphia, 1992, WB Saunders.

Finkler SA, Kovner CT: *Financial management for nurse managers and executives,* Philadelphia, 1993, WB Saunders.

Ford JG, Trygstad-Durland LN, Nelms BG: *Applied decision making for nurses,* St. Louis, 1979, CV Mosby.

Fowler MDM, Levine-Ariff J: *Ethics at the bedside,* Philadelphia, 1987, JB Lippincott.

French WL: *The personnel management process,* ed 6 Boston, 1986, Houghton Mifflin.

Friss L: *Strategic management of nurses,* Owings Mills, Md, 1989, National Health.

Ganong JM, Ganong WL: *Cases in nursing management,* Germantown, Md, 1979, Aspen Systems Corp.

Ganong JM, Ganong WL: *HELP . . . with annual budgetary planning,* Chapel Hill, NC, 1976, WL Ganong.

Garrett TM: *Business ethics,* ed 2, Englewood Cliffs, NJ, 1986, Prentice-Hall.

Goodstein LD, Nolan TM, Pfeiffer JW: *Applied strategic planning: a comprehensive guide,* New York, 1993, McGraw-Hill.

Grove AS: *High output management,* New York, 1985, Random House.

Harrington-Mackin D: *The team building tool kit,* New York, 1994, American Management Association.

Hicks RF, Bone D: *Self-managing teams,* Menlo Park, Calif, 1990, Crisp.

Hampton DR: Contemporary management, ed 2, New York, 1980, McGraw-Hill.

Helfert EA: *Techniques of financial analysis,* Homewood, Ill, 1993, Irwin.

Hickman CR and Silva MA: *Creating excellence,* 1986, New York, New American Library.

Hoffman FM: *Financial management for nurse managers,* Norwalk, Conn, 1984, Appleton-Century-Crofts.

Jacobs P: *The economics of health and medical care,* ed 3, Rockville, Md, 1991, Aspen Publications.

Kaufman R: *Identifying and solving problems: a systems approach,* ed 3, La Jolla, Calif, 1982, University Associates.

Lakein A: *How to get control of your time and your life,* New York, 1989, The New American Library.

Lancaster J, Lancaster W: *Concepts for advanced nursing practice: the nurse as a change agent,* St Louis, 1981, CV Mosby.

Langford TL: *Managing and being managed,* rev ed, Englewood Cliffs, NJ, 1990, Appleton & Lange.

LeBoeuf, M: *Working smart,* New York, 1988, Warner Books.

MacKenzie RA: *The time trap: how to get more done in less time,* New York, 1975, McGraw-Hill.

Mansfield E: *Micro-economics: theory and applications,* ed 8, New York, 1993, WW Norton.

Mark BA, Smith HL: *Essentials of finance in nursing,* Rockville, Md, 1987, Aspen.

McCarthy E, Perreault WD: *Basic marketing: a managerial approach,* ed 11, Homewood, Ill., 1992, Irwin.

Miller WC: *The creative edge,* Redwood City, Calif, 1989, Addison-Wesley.

Naisbitt J, Aburdene P: *Megatrends 2000: ten new directions for the 1990s,* New York, 1991, William Morrow.

National Center for Health Services Research and Development: *Administrative cost determination manual for hospital inpatient-accounting,* Rockville, Md, July, 1972, U.S. Department of Health, Education and Welfare, Public Health Service, Health Services and Mental Health Administration [DHEW publication no. (HSM) 73-3020].

National Center for Health Services Research and Development: *Financial planning in ambulatory health programs,* Rockville, Md, July, 1973, U.S. Department of Health,

Education and Welfare, Public Health Service, Health Services and Mental Health Administration [DHEW publication no. (HRA) 74-3027].

Neal MC: *Nurses in business,* Baltimore, 1985, Williams & Wilkins.

Newman WH, Summer CE, Warren EK: *The process of management,* ed 5, Englewood Cliffs, NJ, 1981, Prentice-Hall.

Pegels CC, Roger KA: *Strategic management of hospitals and health care facilities,* Rockville, Md, 1988, Aspen.

Porter-O'Grady T: *Nursing finance: budgeting strategies for a new age,* Rockville, Md, 1987, Aspen Publishers.

Price M, Franck P, Veith S: *Nursing management: a programmed text,* ed 2, New York, 1980, Springer.

Quinn CA, Smith MD: *The professional commitment: issues and ethics in nursing,* Philadelphia, 1987, WB Saunders.

Rubright R, MacDonald D: *Marketing health and human services,* Rockville, Md, 1981, Aspen.

Rutkowski B: *Managing for productivity in nursing,* Rockville, Md, 1987, Aspen.

Scherubel JC: *Patients and purse strings II,* New York, 1988, National League for Nursing.

Schmied E: *Maintaining cost effectiveness,* Wakefield, Mass, 1979, Nursing Resources.

Schoderbek P, Schoderbek C, Kefalas A: *Management systems: conceptual considerations,* ed 4, Plano, Texas, 1989, Business Publications.

Seawell LV: *Hospital financial accounting theory and practice,* Chicago, 1987, Healthcare Financial Management Association.

Shaffer FA: *Costing out nursing: pricing our product,* New York, 1985, National League for Nursing.

Siegel JG, Shim JK, Hartman SW: *The McGraw-Hill pocket guide to business finance: 201 decision-making tools for managers,* New York, 1992, McGraw-Hill.

Simyar E, Lloyd-Jones J: *Strategic management in the health care sector: towards the year 2,000,* Englewood Cliffs, NJ, 1988, Prentice-Hall.

Stevens BJ: *First-line patient care management,* ed 2, Wakefield, Mass, 1983, Aspen.

Stevens WF: *Management and leadership in nursing,* New York, 1978, McGraw-Hill.

Stone S, et al, editors: *Management for nurses: a multidisciplinary approach,* ed 2, St Louis, 1986, CV Mosby.

Strasen L: *Key business skills for nurse managers,* Philadelphia, 1987, JB Lippincott.

Suver JD, Neumann BR: *Management accounting for health care organizations,* Chicago, 1992, Pluribus Press.

Swansburg RC, Swansburg PW, Swansburg RJ: *The nurse manager's guide to financial management,* Rockville, Md, 1988, Aspen.

Terry GR, editor: *Management: selected readings,* ed 8, Homewood, Ill, 1982, Richard D Irwin.

Thomas JG: *Strategic management: concepts, practices and cases,* New York, 1988, Harper & Row.

Toffler A: *The third wave,* New York, 1984, Bantam.

Vroom VH, Jago AG: *The new leadership: managing participation in organizations,* Englewood Cliffs, NJ, 1988, Prentice-Hall.

Vroom VH, Yetton PW: *Leadership and decision making,* Pittsburgh, 1973, University of Pittsburgh Press.

Ward RA: *The economics of health resources,* Reading, Mass, 1975, Addison-Wesley.

Watson GH: *Strategic benchmarking,* New York, 1993, Wiley.

Watzlawich P, Winkland J, Fisch R: *Change: principles of problem formation and problem resolution,* New York, 1984, WW Norton.

Weeks LE, Burnan HJ: *Economics in health care,* Germantown, Md, 1977, Aspen Systems.

Weinfeld RS, Donahue EM: *Communicating like a manager,* Baltimore, 1989, Williams & Wilkins.

Winston S: *Getting organized,* New York, 1981, WW Norton.

Zielstorff RD: *Computers in nursing,* Rockville, Md, 1982, Aspen.

PART

Two

Organize

Nature and Purpose of Organizing

Organizing is the second managerial function. Having planned, the manager must now organize so that personnel can accomplish the plans with efficiency and effectiveness. Organizing involves establishing a formal structure that provides the coordination of resources to accomplish objectives, establish policies and procedures, and determine position qualifications and descriptions.

Chapter
8

Organizational Structure

Chapter Objectives

◆ Identify at least three principles of organization.

◆ Describe disadvantages of the bureaucratic structure.

◆ Identify at least three adhocracy organizational models.

◆ Describe the corporate model.

Major Concepts and Definitions	
Organization	consolidated group of elements; systematized whole
Structure	formation or pattern of arrangement
Hierarchy	a group of persons arranged by rank, grade, or class
Bureaucracy	administration through departments and subdivisions managed by officials following an inflexible routine
Adaptive	able to change to make suitable to new or changed circumstances
Matrix	the formation of cells
Corporation	a group of employers and employees acting as one body

ORGANIZATIONAL STRUCTURE

Although planning is the key to effective management, the organizational structure furnishes the formal framework in which the management process takes place. The organizational structure should provide an effective work system, a network of communications, and identity to individuals and the organization and should consequently foster job satisfaction. Agencies contain both informal and formal structures.

The informal organization comprises personal and social relationships that do not appear on the organizational chart. This might include a group that usually takes breaks together, works together on a particular unit, or takes a class together. Informal organization is based on personal relationships rather than on respect for positional authority. It helps members meet personal objectives and provides social satisfaction. People who have little formal status may gain recognition through the informal structure. Informal authority is not commanded through organizational assignment. It comes from the follower's natural respect for a colleague's knowledge and abilities.

Informal structure provides social control of behavior. The control can be either internal or external. If pressure is intended to make a member conform to group expectancies, it is internal. Kidding a member about her dirty shoelaces is an example. On the other hand, an attempt to control the behavior of someone outside the social group, such as the manager, is external control.

The informal structure also has its own channels of communication, which may disseminate information more broadly and rapidly than the formal communication system. Unfortunately, the "grapevine" may contain rumors that are not authentic. The best way to correct an invalid rumor is for managers to provide accurate information. It is better not to state that they are correcting the rumor, for in doing so they may strengthen it, and the facts that they give may be seen primarily as a subterfuge to refute the rumor.

The informal organizational structure is important to management. The manager should be aware of its existence, study its operating techniques, prevent antagonism, and use it to meet the agency's objectives.

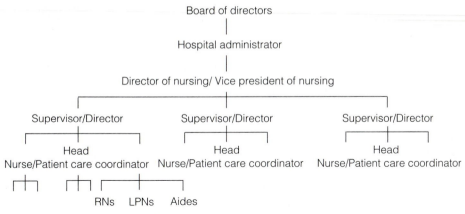

Figure 8-1   Bureaucratic hierarchy.

The formal organizational structure is defined by executive decision determined by planning. It can be diagrammed to show the relationships among people and their positions. It describes positions, task responsibilities, and relationships. The two basic forms of formal organizational structure are the hierarchic, or bureaucratic, model and the adaptive, or organic, model.

Bureaucratic Structure

A hierarchy or bureaucracy is an organizational design to facilitate large-scale administration by coordinating the work of many personnel. It is associated with subdivision, specialization, technical qualifications, rules and standards, impersonality, and technical efficiency. In Figure 8-1, which illustrates a typical bureaucratic hierarchy, the managers are responsible to the director of nursing. The director in turn must answer to the hospital administrator, who is accountable to the board of directors. Managers also have authority over their staff associates, who are accountable to their managers.

Dual management.   Dual management separates technical and administrative responsibilities. It has one hierarchy in which technical professionals make technical decisions and control technical matters and another hierarchy in which management makes decisions about issues such as personnel and budget. This dual hierarchy gives equal status to managers and technical professionals. It provides a set of titles and job descriptions for each hierarchy.

Principles of organization.   Certain principles of organization help maximize the efficiency of the bureaucratic structure. The organization should have clear lines of authority running from the highest executive to the employee who has the least responsibility and no authority over others. There should be unity of command, with each person having only one boss. All employees should know to whom they report and who reports to them. The authority and responsibility of every individual should be clearly defined in writing. This reduces role ambiguity. Employees know what is expected of them and what their limitations are. This prevents gaps between responsibilities, avoids overlapping of authority, and helps determine the proper point for decisions. Although many people do not feel it is necessary to have their responsibilities in writing, it can be revealing to have them write what they believe their functions are and to note the duplicated efforts and jurisdictional disputes. When someone leaves an agency, it is not uncommon for no one to know exactly what that person did. Under such circumstances, it can be difficult to justify replacement and to offer a meaningful orientation.

A clear definition of roles is necessary for effective delegation, but it does not guarantee it. Role clarity allows employees to know what is expected of them, to whom they report, and to whom they should go for help. In contrast, role ambiguity leads to anxiety, frustration, dissatisfaction, negative attitudes, and decreased productivity. Job descriptions increase productivity and satisfaction; however, they should not be so exact that innovation is discouraged.

Patient care coordinators should delegate responsibility to the lowest level within the organization where there is enough competence and information for effective performance and appropriate decision making. Ordinarily, increased delegation and general rather than close supervision increase effective performance, production, and employee satisfaction.

The employee should be given formal authority commensurate with the responsibility delegated. It is not uncommon for managers to delegate authority and then undermine it by making decisions that were supposedly delegated. For example, if patient care coordinators are responsible for the quality of care given on their wards, they should not have to accept members on their team who have been hired by the director without consulting them. In turn, patient care coordinators should not tell patients that they can have a bath at a certain time without consulting the person assigned to give that bath. Preferably, the nurse's aide and the patient will determine when various routines can be performed in accordance with the physician's orders and the manager's rationale.

The delegation of responsibility should be accompanied by accountability. Most effective control systems are probably those that provide feedback directly to the accountable person; this seems to increase motivation and provide direction. When feedback from a manager is given as performance evaluation rather than guidance, it tends to be nonfunctional and only infrequently contributes to improved performance. The delegation of functions with accompanying responsibility and accountability is particularly difficult for managers, because they remain responsible for the actions of their staff associates. They are as responsible as their staff associates for their associates' performance. Consequently, the span-of-control principle becomes important.

There is a limit to the amount of coordination that can be achieved by one person, and it depends on several factors. One can coordinate more similar than dissimilar positions. The more the positions are interdependent, the more coordination is involved. The span of control needs to decrease as the complexity of the staff associate's tasks increases. The stability of the agency should also be considered. If the agency has been functioning in a similar manner for a long time, the problems that arise have probably been solved before, and coordination is less difficult than in a changing situation where many new problems arise. The span of control is not likely to be uniform throughout an organization. Top-level managers of positions that are interdependent and dissimilar will probably have a smaller range of control than lower-level managers who are coordinating people doing similar tasks in a confined area. The span of control should not be so wide that managers do not have time to deal with the human relations aspects, such as giving workers individual attention, communicating information about the agency's policies, and listening to suggestions, grievances, and problems. On the other hand, they need a span of control large enough to keep them busy so they will not interfere with the delegated responsibilities of others.

Three types of divisions are commonly used to define span of control: (1) function or process, (2) product or service, and (3) region. Function is associated with specialization. Specialization may apply both to individuals and to departments or divisions. For example, one nurse may pass medications and give treatments, another may just start IVs, and the nurse's aids may give the baths and change linens. There may be a surgical nursing division with departments for specific types of surgery. It is preferable that if a person is responsible for more than one type of responsibility, they be similar. Efficiency is maximized if employees predominantly perform the tasks they do best and for which their proficiency will consequently continue to increase; they may, however, become bored. It is not uncommon to find individuals within an organization who are assigned several unrelated tasks. Although that may work for some people in given situations, it is not considered good organization, and their replacements are not likely to be successful. It is more viable to hire personnel to fill the organizational structure than to change the structure to fit personnel.

Having individuals perform the same or similar tasks and having divisions with specific functions can help expand the range of control. Similarly, having departments that provide specific services, such as cardiac intensive care, or produce certain products can influence the structure. Organization by geographical location becomes increasingly viable when operations are scattered. Many agencies use a combination of these methods. For instance, a school of nursing may be organized according to campuses (regional division); according to undergraduate, graduate, and continuing education (product division); according to inpatient, outpatient, medical-surgical, maternal-child, or some other service division, or it may assign individual faculty members to teach according to specialization (functional division).

The organizational structure should be flexible enough to permit expansion and contraction in response to changing conditions, without disrupting the basic design. It should also be kept as simple as possible, because additional levels of authority complicate communications and excessive use of committees may impede progress.

Disadvantages of the bureaucratic structure.   There are disadvantages to the bureaucratic model. It may be detrimental to healthy personality patterns by predisposing the authoritarian leadership style, increasing insistence on the right of authority and status, and fostering a pathological need for control. If managers do not have the technical competence of their staff associates, they may feel insecure and fear their associates. Autocratic behavior may become a defense mechanism through the use of power and fear strategies over staff members and the enforcement of norms through arbitrary or rigid rules. The use of reward and punishment to get desired behavior may alienate personnel. Self-serving behavior patterns may develop because of competition for the advancement of individual interests. A certain aloofness can result from the specialization that leads to impersonality. Personnel also may develop a ritualistic attachment to routine, become attached to subgoals, and show resistance to change.

Adhocracy Organizational Models

Adhocracy, or organic, models are newer organizational frameworks that are more free form, open, flexible, and fluid than are older bureaucratic models. Boundaries separating internal and external relationships are more easily penetrated. Temporary affiliations such as consultantships are used.

The underlying assumptions, aims, and structures of adaptive frameworks are different from those of the bureaucratic model. They have resulted from behavioral research to facilitate job satisfaction and creativity as well as efficiency. They give greater recognition to the informal structure and encourage the group to improve its own norms. Adaptive models recognize realities and are designed to meet them. They are less likely to use organizational charts, because the relationships are flexible. Job descriptions are also less meaningful. The models are ambiguous and consequently need to be staffed by independent, self-reliant people who have a high tolerance for ambiguity. They lend themselves to participative management. Motivation is derived from system needs, task-related factors, and peer pressure rather than from supervision. Rewards are based on individual and group results rather than subjective evaluations from managers.

Free form. Free-form organizational design is structured so that the parts can be operated flexibly. It stresses centralized control, decentralized operations, computerized evaluations, profit centers, and dynamic managers who are willing to take risks. The stable part of the organization is composed of planners and a center for control and evaluation. The decentralized operations consist of changing combinations of the various functions, talents, and material resources across lines within the agency. Profit centers rather than budgetary units are used. These centers foster teamwork by organizing all contributors to an objective into a unit so that all will gain or lose by the results. It is an organization that seeks change, development, and expansion by being opportunistic. Managers are expected to manage change. Open communication, consensus, independent judgment, and self-regulation are stressed. Organizational charts, manuals, job descriptions, and position titles are minimized to increase flexibility.

Collegial management. Collegial management restricts monocratic authority by maintaining a division and balance of power among the top management group through collective responsibility. It is most commonly used in Germany and Holland but is also used in Austria, Switzerland, and France. Consequently, it is also referred to as European-style management. The directors usually represent functional areas of the organization. They may or may not have a chairperson. If so, the chairperson may be the first among equals and merely speak for the directors, may coordinate the others, or may be recognized as the general manager or chief executive. The directors may have vice-directors.

The decision-making process varies from one country to another, but in every case, it is the board that makes policy decisions. Essentially, the directors need to persuade each other. Although chairpersons may not have strong decision-making powers, they do have strong veto powers.

Collegial management has several strengths. It limits autocratic leadership, breeds democratic management, and ensures representation of each functional area. Because of their collective responsibility, directors are better informed about the other functional areas; this broadens the approach to problem solving. Collegial management prevents precipitous decisions, encourages long-range planning, and fosters objective appraisal of the functions. Camaraderie is possible.

Collegial management also has limitations. The need for consensus can slow decision making. Consensus based on compromise may be an inferior solution. Logrolling results when directors give reciprocal support to programs that are not viable. Collegial management requires considerable, expensive executive time for what may be relatively minor matters or what may be others' functional affairs; this results in a diffusion of responsibility. The management process may even cease at times, especially when policies and programs are to be determined. Differences of opinions may smolder and lead to rudeness and cold wars. Communications are more likely to be vertical than horizontal. Consequently, coordination is a problem. The encouragement of group action may stifle a strong creative director. Because of the inherent problems in collegial management, some organizations are moving toward committee management with an executive to coordinate policy.

Project management. Project organizational design is used for large, long-range projects where a number of project groups are developed and administered through the various phases of their existence. This method is useful for one-time projects when the task is unfamiliar and complex; when considerable planning, coordination, high-risk research, and development are involved; and when there is a long lead time between planning and production.

There are several types of project units. The general, or functional, management type is the most common. Project activities are done within functional groups that are managed by department heads. The general manager coordinates the activities. With this type of arrangement there is no strong central project authority, and consequently decisions are likely to be made to the advantage of the strongest functional group rather than in the best interests of the project. Lead time and decision-making time are increased because the coordination and approval of all functional groups are required.

Aggregate management has appointed managers who have their own staff and full authority over their projects. All people involved with a project report directly to the manager, giving the manager a high degree of control over each project. This allows rapid reaction time and reduces lead time. Project management is highly regarded by outside sources, and the people involved tend to be loyal to the project because it is their only job at the time.

There are also disadvantages to aggregate management. The people involved are interested in the technology to do the project, but they do not develop the technology, nor do they develop the essential functional organizations. There tends to be little technical interchange between projects and inefficient use of production elements. Because they are managing just one project each, managers cannot keep all production elements in use at all times. With this management method, production elements are not shared with other projects, and there is consequently duplication of functional activities among projects. There is also a lack of career continuity. Anxiety may increase toward the completion of a project, because project personnel do not know where they will be assigned next. It is difficult to balance workloads as projects begin and reach completion. Aggregate management is not often used.

The matrix organization combines concepts from both functional and aggregate organizations. It departmentalizes functions and shares authority among functional heads and project managers. The project manager uses people assigned to functional areas to complete the project while they are still assigned to the functional area. Thus, the worker has two bosses. Reaction time is quite rapid. Matrix organization seems well received by outside contacts. It does not slow down the development of technology; it facilitates the interchange of technology between projects and provides career continuity, because personnel remain in their functional areas. However, conflicts can arise between project and functional managers. Workers have two bosses and accountability becomes diffuse.

In still another design the project manager may monitor the project but serve only in an advisory capacity to the general manager. The project director controls through influence. They have responsibility without authority. The workers once again report to one boss, the general manager.

Project management offers several advantages. It visualizes projects and focuses on results. It produces good control over the project, shorter development time, improved quality, and lower program costs. This yields higher profit margins and good customer relations. Project management facilitates coordination among functional areas and good mission orientation for people working on the project. It can help elevate morale and develop managers.

There are also numerous disadvantages to project management. It requires changes in patterns of interaction and disrupts the established patterns of hierarchy, span of management, unity of control, resource allocation, departmentalization, priorities, and incentives. Work groups are disrupted, and interfunctional groups develop. Duplication is common. Interdepartmental consensus is used and tends to increase fears of invasion from other departments.

Confusion may arise from authority's ambiguity as new patterns for control develop. Power is one's ability to affect the behavior of others. Authority is power derived from one's position. Influence may be power without authority. Sometimes project managers use authority; at other times they have to use influence. Personnel may report to more than one person with varying patterns of authority. Multiple levels of management are more likely to be problems for project than functional management. Authority's ambiguity frequently frustrates personnel.

Project managers tend to depend on functional managers for resources. This dependence can create a conflict over those resources. Hence the project may deplete the functional department of premium professional talent, and the competition for talent may disrupt the stability of the organization and interfere with long-range interests by disrupting traditional business. Some professionals complain that incentives for higher-level ego needs are not met. Project personnel are more likely to be anxious about the loss of their jobs, frustrated by make-work assignments between projects, and confused by a lack of role definitions. They are concerned about setbacks in their careers and upset by the apparent lack of concern about their personal development. Conflicts of allegiance result and undermine loyalty to the organization.

Shifting personnel can disrupt their training. What is learned may not be transferred from one project to another. Long-range planning suffers when people are more concerned with their temporary projects.

Several factors contribute to the failure of project management. The most common include an initially unsound basis for the project, poor selection of the project manager, lack of agency support, use of inappropriate management techniques, poor role and task definitions, and no projected termination date.

Precautions can be taken to prevent failure. Planning is always essential. The project needs to be well conceived with its scope outlined and the end results described. Well-qualified managers should be selected, and their roles defined. It is helpful if their executive rank ensures responsiveness from others. They need the authority to control funds, budgeting, and scheduling for the project; to select subcontractors; and to be able to select, add, or eliminate staff as necessary. They should participate in major managerial activities, especially in policy-making and other decisions related to their projects.

Because functional managers may not wish to take directions from a lesser executive who is suddenly a project manager, top management might select people from high positions of responsibility, assign them impressive titles, support their dealings with functional managers, and have their report to a manager on the same or higher level than the functional managers.

One of the first responsibilities of the project manager is to staff the project. Sometimes several projects compete for the same talent. Functional managers may not be willing to release the requested personnel, or the person may not want to transfer. People may be hesitant to transfer because (1) there is a division of responsibilities between functional and project organizations, (2) the job is less desirable, or (3) they fear unemployment at the end of the project. Management can offer salary increases as incentives. Promotional opportunities may arise from the additional management structure required for the project. Special efforts should be made to relocate people as they are phased out of the project, thus maintaining security. All of these measures, however, are expensive.

Next, the project manager sets time controls. The manager determines what tasks are required from each department to complete the project and what their proper sequence is. Each department itemizes what it needs to know from other departments and then commits itself to an estimate of the time required to do its part. An overall schedule can be developed by use of critical-path scheduling. It should be checked frequently to compare actual progress against the projected deadlines. This network can be the focal point of project implementation. Managers develop information links that serve the project and help them prepare to replan jobs as project dynamics change.

The project manager also needs to determine cost controls. The most sound decisions can be made by dividing the comprehensive cost summary into work packages. Then technical decision makers can offer commitment reports, and the project manager can act on the approximate cost data. After reviewing the detailed estimated costs and current expenses, the manager can switch staff from less productive duties to duties that will reduce costs.

To maintain quality control, the manager defines the project objectives in quality standards, describes performance criteria, and monitors individual and project progress against the standards. It is helpful to reward responsibility and performance and to try to accommodate staff's personal goals while working toward the objectives of the project.

Task forces.   Task forces are sometimes used for special projects. The task force has a mission, a leader, and a projected completion date. To be most successful, the project should be short range. There must be a pool from which to select talent, and task force members should be readily reabsorbed by the organization. Personnel are relieved of their usual tasks and given a temporary assignment, usually to investigate, analyze, research, and plan. They are less often used for decisions and actions. The task force allows personnel with special qualifications to combine their expertise and concentrate on a project in a manner that would not be possible while performing their usual duties. Structural flexibility is accomplished by adding members when their potential contribution is high and removing them when their specific talents are no longer required. It can be an efficient problem-solving method and can offer training opportunities for managers. It can unleash creative energies and introduce innovations.

On the other hand, it can be disruptive to the organization. Key personnel may be away from their jobs for unknown lengths of time. As members experience different qualities of supervision by moving from one team to another, they may become more critical of the less capable manager. Assignment to a task force may make employees consider themselves better than their peers. They may feel independent and detached from their usual work groups. It is not uncommon for personnel to be promoted and removed from their original departments after the task force responsibilities are completed. Reabsorbing the task force member back into the organization is sometimes difficult, and that realization is almost certain to increase the employee's anxiety. Or what began as a short-range, problem-solving task force may become an unwanted permanent arrangement.

Matrix.   Matrix organizational designs try to combine the advantages of project and functional structures. The functional line organization provides support for the project line organization. In a functional organization, the functional manager has the authority to determine and rate goals, select personnel, determine pay and promotions, make personnel assignments, and evaluate personnel and the project. Managers are responsible to their superiors but work independently. In a matrix organization, the functional manager shares those responsibilities with the project manager, because management by project objectives is important to the matrix organization. Initially, the functional manager may experience a sense of loss in status, authority, and control. Therefore, it is important for managers to be able to persuade others by using their personal qualities and knowledge of the program (see Fig. 8-2). The functional and project managers need each other's cooperation for approvals and signoffs. The intent in the matrix organization is to have the decision making as far down in the organizational structure as possible. This encourages group consensus. Most decisions are made at the middle-management level, thus freeing top administration for long-range planning.

The matrix organization increases the amount of contact between individuals, and its complexity makes conflict inevitable. Increased communications are essential. Differences need to be recognized and dealt with, because collaborative behavior is

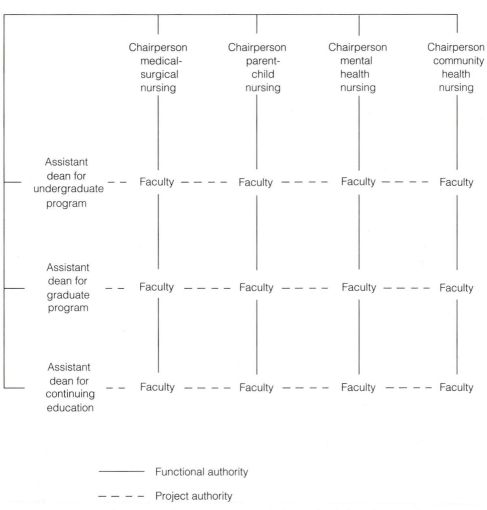

Figure 8-2   Adaptive model: matrix for a school of nursing.

needed. Team building between departments is encouraged, and consultants are used as connections between parts. Managers need human relations training. Organizational charts showing task responsibilities and levels of responsibility may reduce conflict.

Matrix organizations foster flexibility in dealing with change and uncertainty. They enable managers to balance conflicting objectives by maximizing technical excellence through efficient use of resources. By moving decision making down in the organization, opportunities are provided for personal development and motivation. Commitment is improved, and top management is freed for long-range planning.

Because people are more familiar with bureaucratic structures, there is considerable need to orient personnel to the matrix structure and philosophy. Rigid lines of authority, inflexible boundaries separating jobs and divisions, unambiguous resource allocation to divisions, and specific loyalties that exist in bureaucracies are not appropriate in dynamic organizations with overlapping and sometimes contradictory interests and goals. But because of multiple and often ambiguous roles, some personnel may get frustrated and feel insecure.

Systems.   Systems design is an adaptive organizational model. It has been facilitated by the use of computers. The systems approach can be applied to bureaucracies that are considered closed systems or to adaptive models viewed as open systems. The design develops from the flow of work and information. It considers relationships, time, and decision points.

Mixed model.   A mixed model may be the most viable. Bureaucratic design can work very well for routine functions. Adaptive designs may be more useful for research and development. However, the success of any organizational design largely depends on the manager's skills.

Corporate model.   A corporation is any group of people who act as one body. Corporations are required to register their articles of incorporation, which specify the purposes and functions of the organization. Corporations may be private or public and proprietary (for-profit) or not-for-profit. A public corporation is subject to government regulations, may issue and trade stock, and is expected to return a profit to the owners of the stock. Most individual investor-owned hospitals are operated for a profit but are privately owned, not public, corporations. However, many hospital management firms are publicly held corporations that manage both for-profit and not-for-profit individual hospitals. Most private corporations are smaller than public corporations.

Corporate growth leads to mergers, buyouts, and other business transactions to increase the value of the business. Large multihospital corporations have emerged within the health care arena. Nurses have opportunities for leadership and management positions in the corporations and may operate their own corporations (West, 1987).

The physician's share of the health care dollar has increased in the newer delivery systems as the hospital's share has decreased and services have moved out of the hospital. The services still tend to be illness-based, medically dominated, interventive, and expensive. Decentralization using holding companies with multiple subcorporate entities that provide a range of services is the trend. This trend has created a need to restructure nursing.

For nursing service to be a corporate entity it must be able to sustain its own activities without dependence on other units. Nursing practice must be clearly defined and its contribution to profitability clearly identified. The holding company's mission and purposes must be reflected in the philosophy, purpose, and objectives of the nursing service corporate entity. The relationship to the marketplace and plans to meet market demands should be outlined. Remuneration of nurses should reflect the value of their work in the marketplace.

As nursing becomes increasingly decentralized and incorporated it is increasingly important to create a network instead of preserving a pyramid. A coordinating council may centralize the activities of individual councils for practice, education, research, and quality assurance. It is an opportunity for the chairpersons of the individual councils to meet together to discuss issues, coordinate councils, and make decisions that affect the entire corporate nursing entity.

The corporate nursing staff should meet at least once a year to (1) review, revise as necessary, and approve as appropriate the nursing staff bylaws; (2) review, discuss, and revise as appropriate the nursing organization's long- and short-range planning process, goals, and objectives; (3) debate issues of concern and vote on them as appropriate; (4) review, discuss, and approve the coordinating council's activities; (5) provide opportunities for informal networking; and (6) provide education sessions (Porter-O'Grady, 1984).

BIBLIOGRAPHY

Austin NK: The death of hierarchy, *Working Woman* 15:22-25, July 1990.
Barger S, Rosenfeld P: Models in community health care: findings from a national study of community nursing centers, *Nurs Health Care* 14:426-431, October 1993.
Bell RR, Burnham JM: The paradox of manufacturing productivity and innovation, *Business Horizons* 32:58-64, September-October 1989.
Benton P: Developing leaders for managing turbulence, *Canadian Manager* 15:10-11, December 1990.
Chambers GJ: The individual in a matrix organization, *Project Management Journal* 20:37-42, December 1989.
Cooke-Davis T: Return of the project managers, *Management Today* 119-120, May 1990.
Davis AR: Project management: new approaches, *Nurs Manage* 23:62-65, September 1992.
Fielo SB, Crowe RL: A nursing center in Brooklyn, *Nurs Health Care* 13:488-493, November 1992.
Firth G, Krut R: Introducing a project management culture, *European Management Journal* 9:437-443, December 1991.
Heller R: Matrix management muddles, *Management Today* :24, June 1991.
Maritz DG: Management principles and nursing: the inefficiency of efficiency, *Superv Nurs* 11:40-41, March 1990.
Meares W: People smart organization, *Manage* 45:14-15, July 1993.
McCollum JK, Sherman JD: The effects of matrix organization size and number of project assignments on performance, *Trans Eng Manage* 39:75-78, February 1991.
Peters T: Going "horizontal" in your career, *Industry Week* 242:47-50, January 4, 1993.
Regan JD: Focus on criteria for credibility, *Broker World* 12:40,127, January 1992.
Ross A: The long view of leadership, *Canadian Business* 65:46-51, May 1992.
Thomann DA, Strickland DE: Managing collaborative organizations in the 90s, *Indust Manage* 34:26-29, July-August 1992.
Watson L: Materiel management in a changing environment: reactive or proactive? *Hospital Materiel Management Quarterly* 12:33-40, February 1991.
West ME: Nursing and the corporate world, *JONA* 17:22-23, March 1987.
Worley CG, Teplitz CJ: The use of "expert" power as an emerging influence style, *Project Management Journal* 24:31-35, February 1993.

CASE STUDY

Lake View Hospital is adding an ambulatory primary care clinic, hospice, and home care unit to the Director of Nursing Services responsibilities. The administrative title was changed to chief executive officer and directors to vice president for their respective areas. Using the organization chart in the appendix, make the changes.

CRITICAL THINKING AND LEARNING ACTIVITIES

1. Identify the organizational structure for at least one organization.

2. Using Worksheet 8-1, decide whether the principles of organization are implemented in the structure you identified for item 1.

3. Organizations are faced with a rapidly changing environment and greater competition than ever before. The more equalitarian relationships among managers and associates, the growing need for collaboration and shared decision making, and erosion of hierarchy and authority as the basis for influence increase the need for managers to enhance their personal power by acquiring technical knowledge and expertise. Identify what you will do to acquire technical knowledge and expertise.

✍ Worksheet 8-1

Principles of Organization

List principles of organization and check if the structure designed meets or does not meet the principle.

List principles of organization	Met	Not met
1.	_____	_____
2.	_____	_____
3.	_____	_____
4.	_____	_____
5.	_____	_____
6.	_____	_____
7.	_____	_____
8.	_____	_____
9.	_____	_____
10.	_____	_____

Chapter

9

Organizational Concepts

Chapter Objectives

◆ Describe the relationships among span of management, flat or tall structures, and decentralization or centralization.

◆ Describe ways a manager can facilitate adjustments to mergers.

◆ Differentiate between line and staff authority.

Major Concepts and Definitions	
Organizational chart	a drawing that shows how the parts of an organization are linked
Span of management	the number and diversity of people who report to a manager
Centralize	to concentrate power or authority
Decentralize	to distribute power and authority among more places
Mergers	the combination of several companies into one company
Line authority	the formal chain of command
Staff authority	advisory or service-oriented in nature

ORGANIZATIONAL CHARTS

An organizational chart is a drawing that shows how the parts of an organization are linked. It depicts the formal organizational relationships, areas of responsibility, persons to whom one is accountable, and channels of communication.

Managers should consider actual working relationships when drawing an organizational chart. The formal organization may not be functioning as was outlined on an older chart. Rather, an alternate structure may have emerged that operates very effectively. It is essential, then, that the manager know what is happening in actual practice. The process of drawing the chart demands a review of current practices, discovery of relationships not previously examined, and clarification of vague associations.

The organizational chart may be used for outlining administrative control, for policy-making and planning (including organizational change) to evaluate strengths and weaknesses of the current structure, and for showing relationships with other departments and agencies. It also can be used to orient new personnel or to present the agency's structural design to others. The visual diagram of a chart is a more effective means of communicating the agency's organizational structure than is a written description.

Organizational charts are not used by all managers. Autocratic managers who wish to control and manipulate others may feel that their power would be diminished if staff associates understood the working environment. Adaptive structures are more difficult to chart because they are more fluid and subject to change.

Charts become outdated as changes are made. On charts, the informal structure has not been diagramed, the formal structure may be difficult to define, and duties and responsibilities are not described. Charts may foster rigidity in relationships and communications. People may be sensitive about their relative status in the organization and may not want their positions revealed. It can be expensive to develop, disseminate, and store the charts.

Vertical charts, depicting the chief executive at the top with formal lines of

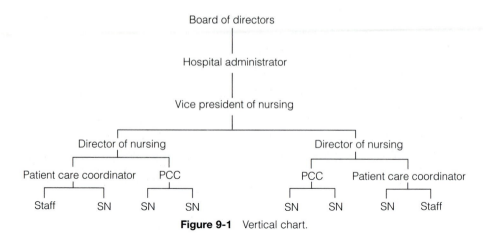

Figure 9-1 Vertical chart.

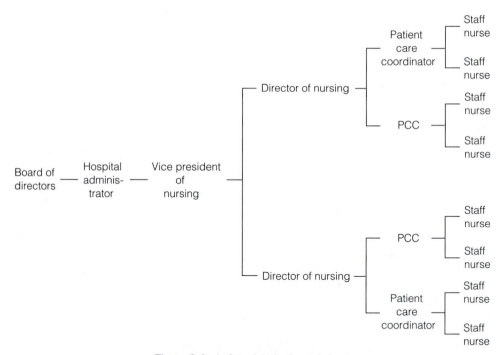

Figure 9-2 Left-to-right horizontal chart.

authority down the hierarchy, are most common, but other modifications are available (Fig. 9-1). A left-to-right, or horizontal, chart depicts the chief executive at the left with lower echelons to the right (Fig. 9-2). It follows the normal reading habit, shows relative length of formal lines of authority, helps simplify the lines of authority and responsibility, and can reveal problems within the structure. A concentric, or circular, chart shows the chief executive in the center with successive echelons in concentric circles (Fig. 9-3). It helps depict the outward flow of formal authority from the top executive and supposedly reduces status implications.

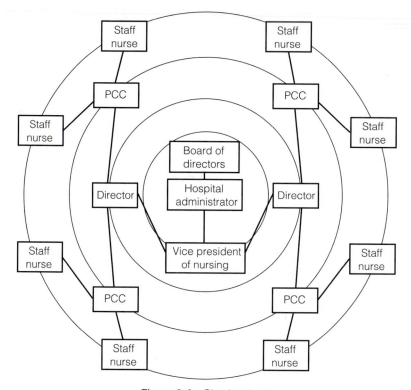

Figure 9-3   Circular chart.

The informal structure can be superimposed on the formal structure or charted through the use of sociograms. Sociograms analyze data on the choice of, communication between, and interaction among members of a small group. Personnel may be asked with whom they prefer to work, or their interactions may be observed and charted. The person with the most relationships is often the leader. Members of the primary group are those most accepted by other group members. Managers should use this information to increase production, because work groups based on sociograms are generally more productive than those arbitrarily designed.

Span of Management

Span of management has been of concern since biblical times. Exodus 18:13-26 is an account of how Moses had to deal with the problem of leading the Israelites out of Egypt. His father-in-law, Jethro, observed Moses counseling people all day long, while others had to wait long periods of time to tell Moses their problems. Jethro suggested that he delegate authority by selecting rulers of thousands, hundreds, fifties, and tens, who would teach the people laws and leave Moses free to deal only with the exceptions.

Initial work with span of management was quantitative and attempted to devise formulas for determining the most desirable number of people reporting to a manager. General Hamilton, a British officer in World War I, concluded that managers at the

Table 9-1 Variable Number of Associates and Resulting Number of Potential Relationships

Number of Associates	Number of Relationships
1	1
2	6
3	18
4	44
5	100
6	222
7	490
8	1,080
9	2,376
10	5,210
11	11,374
12	24,708
13	53,404
14	114,872
18	2,359,602

lower levels could direct more people than those at higher levels. He thought an effective span of control was three to six others, especially at upper levels. Henri Fayol, a French industrialist and early writer about scientific management, used a similar philosophy to develop a hierarchy.

Hamilton's principle has been elaborated on by A.V. Graicunas, a Lithuanian management consultant, whose mathematical analysis of potential relationships illustrates the complex social processes between managers and their staff associates, and among the staff; the complexity especially increases with each additional staff associate. Graicunas demonstrated that as the number of staff associates responsible to a manager increases arithmetically, the number of potential interactions increases geometrically. The geometrical interactions can be classified as direct single relationships, direct group relationships, and cross relationships. If a manager has two staff associates, x and y, the manager may have two direct relationships, one with x and one with y. The manager may speak to either in the presence of the other, forming two group relationships. Two cross-relationships exist between x and y and between y and x. Consequently, there are six possible interactions between one manager and two staff associates—two direct, two group, and two cross. If a third staff associate is added, one direct relationship, seven group relationships, and four cross-relationships are added, making eighteen potential interactions.

Graicunas's formula is $R = n(2n/2 + n - 1)$. R equals all types of relationships and n equals the number of subordinates. The results are presented in Table 9-1.

Graicunas's formula calculates the number of potential relationships. It does not deal with the actual frequency or the importance of the various relationships. In reality, the number of relationships with which a manager must deal is probably not so great. One might question whether the relationship in which the manager speaks to x in y's presence is different from speaking to y in x's presence. Graicunas considers them different psychological situations. It is unlikely that people will engage in all of the relationships that are theoretically possible. Nevertheless, Graicunas's formula illustrates how complex a situation can become as additional staff associates report to a manager.

The optimal span of management depends on many considerations that affect the time requirements for management. Managers' competence and qualifications and those of their staff's affect their time requirements. Some managers, because of their education and personal qualities, can work with more people than others. The better prepared staff associates are for their jobs, the less time managers must devote to teaching, clarifying responsibilities, and correcting mistakes.

Rapidly changing technology, procedures, and policies increase training problems and the need for problem solving. Availability of expert advice and services to managers can free their time and widen their span of management. However, a larger personal staff does not necessarily allow a broadening of the span of control because of the supervision required for those assistants. It may be more economical to increase the responsibilities of lower-level management. The greater the clarity of delegated authority, the less time it will take for managers to explain responsibilities and tasks. There will be less need for them to make decisions staff associates can make. If staff associates' tasks are not clearly defined, are unaccompanied by the necessary authority, or are beyond their competence, there will be an increase in time required for supervision.

Much of a manager's time is spent explaining plans, giving instructions, and receiving information about problems and progress. Clear and concise communications transmit information quickly and accurately. Much communication can be written. However, some situations cannot be handled with planning documents, policy statements, written reports, memoranda, or other written communications. These require personal contact. Some situations, which could be handled by written communications, may be better handled by personal contact. These might include delicate situations and instances where attitudes are involved. Personal contacts require considerable time.

If plans are clear, staff associates will know what is expected of them without frequently checking with the manager. If staff associates do their own planning, they will need more supervision. However, clear policies to guide their planning will reduce demands on the manager. Clear and complete policy statements can also simplify managers' decision making and allow expansion of their span of management. Deciding every problem individually requires more time than making policy decisions that anticipate problems.

The demands on the staff associate vary according to the complexity of functions. Standardization reduces time requirements, because people know what is expected. Routine work requires less time than innovative work. But we can expect that as the degree of difficulty for performing a task satisfactorily increases, so does the demand on the manager. As the variability of functions increases, the manager must consider more factors and interrelationships; this takes more time. Interdependent functions require more management time than independent functions because of the increased need for coordination. The greater the geographical separation of personnel reporting to the manager, the more limiting the span of control. The greater the nonmanagerial responsibilities, the less time the manager has for management. Managers in flat organizational structures have a broader range of management than those in tall structures, and lower-level managers have a broader range than top management.

Flat versus Tall Structures

The flat structure is developed along horizontal dimensions according to the number of organizational functions that are identified separately. There are few levels of management. The tall structure is developed along vertical dimensions by use of the scalar process to define relationships among levels in an organization. Because there are advantages and disadvantages to both the flat and tall structures, it is best to maintain a reasonable balance of dimensions. Changes within the organization bring imbalance over time, so the organizational structure should be reviewed periodically.

The flat structure shortens the administrative distance between top and bottom levels in the organization, thereby minimizing distortions through shorter lines of communication. Communications are direct, simple, fast, and clearly apparent to employees. Another advantage of the flat structure is that large groups have a greater variety of skills available and are capable of solving a greater variety of problems. This structure is believed to contribute to high employee morale and help develop capable, self-confident staff. It lends itself to a democratic approach and general management, which are preferred by many people. This minimal social stratification is consistent with an egalitarian political and social philosophy, which is currently popular.

However, a flat structure may be impractical in large organizations. Large groups have more difficulty reaching a consensus and require more coordination. The flat structure places tremendous pressure on each manager because of the large amount of authority and responsibility and the high penalties for failures. Overburdened managers may not have the time to select, evaluate, and teach subordinates, or the energy to think and plan. They may have difficulty making and communicating decisions. Socializing with staff associates may reduce their authority.

Tall structures lend themselves to authoritarianism, which is most effective in situations requiring rapid changes and precise coordination. In a tall structure, messages from managers are given more attention than those from peers and consequently pass through levels quickly. The narrow range of management allows staff to evaluate decisions frequently. With small groups, decision making takes less time, and there is more opportunity for members to participate and to understand the goals. Such interaction facilitates group cohesiveness.

Levels are expensive because of the large number of executives needed with high salaries. Each additional level makes communication more cumbersome. The more levels that communications pass through, the greater the distortion. Therefore, a tall structure reduces the understanding between higher and lower levels and increases impersonality.

Decentralization versus Centralization

Decentralization is the degree to which decision making is diffused throughout the organization. It is relative, for the degree of decentralization is larger when more important decisions affecting more functions are made at lower levels with less supervision. There are several factors to consider when determining the optimal degree of decentralization for an organization. Top management needs a positive attitude toward decentralization, and they need competent personnel to whom they can delegate authority. The latter need access to the information necessary for decision making.

The number of people who need to interact to solve a problem should be considered. In general, the larger the organization, the greater the number of complex decisions that must be made, and that can overburden top management and delay decision making. Smaller, decentralized units reduce the number of decisions made by each manager and increase the time available to devote to each problem. Usually, agencies tend to be more centralized during their early, formative years. If the agency gradually expands from within, it is more likely to remain centralized. An organization that grows rapidly through acquisitions is more likely to be decentralized; thus, decentralization is more common in organizations with geographical dispersion of operations. Some functions lend themselves more readily to decentralization than do others; production, marketing, personnel, and some purchasing may be readily decentralized. In contrast, finances, accounting, data processing of statistics, and purchase of capital equipment are likely to remain centralized.

The profit center concept has developed from decentralization and has been popular since World War II. It is particularly characteristic of large organizations with multiple product lines. The organization is divided into manageable units called profit centers that are self-contained and have their own management and staff. Each unit competes with others for profits; this arrangement motivates managers to make decisions that will maximize profits. The manager has considerable freedom for making operational decisions. The profit center concept helps give meaning to decentralization by placing the responsibility for profit making on a number of managers instead of just top management.

The advantages of decentralization seem to outweigh the disadvantages. Decentralization increases morale and promotes interpersonal relationships. When people have a voice in governance, they feel more important and are more willing to contribute. This increased motivation provides a feeling of individuality and freedom that in turn encourages creativity and commits the individual to making the system successful. Decentralization fosters informality and democracy in management and brings decision making closer to the action. Thus, decisions may be more effective because people who know the situation and have to implement the decision are the ones who make it. Because managers do not have to wait for the approval of their superiors, flexibility is increased, and reaction time is decreased. Fewer people have to exchange information; consequently, communications are swift and effective. Coordination improves, especially for services, production with sales, and costs with income. Products or operations that are minor to the total production receive more adequate attention. Plans can be tried out on an experimental basis in one unit, modified, and proven before used in other units. Risks of losses of personnel or facilities are dispersed.

Decentralization helps determine accountability. It makes weak management visible through semi-independent and often competitive divisions. Operating on the premise that people learn by doing, decentralization develops managers by allowing them to manage. A management pool can be developed that thereby eases the problem of succession. There is usually less conflict between top management and divisions. Decentralization releases top management from the burden of daily administration, freeing them for long-range planning, goal and policy development, and systems integration.

Nevertheless, several problems can also result from decentralization. An organization may not be large enough to merit decentralization, or it may be difficult to divide the organization into self-contained operating units. Top administrators may not desire decentralization. They may feel it would decrease their status, or they may question the abilities of the people to whom they would delegate. They may feel that most people prefer to be dependent on others and do not want decision-making responsibility. An increased awareness of division consciousness and a decrease in company consciousness may develop. Divisions may become individualized and competitive to the extent that they sacrifice the overall objectives for short-range profitability and work against the best interests of the whole organization. Because of conflicts between divisions, it may be difficult to obtain a majority vote, and compromises may result. If the majority vote is delayed, it may come too late to be effective.

Decentralization involves increased costs. It requires more managers and larger staffs. There may be underutilization of managers. Divisions may not adequately use the specialists housed at headquarters. Functions are likely to be duplicated between divisions and headquarters. Because decentralization develops managers, there are novice managers in the system who will make mistakes. Division managers may not inform top management of their problems. There are problems with control and nonuniform policies. Some restrictions on autonomy remain. Even with decentralization, top management remains responsible for long-range objectives and goals, broad policies, selection of key executives, and approval of major capital expenditures.

Departmentalization. Departmentalization results from span of management, division of work, and need for cooperation. Its primary purpose is to subdivide the organizational structure so that managers can specialize within limited ranges of activity. Organization of the agency influences group behavior and the effectiveness of the group. The objectives of the agency can be met most easily if the group is properly organized. Two common types of departmentalization are input and output. The input, or process orientation, includes function, time, and simple numbers as bases for departmentalization, whereas the output, or goal orientation, includes product, territory, and client divisions.

The input, or process-oriented structure, emphasizes specialization of skills. It reinforces professional skills by uniting people with similar expertise in the same department. For example, the focus may be on cardiac nursing, respiratory nursing, or transplant nursing, depending on the departmentalization. It is possible for professionals to advance within their field of expertise instead of advancing through the administrative hierarchy. Unfortunately, the process-oriented structure emphasizes professional skills over organizational goals. Conflicts increase as communication and cooperation decrease. Input organization provides less favorable training for general administrators than does a goal-oriented structure.

Departmentalization by function groups activities according to similarity of skills or a group of tasks necessary to accomplish a goal. Logical, simple, and commonly used, it facilitates specialization that contributes to economic operations. It groups functions that can be performed by the same specialists with the same type of equipment and facilities. Less demand for one product may be counteracted by a greater demand for another product. Consequently, staff, equipment, and facilities will have optimal utilization. The combination of administrative activities also is economical. One manager is responsible for all related activities; therefore, coordination is improved because it is more easily achieved. The agency benefits from a few people with outstanding abilities, for only top management is able to coordinate the major functions. For example, the hospital may be organized by medical, surgical, and pediatric units.

Functional departmentalization also has its disadvantages. As the size of the agency increases, centralization may become excessive, making effective control more difficult. The necessary additional organizational levels may slow communications and delay decision making. It becomes more difficult to measure performance. Functional departmentalization does not provide good training for general managers. They become expert in their particular function, have little opportunity to learn about other functions, and may emphasize their previous function while deemphasizing others when they become general managers.

Time factors are another basis for organization. Acute care settings need coverage 24 hours a day, 7 days a week, whereas preventive services may only need coverage for 8 to 12 hours a day for 5 to 6 days a week at the most.

Grouping by numbers divides undifferentiated labor into manageable units. A certain number of workers is assigned to each manager. This method is common in underdeveloped countries but is disappearing in industrialized areas.

The output, or goal structure, emphasizes service to the client. It collects all the work for a project under one manager and reduces dependence on other units for needed resources. This allows considerable autonomy, and the client, workers, and goals are readily identified. Systems and procedures are highly standardized. Family planning, pregnancy counseling, and school health are examples of services available from some health departments.

Unfortunately, these units may stress their own goals while deemphasizing agency goals. Duplication of equipment and services may develop. Equipment may not be fully utilized, or smaller-scale equipment may be less effective. The grouping of various skills into one unit can reduce the expertise as professional reinforcement is weakened.

A product or group of closely related products may be the basis of organization for autonomous departments. Emphasis is on the product instead of the process. Improvement, expansion, and diversification of the product is possible because one manager is responsible for all activities affecting that specific product. In a large agency this could result in small, flexible units where functional groupings would be too complex. This method identifies profit responsibilities for specific products. Organization on the basis of products has become increasingly popular. It is common for schools of nursing to organize according to the "products" produced—medical nurses, surgical nurses, obstetrical nurses, pediatric nurses, psychiatric nurses, and community health nurses.

Departmentalization by territories is particularly useful for physically dispersed activities where branches provide similar services at each location. This method serves the local clients with greatest efficiency. Managers consider local circumstances that might be overlooked by a central manager. It uses local people who are familiar with local conditions. It reduces delivery time and may reduce transportation costs related to raw materials and finished products. It is particularly useful for production and sales and when perishability is a problem. However, financial management works best if centralized.

Departmentalization by client makes sense when service is important and the welfare of the client is of primary interest. For example, a clinic may have obstetric, pediatric, and adolescent clinics. Clinics may be open nights and weekends for working people. Schools of nursing may offer night classes for working students. This better uses facilities and is more satisfactory to the client. However, pressure for special consideration and treatment of specific groups may exist, and coordination problems may increase.

Clusters.   Clusters are two or three clinically similar units that share resources such as staff, equipment, and educational materials. Clustering fosters collaboration and consultation among nurses, decreases the isolation of decentralization, and enhances professional marketability by expanding knowledge and skills.

Units forming cluster work groups should develop written agreements describing how the cluster will work, emphasize sharing resources, and arrange for personnel to meet each other through inservices and social events. New staff should know that clustering is an expectation and should be oriented to the cluster units. Staff should be oriented to cluster units before being shared and during nonstressful times. Cross-training facilitates cost-effective, safe, and satisfying nursing services (Ouellette et al. 1989).

Mergers

A merger essentially means that an organization will joint its assets with another. Economics are forcing health care organizations to seek mergers, cut staff, and emphasize cost-effectiveness over patient care and service quality. There are some multiinstitution relationships for sharing assets such as a central laundry service, a purchasing department, or a home health agency. However, mergers usually restructure the relationship of one health care organization with another. These activities can stir many feelings among personnel.

It is appropriate for the nurse manager to assess attitudes toward the merger through a questionnaire, personal interviews, or focus groups. Only personnel who are supportive of the merger should be assigned to leadership positions to accommodate it. Managers need to keep staff informed about the changes. Open communications can help minimize pluralistic views about the merger. Staff may need assistance to understand the new organization culture, and managers can help staff understand the unique qualities of the merging agency. Managers should periodically assess how

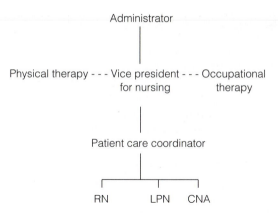

Line authority = solid line

Staff authority = dashed line

Figure 9-4   Line-staff relationships.

personnel are responding to the merger, identify problems, and do problem solving (Kooi, White, and Smith, 1988).

Line-Staff Relationships

Line authority.   Line organization is the oldest type of structure. It is a chain of command, a manager-staff associate or leader-follower relationship. The manager delegates authority to a staff associate, who in turn delegates authority to the staff. This progression is the basis for the term *line authority.* The command relationship is a direct line between manager and staff associate and is depicted by a solid line on organizational charts (see Fig. 9-4). The line positions are related to the direct achievement of organizational objectives. This arrangement fosters quick decision making because managers are given complete charge of their areas and at most would need to consult only with their immediate managers. Buck-passing is reduced, and authority relationships are clearly understood. The manager has the right to give orders, demand accountability, and discipline violators.

Staff authority.   Staff supports line-authority relationships and are advisory or service in nature. Staff authority is depicted by a dashed line on an organization chart. They handle details, locate required data, and offer counsel on managerial problems. Staff function through influence, for they do not have authority to accept, use, modify, or reject plans. Staff make the line more effective, but organizations can function without staff authority.

The two major categories of staff authority are personal and specialist. The personal category includes the assistant and general staff. The specialist staff is composed of advisory, service, control, and functional personnel.

Assistant staff. A personal staff member may be called an assistant, a staff assistant, or an administrative assistant and is responsible to one line manager. The assistant's chief purpose is to extend the line manager's capacity for completing a large amount of work by doing the more routine tasks that the manager would otherwise have to perform. The duties vary widely from one manager to another but might include such activities as mail answering, data collection for decision making, consolidation of information from various reports, preparation of documents, development of budgets, interpreting plans to others, and substitution for the manager at various meetings and functions.

Personal staff members have no specific functions. Their duties vary with the assignments. They do not act on their own behalf but rather as personal representatives of a manager. The only specific authority they have comes from a manager on a limited basis, usually for a specific job over a brief time span. With delegated authority, the personal staff member can give instructions in the manager's name and make decisions that affect the organization. It is important for assistants and the people with whom they work to know the extent of their influence. Misuses of and misunderstanding about the assistant are all too common. Some feel that the assistant is unnecessary and that the duties should be delegated to other line managers. When the assistant takes over tasks that belong to others, misunderstanding and poor cooperation result. Some assistants give the impression that they are the manager instead of just acting for one.

General staff. The general staff is composed of top administrators. The top administrator makes the decision after receiving input from these key people who together have the necessary expertise to make sound decisions for the agency. This is a coordinated group performing to maximize results. They serve in an advisory capacity by collecting and sharing information and are functional through their supervisory activities. The military has used this concept extensively, but it is relatively uncommon in business. Rotating general staff members to various areas and levels within the organization fosters an understanding of line problems.

Advisory staff. Advisory staff counsel line managers. They study problems, collect and analyze data, offer alternatives, and prepare plans. Their work may be accepted, rejected, or modified by the line manager. Although ideas are heard, they are not always implemented. This puts staff on the defensive, because they must sell their ideas. It is important that they counsel rather than suggest or confirm just what the line manager wants. Chances of an idea's being approved are increased when staff have discussed proposed recommendations with line managers who will be affected by the decision and have received their approval before presenting the plan to the top administrator. Careful evaluation of the plan is important. The better prepared the advice, the more likely the staff will be heard and their suggestions implemented. If staff work in seclusion, secretly preparing reports without listening to, or discussing them with, line managers, they are likely to get a suspicious and negative reception from others.

Service staff. Service staff are not advisory. They perform a centralized service that has been separated from the line to prevent duplication and to allow more economical performance and good control. This includes dietary and laundry services in a hospital. Line relies on staff to get the job done. They do not do it themselves.

Control staff. Control staff also do not advise. They control by restraining line authority. They have direct or indirect control over certain line performance. They control directly by acting as an agent for a line manager or indirectly through procedural compliance and interpretation of policies and reports. Quality control personnel and the affirmative action officers are members of the control staff.

Functional staff. Functional authority exists when a specialist is given decision-making authority for specific activities outside the formal chain of command. This authority may be delegated to line, staff, or service managers and may be exercised over line, staff, and service personnel. The functional staff have limited line authority with power to determine standards in their areas of specialization and to enforce them. This authority is usually of an impersonal nature in the form of schedules, inspection reports, and written orders. It breaks the scalar chain and violates the principle that personnel should only be accountable to one superior. Although done in the interest of convenience and efficiency, it should be restricted, because it can damage line authority, destroy departmentalization, and create confusion.

Line-staff conflict.   Conflict is likely to arise in any situation where two or more people must interact to get results. Line-staff conflicts occur when there is a lack of understanding of the roles and functions of others and when their lines of responsibility, accountability, and authority are not clear. Line and staff have different responsibilities and goals. Line is generalized, whereas staff is specialized. Line managers are likely to be pragmatists who have received their positions through competent service. They may not have much formal education but pride themselves on common sense. Staff managers probably consider themselves experts by virtue of their extensive formal education or experience in their areas of competence, or both. In addition to their differences in responsibilities and backgrounds, they also have different loyalties. Line managers identify with their work group; staff managers are inclined to be loyal to their professional colleagues and the company as a whole.

Line may complain that staff is impractical and too academic. Specialists sometimes are not aware of the total picture. Offered from a specialized, narrow viewpoint, their advice is impractical because it ignores the ramifications of a given situation. Staff managers may be viewed as outside interference who do not understand line or technical problems. Consultation causes delay. Line may accuse staff of not keeping them informed in an effort to keep them off balance and to claim credit for good ideas that turn out well, while blaming line for failures. Line may believe that staff lacks responsibility or assumes too much authority and runs the show.

On the other hand, staff complains that line ignores them, resists staff assistance, or does not use them properly. Line may make decisions in specialized situations without consulting them or may seek their consultation too late. Line is often viewed as cautious, conservative, and resistant to new ideas. They want to do things as they have always done them. Staff may feel that line managers do not give them enough authority in their area of expertise and may be concerned about the way line implements staff's ideas and plans.

Improving line-staff relationships.   Certain conditions can be created to foster the integration of line-staff efforts. It is helpful if both line and staff have participated in determining objectives and plans and their implementation. Participation increases everyone's awareness of the overall goals to be accomplished. Each should be briefed on the roles and functions of other team members. The lines of responsibility, accountability, and authority should be clearly established and publicized. A team-effort atmosphere is more likely to prevail in structures that allow line and staff to interact with open communications and that have a problem-solving focus.

BIBLIOGRAPHY

Betts M: Dotted lines and crooked arrows, *Computerworld* 28:16-17, December 27, 1993-January 3, 1993.

Byrne JA: Congratulations. You're moving to a new pepperoni, *Business Week* 3351:80-81, December 20, 1993.

Clark TD: Corporate systems management: an overview and research perspective, *Communications of the ACM* 35:60-75, February 1992.

Hamilton J: Toppling the power of the pyramid: team-based restructuring for TQM, patient-centered care, *Hospitals* 67:38-41, January 5, 1993.

Hattrup GP, Kleiner BH: How to establish the proper span of control for managers, *Indust Manage* 35:28-29, November-December 1993.

Jaques E: In praise of hierarchy, *Harvard Business Review* 68:127-133, January-February 1990.

Kooi D, White RE, Smith HL: Managing organizational mergers, *JONA* 18:10-16, March 1988.

Ouellette JN, Martin LL, Holmes RB et al: Clustering: decentralization and resource sharing, *Nurs Manage* 20:31-35, June 1989.

MacStravic RES: New role-and-feedback system for the supervisor and the organization, *Health Care Superv* 8:23-34, January 1990.

Marriner A: Organizational process and bureaucratic structure, *Superv Nurse* 8:54-58, July 1977.

Marriner A: Adaptive organizational models, *Superv Nurse* 8:44-49, August 1977.

Marriner A: Line-staff relationships, *Superv Nurse* 8:27-29, November 1977.

Reimann BC, Ramanujam V: Acting versus thinking: a debate between Tom Peters and Michael Porter, *Plann Rev* 20:36-43, March-April 1992.

Ross A: The long view of leadership, *Canadian Business* 65:46-51, May 1992.

Sassone PG: Survey finds low office productivity linked to staffing imbalances, *National Productivity Review* 11:147-158, Spring 1992.

Thackray J: Can a good manager manage anything? *Across the Board* 30:13-14, March 1993.

Wellington M: Decentralization: how it affects nurses, *Nurs Outlook* 34:36-39, January-February 1986.

CASE STUDY

After referring to the case study in the Appendix, identify a possible restructuring of units to maximize hospital profits by serving the changing needs of the community. Consider converting Lake View Hospital's underused medical-surgical units to accommodate the increasing demand for geriatric, home health, and ambulatory care services. Develop a new organizational chart, noting span of management, flat or tall structure, decentralization or centralization, and line authority. Using Worksheet 9-1, list the advantages and disadvantages of the new organization and discuss them with your classmates.

CRITICAL THINKING AND LEARNING ACTIVITIES

1. Draw a formal organization chart of the agency where you work. Note the span of management, flat or tall structure, decentralization or centralization, and line authority.

2. Observe the chain of authority and who influences whom where you work. Does the reality match the formal structure?

3. Consider how you would use line or staff authority to improve a procedure where you work.

Advantages and Disadvantages of Structure

List the advantages and disadvantages of the organizational structure.

Advantages	Disadvantages
1. _____	1. _____
2. _____	2. _____
3. _____	3. _____
4. _____	4. _____
5. _____	5. _____
6. _____	6. _____
7. _____	7. _____
8. _____	8. _____
9. _____	9. _____
10. _____	10. _____
11. _____	11. _____
12. _____	12. _____
13. _____	13. _____
14. _____	14. _____
15. _____	15. _____

Chapter

10

Organizational Culture

Chapter Objectives

◆ Identify four factors in organizational culture.

◆ Identify how managers can use heroes.

◆ Describe a cultural network.

◆ Identify at least two rituals.

◆ Explain the relationship between policy and procedure.

Major Concepts and Definitions

Assumptions	suppositions, presumptions, something taken for granted
Values	basic beliefs of the organization about what is desirable or important
Symbols	objects or acts that represent another thing
Language	choice of words and sounds used to express thoughts and feelings
Behaviors	actions or mannerisms
Organizational culture	customary way of thinking and behaving that is shared by members of an organization
Hero	a person honored for outstanding qualities
Cultural network	primary informal means of communication in the organization
Rituals	day-to-day routines
Policy	a governing plan for accomplishing goals and objectives
Procedure	chronological sequence of steps within a process
Protocols	documents of agreement

ORGANIZATIONAL CULTURE

Organizational culture is the customary way of thinking and behaving that is shared by all members of the organization and must be learned and adopted by newcomers before they can be accepted into the agency. Culture is learned, shared, and transmitted. It is a combination of assumptions, values, symbols, language, and behaviors that manifest the organization's norms and values. Objective aspects exist outside the minds of members of the organization and include such artifacts as pictures of leaders, monuments, stories, ceremonies, and rituals. Subjective aspects are related to assumptions and mind-sets such as shared assumptions, values, meanings, and understandings of how things will be done.

Values are the basic beliefs of the organization. Agencies with strong cultures have a complex system of values that are discussed openly by managers and are accepted by members. They establish the standards for achievement in the organization. They are the essence of the organization's philosophy; they provide a sense of direction, guide daily behavior, serve as an informal control system, help set priorities, and plan strategies.

Heroes personify the organizational culture's values. They show that success is attainable, set a standard for performance, preserve what is special in the organization, motivate employees, serve as role models, and symbolize the organization to the outside world.

The cultural network is the primary informal means of communication within the organization that carries the corporate values and heroic mythology. Managers should use this network to understand what is going on and to get things done (Deal and Kennedy, 1982).

Rituals are the day-to-day routines that show employees how they are to behave. Policies and procedures clarify routines. Inductions, promotions, planning retreats, and retirements are rituals that reinforce the values. Ceremonies are extravagant rituals that give visible evidence of the agency's values. Ceremonies keep the values, beliefs, and heroes visible.

Leaders help shape the culture by demonstrating a philosophy, projecting a vision, modeling values, setting policies, creating systems, and supporting a reward system.

Cooke et al. (1987) have identified three culture types: (1) positive, (2) passive-defensive, and (3) aggressive-defensive. In a *positive* culture members are proactive and interactive to meet their satisfaction needs. That culture is based on humanism, affiliative norms, achievement, and self-actualization. In *passive-defensive* and *aggressive-defensive* cultures people protect their security and status in reactive, guarded ways. Passive-defensive culture is based on conventional, approval, dependent, and avoidance norms. Aggressive-defensive culture is based on power, oppositional, competitive, perfectionistic norms. Leaders need to diffuse negativism in oppositional norms and act as role models for desirable behaviors, encouraging a cultural transition to more positive norms.

Leaders help shape the culture by demonstrating a philosophy, projecting a vision, modeling values, setting policies, creating systems, and supporting a reward system. Leaders must ensure congruity between strategic plans and decision-making processes. They need to identify the actual norms, establish desired norms, identify culture gaps, close culture gaps, and sustain culture changes. Leaders help others understand and make sense of events and cope with change, instability, and the unexpected. Leaders need to help members of the organization adapt to the dynamic life cycle of the organization. Open and collaborative interaction between leaders and followers is important.

Policies

Policies and procedures are means for accomplishing goals and objectives. Policies explain how goals will be achieved and serve as guides that define the general course and scope of activities permissible for goal accomplishment. They serve as a basis for future decisions and actions, help coordinate plans, control performance, and increase consistency of action by increasing the probability that different managers will make similar decisions when independently facing similar situations. Consequently, morale is increased when personnel perceive that they are being treated equally. Policies also serve as a means by which authority can be delegated.

Policies should be comprehensive in scope, stable, and flexible so they can be applied to different conditions that are not so diverse that they require separate sets of policies. Consistency is important, because inconsistency introduces uncertainty and contributes to feelings of bias, preferential treatment, and unfairness. Fairness is an important characteristic that is attributed to the application of the policy. Policies should be written and understandable.

Policies can be implied or expressed. Implied policies are not directly voiced or written but are established by patterns of decisions. They may have either favorable or unfavorable effects and represent an interpretation of observed behavior. Courteous treatment of clients may be implied versus expressed. The presence or absence of workers who are over 50 or 55 years of age, minority members, women, or pregnant women may lead to an interpretation of implied policies. Sometimes policies are implied simply because no one has ever bothered to state them. At other times they may deliberately be only implied because they are illegal or reflect questionable ethics. Sometimes implied policy conflicts with expressed policy. These double standards should be prevented.

Expressed policies may be oral or written. Oral policies are more flexible than written ones and can be easily adjusted to changing circumstances. However, they are less desirable than written ones because they may not be known.

The process of writing policies reveals discrepancies and omissions and causes the manager to think critically about the policy, thus contributing to clarity. Once written, they are readily available to all in the same form; their meaning cannot be changed by word of mouth; misunderstandings can be referred to the written words; the chance of misinterpretation is decreased; policy statements can be sent to all affected by them; they can be referred to whoever wishes to check the policy; and they can be used for orientation purposes. Written policies indicate the integrity of the organization's intention and generate confidence in management.

A disadvantage of written policies is the reluctance to revise them when they become outdated. However, even oral policies become obsolete. Managers should review policies periodically, and if that fails, personnel can appeal for a revision.

Policies can emerge in several ways—originated, appealed, or imposed. The originated, or internal, policies are usually developed by top management to guide subordinates in their functions. Strategy for originated policy flows from the objectives of the organization as defined by top management and may be broad in scope, allowing staff associates to develop supplemental policies, or well defined with little room for interpretation. All of the lower managerial decisions should implement the broader policy defined by top management.

Sometimes policies are generated at the operating and first-line manager levels and imposed upward. The extent to which this happens is influenced by the organizational atmosphere and adequacy of policies generated by top management. At times policies may be formulated simultaneously from both directions.

When staff associates do not know how to solve a problem, disagree with a previous decision, or otherwise want a question reviewed, they appeal to the manager for a decision. As appeals are taken up the hierarchy and decisions are made, precedents known as appealed policy develop and guide future managerial actions.

Policies developed from appeals are likely to be incomplete, uncoordinated, and unclear. Unintended precedents can be set when decisions are made for a given situation without consideration for possible effects on other dimensions of the organization. This aimless formation of policy makes it difficult to know what policies exist. Sometimes managers dislike facing issues until forced to do so and consequently delay policy-making until precedents have been set. Appeals policies can be foresighted and consistent, especially when the manager knows that the decision constitutes policy. Nevertheless, when a number of policies are being appealed, it is time to assess policies for gaps and needs for updating and clarification so originated policies can dominate. One can expect health agencies to need policies about patient care assignments, noting physicians' orders, administration of medications, patient safety, charting, and infection control.

Imposed, or external, policies are thrust on an organization by external forces such as government or labor unions. Policies of the organization must conform to local, state, and federal laws. Collective bargaining and union contracts direct labor policies. Professional and social groups—such as the American Nurses' Association, the National League for Nursing, and church, school, and charitable organizations—mold policy.

The planning process involves defining, communicating, applying, and maintaining policies. The development of a policy can originate anywhere in an organization and should involve personnel who will be affected by the policy. They have valuable information for sound policy formation and can ensure that the policy will be implemented. Before writing a policy one must consider whether there are specific, recurring problems, how frequently they occur, whether they are temporary or permanent in nature, and whether a policy statement would clarify thinking and promote efficiency.

When policies are written, the purpose, philosophy, goals, and objectives should serve as guides. Policies should be consistent and help solve or prevent specific problems. Clear, concise statements that establish areas of authority and perhaps include reference to supporting policies minimize exceptions. Managers need sufficient guidance with accompanying freedom for action. It is advisable to have the policy statement reviewed and approved by superiors and the affected managers before the policy is formalized.

Policies are of no use if no one knows of their existence. Oral communication is appropriate to introduce and explain new policies. It is appropriate to send a letter of purpose and a copy of policies to personnel affected by them. The written policies can then be referred to later. Policies should be written in a specific, concise, and complete manner and stored in a policy manual that is easily accessible to all personnel to whom the policies apply. The manual will be well organized if policies are classified, noted in the table of contents, and indexed by topic. Policies should be easily replaceable with revised ones.

Once a policy has been stated and approved, it is applied. Policy formation is a continuous process so the policy is continually reappraised and restated as necessary (see Fig. 10-1). Continuing surveillance to determine that the policy is understood and applied is important. Periodic analysis and evaluation of existing policies can suggest the need for revision. Personnel should be encouraged to help formulate, review, and revise policies. Boxes 10-1 through 10-5 present sample policies for generating and reviewing nursing policies, procedures, and protocols.

Procedures

Procedures supply a more specific guide to action than policy does. They help achieve a high degree of regularity by enumerating the chronological sequence of steps. Procedures are intradepartmental or interdepartmental and consequently do not affect the entire organization to the extent that policy statements do.

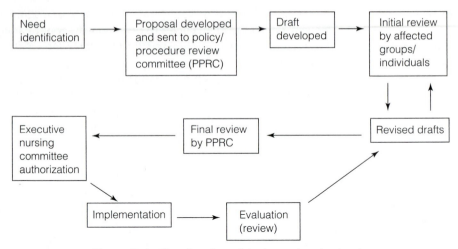

Figure 10-1 Flowchart for policies/procedures/protocols.

Procedure manuals provide a basis for orientation and staff development and are a ready reference for all personnel. They standardize procedures and equipment and can provide a basis for evaluation. Good procedures can result in time and labor savings.

Improvement in operating procedures increases productivity and reduces cost. Waste in performing work can be decreased by applying work simplification that strives to make each part of a procedure productive. First one decides what work needs simplification by identifying problem areas. Next the work selected is analyzed carefully and in detail. Charts that depict the components of the work and the work flow are useful for motion or procedural analysis.

A questioning attitude helps determine why work is done, by whom, when, where, and how. What is the purpose of the procedure? Does it need to be done? Can it be eliminated? For example, are "closed" and "surgical" beds really necessary, or could "open" beds be used for all purposes? Who does the work? Can someone else do it better, or can it be assigned to someone with less skill? Is there duplication of efforts? Can two or more activities be combined? Will changing the time sequence improve the procedure? Can transportation be reduced by changing the location? Once these questions have been answered, work should be simplified by rearranging, combining, or eliminating components. Then the improved methods must be communicated so they can be implemented.

Writing procedures demands a consistent format that considers the definition; purpose; materials needed and how to locate, requisition, and dispose of them; steps in the procedure; expected results; precautions; legal implications; nurse, patient, and physician responsibilities; and appropriate charting. Each step in the procedure leading to the accomplishment of a goal should be necessary and in proper relationship to the other steps. Balance between flexibility and stability should be maintained. As with the policy manual, the procedure manual should be easily accessible, well organized with a table of contents, and indexed. Each procedure should be easily replaceable with a revised one. Because there is a tendency to add new procedures

Text continued on p. 164.

Box 10-1   **PROCESS FOR GENERATION OF POLICY/PROCEDURE/PROTOCOL**

Issue Date July 1989	*PROCESS FOR GENERATION OF A NURSING POLICY/PROCEDURE/ PROTOCOL*	Policy No. A/O QA.08
Review Dates Annually		**Subject** Quality Assurance

POLICY

Written policies, procedures, and protocols that reflect optimal standards of nursing practice will guide the provision of nursing care.

SCOPE

This policy applies to all of Nursing Services.

PURPOSE

To provide a consistent format for the writing and processing of policies/procedures/protocols (P/P/P): identify resources for creating, reviewing, and changing P/P/P for Indiana University Hospitals Nursing Services; to eliminate duplication of efforts and ensure current and consistent practice.

PROCESS

1. A written P/P/P may be initiated by any nurse with approval of the Unit Director of Associate Director when appropriate. A self-study packet is available to assist with this process.

2. A proposal for all new P/P/Ps will be sent to the Nursing Service Policy/Procedure Review Committee (PPRC). (See attached form.) The proposal includes the topic/title, patients affected by the procedure, why it is needed, resource persons who will be used to write or consult, appropriate signature(s).
   In some cases a proposal may not be necessary, but the intent to write a P/P/P should be communicated to the PPRC. The committee will then serve as a resource for format, other resources, and for distribution. Exceptions for the initial proposal might be direction from the Executive Nursing Council or the hospital system.

3. Approval/disapproval to write will then be communicated to the initiating individual(s) by the PPRC after considering the possible overall need, already existent P/P/P, and additional resources. A member of the PPRC will be assigned to each approved proposal to ensure consistency of format. (See attached format guidelines.)

Associated Director of Hospitals for Nursing	Date
Sonna Ehrlich	7/11/89

Used with permission from Indiana Hospitals.

Box 10-2   **PROPOSAL FOR POLICY/PROCEDURE**

Proposal for Policy/Procedure

This form is submitted to the Policy/Procedure Committee of Nursing Services to request a written Policy/Procedure designed to implement policy and maintain policy standards in regard to the following nursing care:

Topic: _____

Patients affected by the policy/procedure: _____

Explanation of the policy/procedure: _____
_____

Problems that arise as a result of not having a written policy/procedure: _____
_____

Resources that you will use to write and document the validity of this policy/procedure:
_____

Name _____

Unit Director _____

Associate Director _____

****

For use by Policy/Procedure Committee

Date Received: _____

      Approval for writing of policy/procedure.   Yes   No

      Contacts within Nursing Services and Medicine that must be made for coordination of the writing of this procedure: _____
_____

Committee member assigned to supervise project: _____

Guidelines for Procedure Format

Title
Policy Statement
Scope
Purpose (optional)
Assessment and Planning
   Nursing Considerations
   Cautions
   Resources
Implementation
   Sequence of Interventions/Rationale
   Cautions
Evaluation
Documentation
Authorization Signature
References:
Written By:
Date of Revision(s):
Date of Review(s):

Used with permission from Indiana Hospitals.

Box 10-3   **REVIEW PROCESS FOR POLICIES/PROCEDURES/PROTOCOLS**

Issue Date November 1987	*PROCESS FOR GENERATION OF A* *NURSING POLICY/PROCEDURE/* *PROTOCOL*	Policy No. A/O QA.07
Review Dates Annually		Subject Quality Assurance

POLICY

All policies, procedures, and protocols (P/P/P) will be reviewed annually and re-vised as necessary.

SCOPE

This policy applies to all Nursing service policies, procedures, and protocols.

PROCESS

1. Reviews of P/P/P will be conducted in quarterly periods (Jan-Mar, Apr-Jun, Jul-Sept, Oct-Dec).

2. Before the beginning of the upcoming quarter, the Policy/Procedure Review Commit-tee (PPRC) will receive notice of which P/P/Ps are due for review. Members of the PPRC will be assigned accountability for the review of specific P/P/Ps.

3. The accountable PPRC member will review the P/P/P and will solicit feedback from appropriate content experts, using the appropriate Policy or Procedure Review Questionnaire. (See attached.)

4. The content experts will complete the Review Questionnaire after obtaining input from most affected groups or individuals. The completed questionnaire and a draft of the revised P/P/P will be returned to the accountable PPRC member by the deadline date indicated.

5. On receipt of the questionnaire and draft, the accountable PPRC member will sub-mit the final draft of the revised P/P/P to the PPRC.

6. Upon approval by the PPRC, the final draft will be submitted to the Executive Nurs-ing Council for authorization and signature.

7. Revised P/P/P will then be distributed to all holders of Nursing Service Policy/ Procedure Manuals.

8. Requests to review P/P/Ps can be made at any time during the year to the PPRC. (See attached flowchart.)

Date of Revision(s): 7/89
Date of Review(s): 7/90

Associated Director of Hospitals for Nursing	Date
Sonna Ehrlich	7/21/89

Used with permission from Indiana Hospitals.

Box 10-4

PROCEDURE REVIEW QUESTIONNAIRE

Procedure Review Questionnaire

Name of Procedure _____

Date of Review _____

Reviewer(s) _____

       (Name)   (Title)   (Service/Unit)

       (Name)   (Title)   (Service/Unit)

(Note: The reviewer may wish to carry out the procedure exactly as written before addressing the questions below.)

Please circle the number that most accurately reflects your response to the following response.

*Where procedure differs from practice, please note discrepancies on separate sheet of paper. Please write recommended revision on separate sheet of paper and return to _____ by _____.

	Yes	No	Uncertain	Comments
1. Does the procedure accurately reflect all equipment/materials necessary to carry out the procedure				
a) safely?				
b) competently?	1	2	3	
2. Does the procedure reflect equipment used at IUHs?	1	2	3	
3. Is the sequence of steps correct?	1	2	3	
4. Is the sequence of steps complete?	1	2	3	
5. Are the contraindications, if any, clearly identified?	1	2		
6. Does the scientific rationale provide a meaningful reason for each intervention?	1	2	3	
7. Does the procedure reflect results of current research and state-of-the-art clinical nursing practice?	1	2	3	
8. Does the procedure reflect current clinical practice at IUHs?	1	2	3	
9. Is the procedure in conflict with any other hospital or Nusing Services' policies/procedures? If so, please list.	1	2	3	

Additional Comments:

RECOMMENDED ACTION

___ The procedure is correct as written. Recommend adoption of procedure.

___ Discrepancies noted. Recommended revision attached.

___ Recommend procedure not be adopted.

12/84

Used with permission from Indiana Hospital.

Box 10-5   **POLICY REVIEW FORM**

Policy Review Form

Name of Policy _____

Date of Review _____

Reviewer _____

          (Name)   (Service)

INSTRUCTIONS: Please circle the number that most accurately reflects your response to the following questions. Please check at the bottom your recommended action.

	Yes	No	Comments
1. Is there a need for the policy?	1	2	
2. Is the policy relevant to this institution and staff?	1	2	
3. Is the policy consistent with Indiana University Hospitals Nursing Services philosophy?	1	2	
4. Is the policy in conflict with any other hospital or nursing policies?	1	2	
5. Does the policy create any inequities among hospital staff or patients?	1	2	
6. Is the policy reasonable (i.e., can compliance be enforced)?	1	2	
7. Is the policy clearly written so that anyone unfamiliar with the subject can understand it?	1	2	
8. Is the information accurate?	1	2	
9. Is the policy complete (i.e., does it include the scope, purpose, and any related information)?	1	2	

ADDITIONAL COMMENTS:

RECOMMENDED ACTION:

___ No Action Required   ___ Revision Required   ___ Remove from Manual
    Approved as Written   (Changes Attached)   (Justification Attached)

Used with permission from Indiana University Hopsitals.

Box 10-6   PROCEDURE

PROCEDURE

Blood Pressure Measurement

A. Definition: Amount of pressure exerted against the arterial wall as the blood is forced by the pumping action of the heart

B. Purpose: To determine the changes in the arterial walls, the condition of the heart, and the volume of the blood

C. Materials needed
   1. Stethoscope
   2. Mercury sphygmomanometer
   3. Cuffs (12 to 14 cm for adults; 18 to 20 cm for large adults; 2.5 to 9.5 cm for children)

D. Location of materials
   1. Stethoscope, sphygmomanometer, and cuffs are located at the nursing stations.
   2. Materials do not need to be requisitioned.

E. Steps in procedure

Steps in procedure	Key points
1. Collect equipment and check to see that it is in working order.	Be sure that all connections are right. Examine rubber bladder and pressure bulbs for leaks. Check that the edge of the meniscus of the mercury manometer is at the zero mark.
2. Cleanse earpieces of stethoscope with a Zephiran or alcohol sponge.	
3. Wash your hands.	
4. Enter patient's room and verify name.	Assess environmental conditions that may influence pressure.
5. Explain procedure to patient.	It is very important to gain the cooperation of the patient because distress will alter the reading of the blood pressure. Identify other factors that may affect the blood pressure reading (such as exercise, eating, weight, changes in posture, full bladder
6. Position patient in a relaxed, reclining, or sitting position with the arm flexed, palm up, and with the whole forearm supported at heart level (fourth intercostal space) on a smooth surface.	If arm is placed above the level of the heart, the reading will be falsely low; if placed below the level of the heart, the reading will be falsely high. Quiet must be maintained to allow hearing the blood pressure sounds.
7. Position yourself no more than 3 ft away from the sphygmomanometer with the meniscus of the mercury model at eye level.	
8. Select correct cuff size.	Average adult size is 12 to 14 cm; large adult, 18 to 20 cm; child, 2.5 to 9.5 cm.

9. Measure length of bladder to fit two thirds distance between shoulder and elbow. It should be 20% wider than the diameter of the arm, or 40% wider than its circumference.

If cuff is too narrow, pressure reading will be abnormally high; if too wide, the reading will be falsely low.

10. Palpate brachial artery in the medial surface of the arm and place the center of the bladder directly over the brachial artery 2.5 cm above the antecubital space.

11. Apply cuff snugly and smoothly.

If cuff is wrapped too loosely, the results will be falsely high.

12. Palpate radial pulse by placing index and middle finger on radial pulse. Inflate cuff rapidly until radial pulsation disappears. Identify this reading as the palpatory systolic reading.

13. Wait 30 to 60 sec before reinflation of cuff to 30 cm above the palpatory systolic reading.

This waiting period is necessary to allow time for the release of blood trapped in the veins. Failure to do so may prevent recognition of auscultatory gap (sound initially appears at a high level, fades completely, and reappears 10 to 40 mm later), accounting for falsely low systolic pressure.

14. Position stethoscope with ear tips forward.

15. Place diaphragm or bell of stethoscope over brachial artery in antecubital fossa with as little pressure as possible and with no space between skin and stethoscope.

Heavy pressure distorts the artery, and sounds are heard below the diastolic pressure.

16. Tighten screw on bulb and inflate cuff rapidly to 30 mm above palpatory systolic pressure.

Column of mercury (Hg) must be in a vertical position. If it is tilted, results will be falsely high. The edge of the mercury meniscus should be exactly at zero.

17. Deflate cuff 2 to 4 mm Hg per heartbeat to zero levels.

Deflating too slowly will cause a falsely high reading.

18. Note reading at the meniscus on the mercury column at which the first two regular tapping sounds (Korotkoff phase I) are heard. This is the systolic pressure.

If sounds are difficult to hear, raise the arm a few seconds to drain venous blood before inflating cuff; inflate cuff, then lower the arm, deflate, and listen for sounds; or have patient open and close fist 10 times after the systolic level has been obtained.

19. Deflate cuff at an even rate of 2 to 4 mm while the sounds change from faint and clear tapping sounds (Korotkoff phase I), to a swishing quality (Korotkoff phase II), to crisper and louder sounds (Korotkoff phase III), to abrupt muffling of sound (Korotkoff phase IV), to the point at which sounds disappear (Korotkoff phase V).

The best index of diastolic pressure in adults is the point at which the sounds disappear. The onset of muffling (fourth phase) is the best index of diastolic pressure in children.

20. Expel any air in cuff and remove from patient's arm.
21. Return equipment to nursing station.

F. Charting
   1. Chart systolic pressure over diastolic pressure on graphic sheet at foot of patient's bed.
   2. Chart systolic pressure over diastolic pressure on flow chart in patient's chart. If sounds were heard to zero, chart systolic, fourth phase (muffling sound), and disappearance of sound (for example, 148/72/0 or 10/60/50).
   3. Specify position of patient: "L" (lying), "ST" (standing), "SIT" (sitting), "RA" (right arm), or "LA" (left arm).

instead of revising existing ones, it is important to review and revise the procedure manual periodically.

In reviewing, check the effectiveness and workability with personnel to determine whether the procedure has been followed. Procedures should be realistic and written in simple language that is easy to understand. Changes should be dated and provided to all appropriate personnel.

Before spending valuable time writing procedures, one must consider whether a procedure is actually needed. With preservice and on-the-job preparation, is there really a need to have on each unit procedures on how to feed a patient and how to make a bed? Goals can be reached in a variety of ways, and consequently nursing students are taught principles rather than procedures. There are textbooks with bedside nursing procedures, and many disposable products with directions are available. It seems most important for the procedure manual to contain information that may vary from institution to institution. Not all parts of the procedure format may be necessary for each procedure. New personnel and float nurses can serve as valuable resources for nursing managers to consult when they are determining what content is important for the procedure manual. Box 10-6 presents a sample procedure for taking a blood pressure measurement.

BIBLIOGRAPHY

Bass BM, Avolio BJ: Transformational leadership and organizational culture, *Public Administrative Quarterly* 17:112-121, Spring 1993.

Brown A: Organizational culture: the key to effective leadership and organizational development, *Leadership and Organizational Development Journal* 13:3-6, 1992.

Caroselli C: Assessment of organizational culture: a tool for professional success, *Orthopaedic Nursing* 11:57-63, May-June 1992.

Coeling HVE, Simms LM: Facilitating innovation at the unit level through cultural assessment part 2, *J Nurs Adm* 23:13-20, May 1993.

Coeling HVE, Wilcos JR: Using organizational culture to facilitate the change process, *ANNA Journal* 17:231-236, June 1990.

Cooke R, Rousseau D: Behavioral norms and expectations: a quantitative approach to the assessment of organizational culture, *Group Organ Stud* 13:245-273, 1987.

Covey SR, Gulledge KA: Principle-centered leadership, *Journal for Quality and Participation* 15:70-78, July-Aug 1992.

Curran CR, Miller N: The impact of corporate culture on nurse retention, *Nurs Clin North Am* 25:537-549, September 1990.

Grigsby KA: Perceptions of the organization's climate: influenced by the organization's structure, *J Nurs Educ* 30:81-88, February 1991.

Hall DT: Promoting work/family balance: an organization-change approach, *Organ Dyn* 18:5-18, Winter 1990.

Heerema DL, Giannini R: Business organizations and the sense of community, *Business Horizons* 34:87-91: July-August 1991.

Hern-Underwood MJ, Workman LL: Group climate: a significant retention factor for pediatric nurse managers, *J Professional Nurs* 9:233-238, July-August 1993.

Hollander SF, Allen KE, Mechanic J: The intrapreneurial nursing department: nature and nurture, *Nurs Econ* 19:5-9, January-February 1992.

Hughes L: Assessing organization culture: strategies for the external consultant, *Nurs Forum* 25:15-19, 1990.

Lawton R: A service quality strategy that will work for you, *Journal for Quality and Participation* 15:38-44, June 1992.

Manion J: Chaos or transformation? Managing innovation, Journal of Nursing Administration 23(5):41-48, May 1993.

McDaniel C, Strump L: The organizational culture: implications for nursing service, *J Nurs Adm* 23:54-60, April 1993.

Mills DQ, Freisen B: The learning organization, *European Management Journal* 10:146-156, June 1992.

Oyeleye BA: Faculty/student perception of organizational climates in the schools of nursing, Oyo State, Nigeria, *International Journal of Nursing Studies* 29:341-344, November 1992.

Pratt KH, Kleiner BH: Towards managing by a richer set of organizational values, *Leadership & Organization Development Journal* 10:10-16, 1989.

Sanzgiri J, Gottlieb JZ: Philosophic and pragmatic influence on the practice of organization development, *Organizational Dynamics* 21:57-69, Autumn 1992.

Sovie MD: Hospital culture—why create one? *Nurs Econ* 11:69-75, March-April 1993.

Shortell S, Rousseau D, Gillies R et al: Organizational assessment in intensive care units (ICUs): construction, development, reliability, and validity of the ICU, nurse physician questionnaire, *Med Care* 29:709-726, August 1991.

Thomas C, Ward M, Chorba C et al: Measuring and interpreting organizational culture, *J Nurs Adm* 20:17-24, June 1990.

CASE STUDY

Primary nursing with all nursing care given by registered nurses has been practiced for the past several years on the unit where you are the patient care coordinator. In an effort to cut costs the hospital is going to hire technicians to work with registered nurses and implement a "partners' in practice" model. What will you do as a patient care coordinator to help change the organizational culture?

CRITICAL THINKING AND LEARNING ACTIVITIES

1. All organizations express cultural traits in rituals and symbols that serve to communicate and perpetuate the values, beliefs, and behaviors of the organization's members. Within organizations, subcultures develop that reflect more specific traits of specific occupational groups. Registered nurses form an occupational group because they engage in the same sort of work, and get their professional identity from that work. They may do activities together outside the work area. Using Worksheets 10-1 and 10-2, identify some rituals and symbols of the organization in general and registered nurses more specifically in an organization with which you are familiar.

2. Write a policy for Lake View Hospital (see the organizational chart in the appendix).

3. Write a procedure for Lake View Hospital (see appendix).

✍ **Worksheet 10-1**

Rituals

List rituals in general and registered nurse–specific rituals:

Rituals in general	RN-specific rituals
1.	1.
2.	2.
3.	3.
4.	4.
5.	5.
6.	6.
7.	7.
8.	8.
9.	9.
10.	10.

✍ Worksheet 10-2

Symbols

List symbols of the organization in general and registered nurse–specific symbols:

Symbols in general	RN-specific symbols
1.	1.
2.	2.
3.	3.
4.	4.
5.	5.
6.	6.
7.	7.
8.	8.
9.	9.
10.	10.

Organizational Change

Chapter Objectives

◆ Define three strategies for effecting change.

◆ Define at least three types of change.

◆ Describe the five tracks that must be carefully planned to facilitate complex organizational change.

◆ Identify the three developmental stages of an organization and discuss what occurs in each stage.

◆ Describe features of job descriptions.

◆ Describe advantages and disadvantages of career ladders.

Major Concepts and Definitions

Change	to become different
Change agent	one who helps bring about change
Organizational development	stages of birth, youth, and maturity of organizations
Job analysis	the study of a position to determine what knowledge, skill, aptitude, and personal characteristics are needed to perform certain responsibilities
Job evaluation	process of measuring the remunerative worth of a job in relationship to other positions
Job design	specifies what the job requires, job methods, and the relationship between the organizational, social, and personal needs of the worker
Job rotation	a horizontal job enlargement technique
Job enrichment	vertical approach to job design that uses more abilities and skills of personnel
Job descriptions	specifications that are the requirements for the job
Career ladder	vertical clinical advancement

MANAGEMENT OF CHANGE

Strategies for Effecting Change

Whether working with individuals, groups, or systems, the nurse manager is sure to be involved with management of change. Several strategies for managing change have been identified.

Empirical-rational strategies. Empirical-rational strategies are based on the assumption that people are rational and behave according to rational self-interest. It follows then that people should be willing to adopt a change if it is justified and if the people are shown how they can benefit from the change.

Nurse managers who use empirical-rational strategies are likely to want the appropriate persons for specific positions. Desirous of having well-qualified people performing jobs for which they are well qualified, nurse managers give considerable attention to recruitment and selection of personnel. Staff development through independent study, in-service education, continuing education, and formal degree programs is encouraged. Systems analysis, operations research, and implementation of research findings are consistent with the empirical-rational philosophy, as is long-range futuristic planning.

Normative reeducative strategies.   Normative reeducative strategies are based on the assumption that people act according to their commitment to sociocultural norms. The intelligence and rationality of people are not denied, but attitudes and values are also considered. The manager pays attention to changes in values, attitudes, skills, and relationships in addition to providing information.

Believing that the basic unit of the social organization is composed of individuals, the manager fosters the development of staff members through means such as personal counseling, training groups, small groups, and experiential learning because people need to participate in their own reeducation. Organizational development programs are fostered, and it is typical to collect data about the organization, give data feedback and analysis to appropriate people, plan ways to improve the system, and train managers and internal change agents. The relationships of internal change agents with other personnel can be a major tool in reeducating others.

Power-coercive strategies.   Power-coercive strategies involve compliance of the less powerful to the leadership, plans, and directions of the more powerful. These strategies do not deny the intelligence and rationality of people or the importance of their values and attitudes, but rather they acknowledge the need to use sources of power to bring about change. Use of strikes, sit-ins, negotiations, conflict confrontation, and administration decisions and rulings are power-coercive strategies.*

Process of Change

Unfreezing, moving, and refreezing are the three phases of change (see Fig. 11-1). Unfreezing is the development through problem awareness of a need to change. Even if a problem has been identified, people must believe there can be an improvement before they are willing to change. Coercion and the induction of guilt and anxiety have been used for unfreezing. Removal of people from the source of their old attitudes to a new environment, punishment and humiliation for undesirable attitudes, and rewards for desirable attitudes effect change.

Stress may cause dissatisfaction with the status quo and become a motivating factor for change. Points of stress and strain should be assessed. Change may begin at a point of stress but ordinarily should not be started at the point of greatest stress. It is most appropriate for it to start with a policy-making body that considers both formal and informal structures. The effectiveness of the change may depend on the amount of involvement in fact finding and problem solving of all personnel.

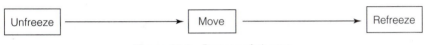

Figure 11-1   Process of change.

---

* Discussed in detail in Chin R, Benne KD: General strategies for effecting changes in human systems. In Bennis W, Benne KD, Chin R, editors: *The planning of change,* New York, 1969, Holt, Rinehart & Winston, pp. 32-59.

Moving is working toward change by identifying the problem or the need to change, exploring the alternatives, defining goals and objectives, planning how to accomplish the goals, and implementing the plan for change.

Refreezing is the integration of the change into one's personality and the consequent stabilization of change. Frequently, personnel return to old behaviors after change efforts cease. Related changes in neighboring systems, momentum to perpetuate the change, and structural alterations that support the procedural changes are stabilizing factors.

Types of Change

The variables of mutual goal setting, the power ratio between the change agent and the client system, and the deliberativeness of change are differentiating factors in the change process.

Coercive change. Coercive change is characterized by nonmutual goal setting, imbalanced power ratio, and one-sided deliberativeness.

Emulative change. In this case, change is fostered through identification with and emulation of power figures.

Indoctrination. Indoctrination uses mutual goal setting, has an imbalanced power ratio, and is deliberative. Subordinates are instructed in the beliefs of the power sources.

Interactional change. This is characterized by mutual goal setting, fairly equal power, but no deliberativeness. Parties may be unconsciously committed to changing one another.

Natural change. These changes include accidents and acts of God. They involve no goal setting or deliberativeness.

Socialization change. This has a direct relationship with interactional change. One conforms to the needs of a social group. When there is greater deliberativeness on the power side, change becomes indoctrination.

Technocratic change. Change is brought about by collecting and interpreting data. A technocrat merely reports the findings of the analysis to bring about change.

Planned change. Planned change involves mutual goal setting, an equal power ratio, and deliberativeness.

Seven phases of planned change have been identified. First, the client must feel a need for change. The manager, as the change agent, can stimulate an awareness of the need to change, help the client become aware of the problems, and indicate that a more desirable state of affairs is possible. Thus, unfreezing occurs.

Next, the helping relationship must be established, and the moving process begun. Managers as change agents must identify with clients' problems while remaining neutral so that they can remain objective. The change agent needs to be viewed as an understandable and approachable expert. The success or failure of most planned action will depend largely on the quality and workability of the relationship between the change agent and the client.

Third, the problem must be identified and clarified. Collecting and analyzing data can facilitate this process. Fourth, alternative possibilities for change should be examined. Goals and objectives are planned. The client's emotional and material resources are examined. Strategies for change are determined. The success of planned change is evaluated by the implementation of the plans. The fifth phase is the active work of modification, which completes the moving process.

The refreezing process occurs during the sixth phase—generalization and stabilization. All too often clients slip back to their old ways after change efforts cease. The spread of change to neighboring systems and to subparts of the same system aids the stabilization process. Change momentum, positive evaluation of the change, rewards for the change, and related procedural and structural changes increase the stabilization.

The helping relationship ends, or a different type of continuing relationship is established in the last phase. Dependency is the major factor determining when the relationship will end.*

Role of the Manager as Change Agent

As a change agent, the manager identifies the problem, assesses the client's motivations and capacities for change, determines alternatives, explores ramifications of those alternatives, assesses resources, determines appropriate helping roles, establishes and maintains a helping relationship, recognizes the phases of the change process and guides the client through them, and chooses and implements techniques for planned change (Lippit, Watson, and Westley, 1958).

Force-Field Analysis

Kurt Lewin's force-field analysis provides a framework for problem solving and planned change. Status quo is maintained when driving forces equal the restraining forces (see Fig. 11-2), and change will occur when the relative strength of opposing forces changes. Consequently, when planning change, the manager should identify the restraining and driving forces and assess their strengths.

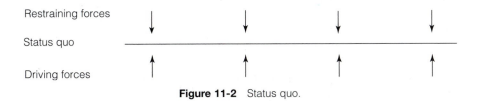

Figure 11-2 Status quo.

---

* Planned change is discussed in more detail in Lippit R, Watson J, Westley B: *The dynamics of planned change,* New York, 1958, Harcourt, Brace & World.

Box 11-1   **DRIVING AND RESTRAINING FORCES**

Driving forces		Restraining forces	
Rank	**Factor**	**Rank**	**Factor**
1	Pressure from manager	4	Conformity
4	Please manager	4	Security
2	Improve self-image	2	Economic threat
2	Improve situation	3	Threat to prestige

Scale:
1 = Little strength
2 = Moderate strength
3 = Important strength
4 = Major strength

Adapted from Lippitt R, Watson J, Westley B: *The dynamics of planned change,* New York, 1958, Harcourt, Brace & World, p. 126.

Driving forces may include pressure from the manager, desire to please the manager, perception that the change will improve one's self-image, and belief that the change will improve the situation. Restraining forces include conformity to norms, morals, and ethics; desire for security; perception of economic threat or threat to one's prestige and homeostasis; and regulatory mechanisms for keeping the situation fairly constant.

Once the driving and restraining forces have been identified, the manager determines their relative strengths. Which are the major factors toward or resisting change? Which are important or moderately important? Which have little effect for or against change? These might be listed in columns under "driving" and "restraining" and ranked (see Box 11-1).

To help visualize these forces, the manager can draw a diagram as shown in Figure 11-3, write in key words to identify the forces, and draw arrows toward the status quo line to represent the strength of the forces. The longer the line, the stronger the force.

Next the manager plans strategies for reducing the restraining forces and strengthening the driving forces. Managers may do some experiential learning exercises to facilitate the change of group norms, explain each person's role in the change with emphasis on security, and provide some status symbols to reduce the threat to people's prestige. They should also help the workers identify how the change will improve their situation. Steps should be taken to improve self-images. For instance, people may be taught new tasks to prepare themselves for the change, to reduce the threat to their prestige and their fear of making fools of themselves when doing something new, and to improve their self-images. If managers perceive that the workers want to please them, they may inform the workers that they desire the change and give positive reinforcement for the desired changes. Keeping the goals in mind, the

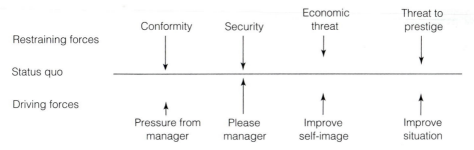

Figure 11-3 Strength of driving and restraining forces.

manager should assess the results of implementing the strategies and revise plans as necessary.

MAPS Design Technology

MAPS is an acronym for multivariate analysis, participation, and structure. It facilitates the organization's development by applying theories of motivation to create organizational structures. First, the organization is designed to determine whether the organization's structure is a cause of performance problems. Second, the focus of the change effort must be determined. Will only selected work-group structures or will the whole organization structure be changed? Third, the objectives of the project must be identified and stated. Fourth, strategies to deal with diagnosed problems and to meet the objectives must be determined. Fifth, a questionnaire that identifies the total range of tasks necessary to achieve the change and a list of the members of the organization or group involved must be composed. Participative collaboration from organizational members and possibly from clients is recommended. Next the questionnaire is administered to all members of the targeted group. They identify their qualifications and preferences for tasks and identify with whom they would prefer to work. Then the questionnaire is analyzed by use of multivariate statistics to identify clusters of tasks and people that reflect sociometric choice. A specific cluster of tasks and people is selected. Resources and support are provided to help the new group develop and do the tasks. The implementation process is monitored so that problems can be detected and resolved easily. Results are evaluated in terms of meeting the objectives. The new structure will then need to be redesigned, because solutions to old problems create new problems.

Cultural Change in Organizations

In an adaptive culture, members of an organization support each other's efforts to identify and solve problems. The members believe they can manage the problems; have confidence and enthusiasm; and are receptive to change. In a dysfunctional culture, members continue behaviors that have worked in the past but are no longer effective. Culture rut occurs when members do not adapt to change and continue to function out of habit even when success is not forthcoming. Culture shock happens when the members realize that the organization is out of touch with its setting, mission, and assumptions.

FIVE STAGES OF ORGANIZATIONAL PLANNED CHANGE

Initiate the integrated program of cultural change
Diagnose the problems
Schedule the tracks
Implement the tracks
Evaluate the results

 FIVE TRACKS FOR CULTURAL CHANGE

Culture
Management skills
Team building
Strategy structure
Reward system

Kilmann (1991) identified five stages of organizational planned change: (1) initiate the integrated program for cultural change, (2) diagnose the problems, (3) schedule the tracks, (4) implement the tracks, and (5) evaluate the results (see Box 11-2).

The five tracks are (1) culture, (2) management skills, (3) team building, (4) strategy structure, and (5) reward system (see Box 11-3). They need to be implemented in that order to be most successful. The culture track helps explain organizational differences in decision making and actions much as personality explains differences in individuals. The culture track reveals the norms of the organization. It exposes the old culture and helps create a new culture. Without an adaptive culture it can be impossible to make improvements, so removing the cultural barriers has to be accomplished before proceeding to another track.

First, one needs to clarify the actual norms. For instance, one could ask members to list current do's and don'ts. The members can then list what they want the norms to be and identify the culture gaps. Culture gaps are often related to (1) task support-norms related to helping others, information sharing, and concern for efficiency; (2) task innovation-norms related to performing new activities, trying different approaches, and being creative; (3) social relationship-norms about mixing business with pleasure and socializing with co-workers; and (4) personal freedom-norms for pleasing oneself, using self-expression, and exercising discretion (see Box 11-4). Culture gaps are generally largest at lower levels in the organization.

Closing the culture gaps then becomes the issue. If the managers and associates decide that changes should occur, they can. Adaptive cultures have internal control. Control is a social reality but not necessarily an objective one. To establish desired norms, members can be asked to list norms they think would lead to organizational

**Box
11-4**   **CULTURE GAPS**

> Task support-norms
> Task innovation-norms
> Social relationship-norms
> Personal freedom-norms

**Box
11-5**   **MANAGEMENT SKILLS TRACK**

> Sensing problems
> Defining problems
> Deriving solutions
> Implementing solutions
> Evaluating outcomes

success. Then work groups need to develop a sanctioning system to monitor and enforce the new norms. Work groups should decide what will be done if a member violates a new norm or performs the desired behavior. The open sanctioning system is probably more equitable than the old unconscious sanctions.

Now it becomes important to sustain the cultural change. If the new culture is not supported by the remaining four tracks it is likely that the culture will revert to the dysfunctional ways. The management skills and team-building tracks develop leadership to support the adaptive culture. The strategy-structure track will document the new systems, and the reward system track will support the new norms.

In the management skills track, managers are taught the five steps of problem management: (1) sensing problems, (2) defining problems, (3) deriving solutions, (4) implementing solutions, and (5) evaluating outcomes (see Box 11-5). Next, managers examine their personality types. Because one's personality type determines how one will assimilate information and make decisions, managers should be aware of their style and the style of associates so they can compensate for their natural inclinations and acknowledged limitations and develop strong work teams.

Managers also need to learn assumptional analysis: how to surface, classify by amount of certainty and importance, and synthesize assumptions. Outdated assumptions can lead to the wrong strategy-structure and reward systems. In a climate of trust and openness, associates should be able to examine previously unstated assumptions so they are not held back by faulty assumptions.

The team-building track activates the new culture and skills through the entire organization. Team building involves (1) reuniting the work group, (2) identifying work group problems, (3) identifying solutions and developing action plans, (4) implementing the plans, and (5) evaluating and monitoring the outcomes (see Box

TEAM BUILDING

Reuniting the work groups
Identifying work-group problems
Identifying solutions and developing plans
Implementing the plans
Evaluating and monitoring the outcomes

STRATEGY-STRUCTURE TRACK

Operationalizing strategy
Designing subunits
Implementing structure

11-6). Interteam building is also included in this track. Everyone in the organization needs to learn how to cope with difficult people, understand their own personality style, and appreciate the styles of others.

In the strategy-structure track, strategy sets the direction and structure organizes the goals, tasks, people, and other resources to accomplish the plans. This involves operationalizing strategy, designing subunits, and implementing structure (see Box 11-7). The reward-system track ensures that associates are rewarded for doing the right things for the right reasons.

ORGANIZATIONAL DEVELOPMENT

Organizations progress through developmental stages—birth, youth, and maturity (see Box 11-8). The creation of a new organization and its survival as a viable system are primary concerns during the birth stage. Gaining stability and developing a reputation and pride are the focuses of the youth stage. The maturity stage involves achieving both uniqueness and adaptability and contributing to society.

As organizations are born and grow, they pass through increasingly complex stages of life. They must develop internally and generate new control processes to fit the amount of turbulence and complexity in the environment. At each stage, the environment can become more unknown, unsettled, and difficult. A crisis develops in each stage. The organization needs to change its organizational and decision-making structure to fit this new complexity. The new organization copes by developing job descriptions, programs, policies, and procedures.

However, as the organization grows and becomes more complex, these policies do not cover the exceptions. As a result, the organization develops a set of hierarchical positions to make judgments about the exceptions to the existing job descriptions and

**Box
11-8** **DEVELOPMENTAL STAGES OF AN ORGANIZATION**

Birth—creation and survival as a viable system
Youth—stability, reputation, pride
Maturity—uniqueness, adaptability, contribution to society

---

policies. As the organization becomes larger and more complex, the managers in the hierarchy become overloaded. They do not have time to deal with all the exceptions and cannot make sense out of the situation.

Consequently, in the third stage, the organization needs to accomplish orderliness by developing broader goals. However, as the organization becomes increasingly complex, conflicts arise among factions, and the organization regresses to hierarchical referral again.

A decentralized system of departments reduces the interconnections between divisions and reduces the number of communications necessary to make decisions. But as the revolutionary cycle continues, conflict between decentralized departments develops.

In the last stage, a vertical information system is developed so that standardized accounting and statistical reporting systems from each department are consolidated at the top, and then resources are allocated among departments. Because all the complex information in turbulent systems cannot be reduced to numbers, human contacts made among department members become a major coping mechanism. Liaisons, teams, committees, task forces, and integrator roles are used.

BEHAVIORAL ASPECTS OF ORGANIZATIONAL CHANGE

Many people are unaware of the factors that initiate change or influence its direction. Even when known, some forces are beyond their control. Some factors that effect change in an agency stem from society, such as new knowledge and technology, new social requirements, changing client needs and demands, and increased competition. Even when known in advance and anticipated, they cannot be controlled by an agency.

The efficiency of an organizational structure is hard to measure, and the factors contributing to success or failure may be impossible to isolate. Organizational structure may not be the problem. A few ineffective people can disrupt an otherwise sound structure, and good people can make a bad structure work. High labor costs, inadequate equipment, ineffective advertising, changing client needs, and increased competition may contribute to inadequate profits.

Some symptoms reflect inefficiencies within the organization and indicate a need for change. If slow and erroneous decision making is a problem, one may question the qualifications of the person making decisions, the level at which responsibility is placed, and access to necessary information. Poor communications, a dearth of innovation, and failure in functional areas are other symptoms indicating a need for change. Diagnosis of the problem is extremely important for planned change. Some problems may be corrected by minor adjustments rather than major reorganizations. However, even a small change in one part of an organization can cause a chain reaction throughout the agency. This domino effect creates problems with coordination and control and brings about a need for comprehensive planning.

Change disrupts equilibrium. Equilibrium can be maintained only when opposing forces are equal. Production may be maintained when the forces fostering production, such as pressure of the manager to produce, desire for favorable attention from the manager to foster one's own gain, and desire to earn more through the incentive plan, equal the forces limiting production, such as the informal group's standard against rate busting, resistance to training, and the feeling that the job and product are not important. However, when the forces in one direction or the other change in relation to each other, a new grouping forms, and change is inevitable.

Resistance to Change

Caution should be used when making organizational changes. Changes are disturbing to those affected, and resistance often develops. Giving the structure a chance to work may be better than changing it. Although changing the organizational structure may appear easy on paper, it is quite complicated in reality. It affects the attitudes and effectiveness of personnel whose prestige and status are threatened. Resistance to change is a common phenomenon whether it is initiated by positive stimuli, such as growth or promotion of an employee, or negative forces, such as poor management. Personnel develop vested interests, preferences, habits, and rigidities that attract them to the existing structure. People tend to consider the effects of the change on their personal lives, status, and future more than on the welfare of the agency. Change introduces the risk of error, fear of failure when trying something new, resistance to admission of weakness, fear of losing a current satisfaction, or a fatalistic expectation based on previous unsuccessful attempts to change. Change is most threatening in the presence of insecurity. Even logical, needed changes produce resistance.

Gradual changes made in progressive phases are usually less disturbing than radical, sweeping, unpredicted changes. Changes in the structure resulting from sharply defined events that have already been planned—such as changes in size, scope, or objectives—are easier to execute than shifts in personnel, which involve infinitely complex human relations. Careful planning, appropriate timing of communications, adequate feedback, and employee confidence in management can reduce resistance to change.

Resistance can be further reduced by informing personnel of the reasons for change, especially when the advantages of the change are stressed. Personnel can be involved by requests for their input, including feelings, suggestions, and talents; their negative as well as positive feelings should be respected. Communicating honestly about the changes, giving specific feedback, asking what assistance is needed to help them cope, and recognizing their contributions to the implementation of the change can further minimize resistance.

Types of Change

Organizational structure usually grows vertically, then horizontally, and from functional to divisionalized type. Initially there is vertical growth, but as the amount of work and its complexity increases, horizontal growth develops. Usually organizations develop from a functional type, which is departmentalized by major functions, to one divisionalized by product or territory.

Planning for Change

Plans for change begin with an evaluation of the existing organization. An organizational audit provides a detailed analysis of the organization, reveals the extent to which goals are accomplished, and examines the use of personnel and the growth of individuals. One begins an organizational audit by collecting and reviewing all available written material about the organization, including statement of the mission or purpose, scope of the agency, goals and objectives, organizational chart, job descriptions, annual reports, performance appraisals, and qualifications needed and not needed by personnel in their present positions. The planner notes whether the reviewed materials are consistent, looks for gaps and overlapping of functioning, and determines that all activities contribute to the major goals of the agency.

Departmentalization, span of management, and balance and emphasis are analyzed. Authority relationships are studied. Leadership patterns, delegation, decentralization, use of committees, and provision of controls are considered. The agency may be compared with what is visualized as an ideal agency or with competitors to identify areas of need and to propose recommended changes. Personnel may be surveyed to identify areas needing improvement. The quantitative approach may be used where ratios are appropriate, such as figuring range of management. Then various organizational patterns are designed, and position breakdown using existing personnel is developed. Personnel needed who are not presently available and people available who are not qualified or needed are identified.

A job description and requirements are necessary for each position. Each person's qualifications can be compared with the job requirements. Notations are made of job requirements for which skills are not possessed. Those qualities that can be developed on the job within reasonable time limits should be separated from required skills that cannot be acquired. Unused abilities should be related to requirements of other jobs for which the individual may be better qualified.

Changes in personnel are normal, but they are accelerated during organizational changes. Unless managers are to become obsolete, they must change with the times. Some quickly increase their managerial knowledge and skills. Unfortunately, others are inflexible, overly conservative, and negative. Executive obsolescence is increasingly common with the rapid changes in our society. Managers who previously performed competently may be overwhelmed with increasingly complex duties, or they may have been promoted during an emergency to a position for which they were inadequately prepared.

What can one do about an unqualified incumbent? In developing a strategy, one should consider the ramifications of the action on the individual and on the group. The strategy should depend on the particular circumstances. An incompetent staff associate may be counseled toward satisfactory performance. Weaknesses should be identified and means to overcome them defined. On-the-job training, in-service education, college courses, and independent study may be explored. A contract may be written between the employer and the incompetent subordinate, specifying what skills are to be developed to what level of achievement and in what time frame.

Incompetent executives may be transferred to positions for which they are more qualified. They may be moved from line to staff authority. The change is most attractive when the advisory staff position is at a higher organizational level than the present line responsibilities, carries prestige, and maintains the current salary. Executives may be told there is a problem in the new area that they are to solve. This method fosters high morale and loyalty. It removes incompetence from line authority when damage could be done but uses the executive's knowledge and skills to solve specific problems. This is an expensive method.

Termination is the most extreme way to handle incompetence. It is either direct or indirect. In the direct method employees are informed that their work does not meet the minimal criteria and they are expected to leave the agency. The indirect method may involve giving incompetent employees nothing to do, withholding information from them, leaving their names off memoranda, excluding them from conferences, and generally making them so miserable they will voluntarily resign.

New managers may be hired, particularly when new positions become available during reorganization. They often bring new ideas, objectivity, and enthusiasm to the job. Recruitment is important for development of an executive pool. The best managers do not need to hunt for jobs. The jobs hunt for them. The agency needs to let its need be known and to seek good managers aggressively. Similar agencies may be a resource for managers with new ideas and different approaches. Graduates may be recruited from university programs. Recruiting advertisements in professional journals and through employment agencies are useful for locating potential managers and well-qualified staff.

Promotions within the agency provide incentives and supply the executive pool. However, some personnel may not be interested in managerial work, and competent, satisfied employees may lack managerial potential.

After the revised organization is decided, operational procedures to expedite changes need to be developed. They define activities that are necessary for specific work and identify changes needed. The revised operational procedures should be inclusive, show all details, and ensure coordinated change. Work flow should be maintained and standards upheld. Special activities are likely to be needed during a transitional period. The revised operational procedures should be perceived as carefully thought-out, planned changes and not just as stopgap actions.

Strategies for Change

Visions of what the organization can become, instead of what it is or has been, allow for organizational change. To this end, managers need to create an open atmosphere where questions can be asked. Welcoming criticism instead of forbidding it helps personnel be adequately self-critical. Denying problems has serious consequences. A good recruitment plan is needed for hiring competent, highly motivated personnel. Career development programs should be provided. All employees need to feel that what they achieve is important to the agency and that needed change for the continuing vitality of the organization overrides their vested interests.

Job Analysis

Job analysis affects employee recruitment, hiring, orientation and training programs, performance appraisal, placement, transfers, and promotions; it consequently influences nursing care. It can determine equitable rates of pay and grade nursing positions within the total agency personnel system. By reviewing national, state, regional, and local wage surveys and using wage scales and performance appraisal, nursing personnel can be compensated satisfactorily for performance. It is the nurse administrator's responsibility to inform the analyst of the scope of authority in nursing positions so that they might be upgraded. This is especially pressing in the nursing profession, because nursing positions have long been rated lower than those of other professionals with comparable education, experience, and responsibility.

Job analysis is the study of a position to determine what knowledge, skill, aptitude, and personal characteristics are needed to perform certain responsibilities successfully. Analysis does not include any attempt to change the task. Rather, one starts by locating or developing a job description and position requirements. Questionnaires, interviews, observation, and logs furnish information about the job title and summary, duties performed, type of supervision given and received, equipment used, working conditions, and relationship to other positions. Job analysis determines minimum requirements (type and level of knowledge, skill, aptitude, and personal characteristics) and consequently sets standards for such factors as education, experience, intelligence, personality, and physical strength.

Job Evaluation

Job evaluation is a process of measuring the remunerative worth of a job in relation to other positions, both internal and external to the organization. On the assumption that workers will be more satisfied if they perceive pay rates as consistent, the objective of evaluation is to compare jobs and establish a consistent pay base, providing employees in responsible positions with more pay than those with less demanding jobs. A point system, ranking of jobs, job grading, and job-to-job comparison are used. Consideration is given to education, mental and manual skills, responsibility for resources (personnel, materials, and finances), mental and physical effort, and working conditions, such as exposure to dangerous or disagreeable elements.

With the point system the nurse manager assigns numerical values to specific qualifications. An example appears in Box 11-9.

Once point values have been assigned to various job factors, they can be added to determine a grade. The grades for various jobs can be ranked, and job-to-job comparisons can provide a basis for determining pay.

Job evaluation is a systematic rather than a scientific process, and its high reliability does not ensure validity. The management values used to choose and weight factors may not be consistent with the values of other personnel, or the selected values may be different among work groups. Although relative pay rates can be determined by job evaluation, the absolute levels are often negotiated by the individual or unions.

Box 11-9   JOB EVALUATION

Qualifications	Points
Education	
Less than a high school diploma	10
High school diploma	20
High school diploma plus a special training course	30
Associate degree or three years in work study program and passage of accrediting examinations	40
Baccalaureate degree and passage of accrediting examinations	50
Master's degree in area of speciality needed for the position	60
Doctorate in area of specialty appropriate for the position	70
Mental skills	
Work is simple and repetitive and is performed according to instructions	10
Work involves a variety of duties that are performed according to procedures but require alertness to identify needed changes	20
Work involves a variety of complicated duties and some independent actions in adapting procedures to specific situations	30
Work involves planning, organization, implementing, and evaluating actions related to patient care	40
Work involves development of policies and procedures, organization of functions, development of staffing patterns, and budget preparations	50
Manual skills	
Work involves the normal manual skills, such a lifting, pushing, folding, writing, filing	10
Work involves about-normal manual skills, such as accurate measurements, administration of medications and treatments, manipulation of instruments, typing, bookkeeping	40
Work involves considerable manual skill, such as administering complex treatments and manipulation of complex equipment	50
Responsibility for resources	
Personnel	
Supervises no one	10
Supervises fewer than 10 people	20
Directs up to 25 people	30
Directs up to 50 people	40
Directs up to 100 people	50
Directs more than 100 people	60
Finances	
No responsibility for budget	10
Responsible for budget up to $10,000	20
Responsible for budget up to $25,000	30
Responsible for budget up to $100,000	40
Responsible for budget over $100,000	50
Effort	
Mental	
Requires little thinking or judgment	10
Requires some alertness while performing repetitious tasks according to directions	20
Requires mental effort for problem solving	30

Requires considerable mental effort for decision making and problem solving	40
Requires continuous mental effort for dealing with the most difficult situations	50
Physical	
Light work requiring little physical effort, usually seated	10
Light physical effort, use of light materials, frequently seated	20
Sustained physical effort, seldom seated, continuous activity	30
Considerable physical effort, continuous activity, lifting	40
Working conditions	
Good working conditions—light, ventilation, freedom from disagreeable elements such as dirt, heat, wetness, odors, noise	10
Average working conditions with occasional exposure to disagreeable elements and danger	20
Fair working conditions with frequent exposure to disagreeable elements and danger	30
Poor working conditions with continuous exposure to disagreeable elements and danger	40

The number of grievances related to pay rates commonly increases after the introduction of job evaluation because personnel now have an objective basis for a grievance. Before job evaluation, employees had little concrete justification on which to file grievances. They complained that they were not getting paid enough; management insisted that they were. With job evaluation, employees have criteria on which to base grievances.

The transition period is especially troublesome. Problems related to adjusting the worker's present pay to the new pay structure may interfere with traditional lines of promotion. Adjusting a worker's pay upward to the new rate is acceptable to employees, but some may then file grievances for back pay. Back pay, however, could undermine the agency's budget. Therefore, management may decide that back pay is retroactive only to a specified date. The case of an employee who has previously been overcompensated creates a more difficult situation. To prevent dissatisfaction, personnel can be assured that no one's pay will be reduced as a result of the new pay schedule. However, it is possible to deny any pay increase to the individual who was overcompensated until others' salaries have been raised and all have been realigned to the new pay schedule. That, of course, can be demoralizing to the overpaid individual, but the previous situation is demoralizing to other employees. More acceptable options may be to promote the individual to a job commensurate with the pay or give the overpaid employee additional responsibilities in the present position to make the current job commensurate with the salary. After the individual vacates the position, the salary for the job can be realigned at a lower salary level according to the pay schedule.

Job Design

Job design specifies the job content (what the job requires), job methods (how to do it), and the relationship between the organizational, social, and personal needs of the worker. It involves observation, recording, and analysis of current jobs to make work more efficient and to provide incentives for the workers, thereby reducing costs and improving job satisfaction.

Time-and-motion studies.   Time-and-motion studies were the first techniques used to study job designs. Time studies are observations that determine the amount of time it takes to do a job under certain circumstances. After the activity is timed with a stopwatch and the times recorded, the normal time and the standard time are determined. In this way the most expedient way to do a job and a fair day's work are calculated.

Motion studies help determine the one best way to do a job. Process charts are useful in recording movements so the analyst can identify wasteful activity. Micro-motion study uses a slowly projected movie to allow one to analyze and time each motion. Sociotechnical studies, which analyze the relationship between social needs and task performance, became popular after World War II. Suggestive and detailed questions asking who, what, when, where, why, and how became a method for analysis.

Methods improvement.   Methods improvement is an organized approach to deter-mine better ways to accomplish a goal in less time, with less effort, and at a lower cost, while maintaining or improving the results. It is also called job improvement, work simplification, and methods engineering.

First one selects the job to improve and then collects related information such as policies, procedures, statistical reports, accounting data, work schedules, pertinent records, and architectural drawings. Next the manager analyzes how the task is currently being done.

A flow process chart helps analyze how a task is being performed (Fig. 11-4). Flow process chart symbols include ○ for operation, → for transportation, □ for inspec-tion, **D** for delay, and △ for storage. An operation is the actual performance of the work, such as giving an injection. Transportation represents physical movement—the relocation of a person or thing from one place to another, such as movement of the syringe from the medication room to the patient's bedside. Inspection is to determine whether the necessary work has been properly performed. Nurses make sure that they are giving the right medication and using the right mode at the right time, to the right patient. A delay is an unplanned interruption in the flow of the process. Storage is an anticipated interruption in the process or at the end of it.

When making a flow process chart, one must decide whether to follow the flow of material or the activities of the worker, because they may not be the same. A flow diagram is an architectural drawing to scale. Lines are used to show material flow or paths of personnel movement (Fig. 11-5).

As a result of methods improvement, one should eliminate activities or combine steps when possible and change the sequence of activities as necessary to improve the performance of various steps. The proposed method is then analyzed using flowchart-ing. The potential impact on people is considered. Trial runs are conducted, and debugging is done.

To reduce the boredom of workers, management turns to job enlargement—a horizontal approach to job design that makes a job structurally larger and challenges

Procedure: Injection	Distance traveled	Present ☐ Proposed ☐

Person ☐

Material ☐

	Present		Proposed		Savings	
	No	Hr	No	Hr	No	Hr
Operation	8					
Transportation	2					
Inspection	2					
Delay	0					
Storage	1					

Steps in procedure	○ → ☐ D △	Distance (ft)	Time (hr)	Remarks
Read medication order	○ → ☐ D △			
Collect vial and syringe	○ → ☐ D △			
Open vial	○ → ☐ D △			
Open disposable syringe	○ → ☐ D △			
Draw up solution	○ → ☐ D △			
Recheck medication order	○ → ☐ D △			
Put vial in medication drawer	○ → ☐ D △			
Take shot to patient	○ → ☐ D △			
Check patient identification	○ → ☐ D △			
Administer shot	○ → ☐ D △			
Return to medicine room	○ → ☐ D △			
Dispose of syringe	○ → ☐ D △			
Chart medication	○ → ☐ D △			
Store chart	○ → ☐ D △			

Key:
○ operation
→ transportation
☐ inspection
D delay
△ storage

Figure 11-4 Flow process chart.

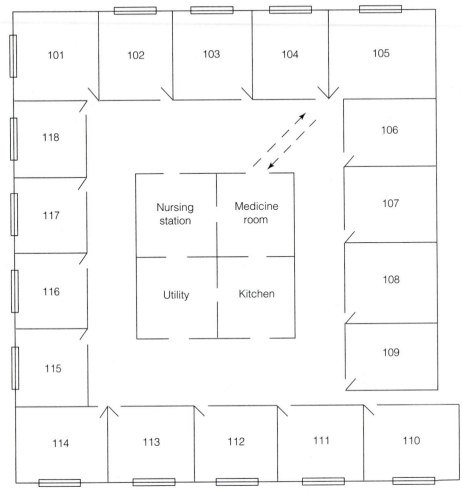

Figure 11-5 Flow diagram.

the employee. If nurses have been taking care of an average of five patients, they are asked to attend seven. Similarly, nursing educators might be challenged to teach an additional two hours a week or to add three more students to their clinical group. Not surprisingly, this method frequently fails. Nurses commonly respond, "Why should I?" Many employees are already doing large amounts of work or already do not like their work.

Job simplification. Another technique, job simplification, removes the more difficult parts of the job so that the worker can do more of what remains. For example, a nurse can be hired to start all IVs. The treatment nurse, team leader, and primary nurse, then, do not have to start any IVs but can give other medications and treatments to more patients. Work simplification, however, tends to lead to further boredom.

Personnel may also be assigned more tasks. For instance, staff nurses can teach aides to do additional treatments. This may relieve some monotony, but many workers are already very busy, and the new tasks may prove to be no more meaningful than the others.

Job rotation.   Job rotation is another horizontal job-enlargement technique. Nurses may rotate shifts and assignments among different units and different patients on the units, but this practice complicates continuity of care and often leads to additional frustration. Community health nurses may be rotated through clinic assignments. For instance, a nurse may work well-baby clinics one month; family planning the next; and immunization, tuberculosis, or venereal disease clinics at other times. Again, this can disrupt continuity of care.

Job enrichment.   Job enrichment is a vertical approach to job design that uses a fuller range of abilities and skills of the personnel. When planning job enrichment, one should consider skill variety—the number of different talents and skills needed to do a job; task identity—the degree to which one can do a job from beginning to end with a visible outcome; task significance—the degree to which the job has an impact on others; autonomy—the degree of independence and discretion one has to plan and implement the job; and feedback—the degree to which one receives clear feedback about the effectiveness of one's performance. These core job dimensions contribute to the psychological states that affect the work outcomes. Skill variety, task identity, and task significance contribute to the experience of meaningfulness of work. One may experience responsibility for outcomes through autonomy and knowledge of the results through feedback. That should contribute to motivation, high-quality work performance, and satisfaction, which in turn contribute to lower absenteeism and turnover.

For example, community health nurses may have "their own" assortment of clinics in addition to their family case load. Continuity is preserved because nurses are always at that clinic. They need to develop their expertise, knowledge, and skill in all of the clinical areas. A hospital unit may switch from functional or team nursing to primary nursing so each nurse can give total patient care and consequently assume additional responsibility and accountability.

Job enrichment is intended to increase motivation and productivity while reducing absenteeism and turnover. It can, however, increase anxiety, conflict, and feelings of exploitation. Skill levels of personnel limit the amount of job enrichment possible, because some workers lack managerial skills and may not be able or willing to plan and control their jobs. Supervisors may not be willing to trust workers, and personnel may feel they are being exploited.

Job Descriptions

Job descriptions are derived from job analysis and are affected by job evaluation and design. They generally contain specifications that are the requirements for the job, major duties and responsibilities, and the organizational relationships of a given position. The title of the job indicates the major responsibilities and sets that job apart from others. The job description is a summary of primary duties in a complete but not detailed fashion. Job relationships and professional affiliations may be cited. Education, experience, and worker traits such as aptitude, interests, and temperament may be included. The physical demands and working conditions of the job may be mentioned. Job descriptions should be up to date, accurate, and realistic in terms of the resources available. Standard forms for all jobs within a category facilitate comparison.

Job descriptions should arrange duties in a logical order, state them separately and concisely, and use verbs to describe the action. They should be specific rather than vague and should avoid generalizations by using quantitative words whenever possible. To indicate frequency, one can note *daily, periodically,* or *occasionally* when the percentage of total time spent on a specific activity cannot be determined.

Job descriptions are useful for recruitment, placement, and transfer decisions. They can also be used to guide and evaluate personnel. Job descriptions help prevent conflict, frustration, and overlapping of duties. See Box 11-10 for a sample of a job description.

Career Ladders

Zimmer designed a career ladder to create a work environment that would nurture and challenge professional growth and recognize clinical excellence to meet the professional's need for growth and recognition and the institution's need for a stable, experienced nursing staff. It was a ladder for clinical advancement with rungs for vertical advancement, which provided recognition of nurses who chose to stay at the bedside. Career ladders proliferated during the 1970s and early 1980s.

Ladders were designed in various sizes and shapes. Most initially had three to five rungs for vertical clinical advancement. Now ladders may have one to five tracks and are more likely to be called career ladders. Career programs may vary from a simple two-level clinical ladder to multitrack and multileveled systems that include provisions for evaluation.

Practice Alternatives for Career Expansion (PACE) is a six-level, four-track career mobility program that includes clinical, research, education, and administration tracks. Special aspects include a residency program, a PACE consultation team, a performance appraisal system, and a career consultant. The residency program is a course developed to groom nurses for advancement to higher levels. Advancement to level four is mandatory on any track. It has structured didactic classes and individually designed practical experiences. The PACE consultation team is composed of a nursing director, patient care coordinator, and several staff nurses who respond to a unit's invitation for consultation about the PACE program. The PACE program stimulated the development of new job descriptions and performance appraisal systems. Job descriptions are behaviorally defined for each level of each track and serve as the performance evaluation tool. The career consultant is available to discuss career opportunities within the institution, aspects of the career development program, educational opportunities, and general issues of concern about upward mobility (Vestal, 1983).

Advantages of career ladders include potential to increase positive self-image, increase motivation, improve personal and professional satisfaction, provide oppor-

Box 11-10 **SAMPLE JOB DESCRIPTION**

SAMPLE JOB DESCRIPTION

Nursing service director
Description of work
    General statement of duties: Performs administrative work in planning, coordinating, and directing the nursing service.
    Supervision received: Works under general direction of the hospital administrator.
    Supervision exercised: Supervises assigned personnel as a significant part of the duties.
Examples of duties
    (Any one position may not include all of the duties listed, nor do the listed examples include all tasks that may be found in positions of this class.)
    Directs and administers the nursing service, including inpatient and ambulatory care; develops and implements policies and patient care standards for all nursing service areas.
    Participates in the planning and development of hospital policies and practices; works closely with administrative and medical personnel in coordinating nursing service functions with those of all other hospital departments and services.
    Develops and implements staffing and ratio patterns to meet patient care and medical service needs; directs the broad planning of in-service training and orientation programs for nursing staff; directs research activities for continuing education and coordinates the clinical experience of nursing students.
    Develops nursing service philosophies and goals in accordance with hospital policies; encourages and provides channels for staff participation in achieving these goals; interprets nursing service objectives to administrative and medical staff.
    Serves on various hospital and community committees for the coordination of nursing services with other patient care and educational services; participates in professional organizational activities and represents the hospital in working with various service agencies and volunteer groups.
    Directs the preparation of budget for nursing service staffing, equipment, and supplies; develops systems and standards for patient care records and reports.
    Directs the recruitment, selection, transfer, and promotion of nursing personnel and the maintenance of personnel records.
    Performs related work as required.
Qualifications for appointment
    Knowledges, skills, and abilities: Extensive knowledge of professional nursing theory and practice. Extensive knowledge of modern principles and practices of hospital operation and nursing administration. Ability to plan, organize, and direct large-scale and comprehensive nursing activities. Ability to supervise, train, and motivate employees. Ability to communicate effectively orally and in writing. Ability to establish and maintain effective working relationships with administrative and medical personnel, employees, the public, and other agencies.
    Education: Graduation from a four-year college with attainment of a master's degree in nursing and major course work in nursing administration or education.
    Experience: Five years' professional nursing experience including three years in an administrative capacity.

Necessary special requirement: Possession of a license or permit to practice as a registered nurse as issued by the State Board of Nursing, permit to be used only until such time as a decision on licensure is made.

Clinical specialist I
Description of work
General statement of duties: Performs advanced professional nursing work in a recognized medical specialty field.

Supervision received: Works under the general supervision of an administrative superior.

Supervision exercised: Supervises personnel as assigned, or full supervision incidental to the other duties.

Examples of duties
(Any one position may not include all of the duties listed, nor do the listed examples include all tasks that may be found in positions of this class.)

Performs advanced professional nursing work in specialized medical fields such as mental health, respiratory care, and other recognized medical specialities in accordance with standard nursing procedures and medical direction.

Interviews patient to obtain general background information and problem identification; evaluates patient's behavior and assesses immediate and long-range needs; schedules and conducts individual and group psychotherapy sessions.

Participates as a member of a professional medical, psychiatric, social public health team in evaluating, developing, and implementing health care plans.

Makes rounds with physician to review condition of patients; develops nursing care plans; participates in the care of the critically ill.

Participates in the orientation and in-service training of professional nursing personnel in teaching new, advanced, or complicated methods and procedures; interprets nursing services to patients and hospital personnel.

Performs related work as required.

Qualifications for appointment
Knowledge, skills, and abilities: Thorough knowledge of professional nursing theory and practice. Thorough knowledge of modern nursing care principles and practices in a recognized medical specialty. Ability to motivate and train employees. Ability to communicate effectively orally and in writing. Ability to establish and maintain effective working relationships with patients, employees, the public, and other agencies.

Education: Attainment of a Master's degree in nursing.

Experience: Two years' experience in an appropriate nursing clinical specialty.

Necessary special requirement: Possession of a license or permit as a registered nurse by the State Board of Nursing, permit to be used only until such time as a decision on licensure is made.

Graduate nurse I
Description of work
General statement of duties: Performs professional general duty nursing work.

Supervision received: Works under direct supervision of a higher-level nurse.

Supervision exercised: Supervises personnel as assigned, or full supervision incidental to the other duties.

Examples of duties
(Any one position may not include all of the duties listed, nor do the listed examples include all tasks that may be found in positions of this class.)

Performs professional nursing care in accordance with standard nursing procedures and medical direction.

Evaluates patient care needs; initiates nursing care plans; coordinates patient services.

Takes temperature, pulse, respiration, and blood pressure; administers prescribed medication and reports symptoms, reactions, and condition of patients; assists physicians with examinations, treatments, and diagnostic tests; prepares and applies dressings, compresses, and bandages; instructs patients in health measures and self-care; instructs nonprofessional nursing personnel and hospital attendants.

Performs related work as required.

Qualifications for appointment

Knowledge, skills, and abilities: Working knowledge of professional nursing theory and practice. Ability to communicate effectively orally and in writing. Ability to establish and maintain effective working relationships with patients, employees, the public, and other agencies.

Education: Graduation from a school of nursing.

Experience: None.

Necessary special requirement: Possession of a license or permit to practice as a registered nurse as issued by the State Board of Nursing, permit to be used only until such time as a decision on licensure is made.

Adapted from Job Descriptions, Denver General Hospital, Denver, Colorado.

tunity for professional growth, provide a system of rewards for accomplishments, encourage development of peer review, improve recruitment and retention, and improve cost-effectiveness through lower attrition rate and retention of experienced nurses.

Potential problems with career ladders include the difficulty of designing them and their potential negative psychological effect. A newly hired experienced nurse may enter the career ladder at the same level as an inexperienced, newly graduated nurse; there may be fewer monetary rewards between clinical levels than administrative levels. Competency is difficult to define, and nurses on tracks may be evaluated by administrators instead of peers (McKay, 1986).

BIBLIOGRAPHY

Barker ER: Use of diffusion of innovation model for agency consultation, *Clin Nurse Spec* 4:163-166, Fall 1990.

Bhola HS: The cler model: thinking through change, *Nurs Manage* 25:59-63, May 1994.

Bourcier M: The right-brain way to manage change, *CMA Magazine* 67:10-12, June 1993.

Boyd MA, Luetje V, Eckert A: Creating organizational change in an inpatient long-term care facility, *Psychosocial Rehabilitation Journal* 15:47-54, January 1992.

Brett JLL: Organizational integrative mechanisms and adoption of innovations by nurses, *Nurs Res* 38:105-110, March-April 1989.

Dienemann J, Gessner T: Restructuring nursing care delivery systems, *Nurs Econ* 10:253-258, July-August 1992.

DiSogra L, Glanz K, Rogers T: Working with community organizations for nutrition intervention, *Health Educ Res* 5:459-465, December 1990.

Flarey DL: The social climate scale: a tool for organizational change and development, *JONA* 21:37-44, April 1991.

Fleeger ME: Assessing organizational culture: a planning strategy, *Nurs Manage* 24:39-41, February 1993.

Hagerman ZJ, Tiffany CR: Evaluation of two planned change theories, *Nurs Manage* 25:57-60, April 1994.

Hall LW: Six elements for implementing and managing change, *Leadership and Organization Development Journal* 12:24-26, 1991.

Hibberd JM: Implementing shared governance: a false start, *Nurs Clin North Am* 27:11-22, March 1992.

Lasater ME: Strategies for organizational change in home healthcare, *Home Healthcare Nurse* 11:38-42, March-April 1993.

Lawrie J: The ABCs of change management, *Training and Development Journal* 44:87-89, March 1990.

Lutjens LRJ, Tiffany CR: Evaluating planned change theories, *Nurs Manage* 25:54-57, March 1994.

Manz CC, Keating DE, Donnellon A: Preparing for an organizational change to employee self-management: the managerial transition, *Organ Dyn* 19:15-26, Autumn 1990.

McKay, DI: Career ladders in nursing: an overview. *Am J Nurs* 12:272-278, September-October 1986.

Minnen TG, Berger E, Ames A et al: Sustaining work redesign innovations through shared governance, *JONA* 23:35-40, July-August 1993.

Murphy R, Pearlman F, Rea C et al: Work redesign: a return to the basics, *Nurs Manage* 25:37-46, Feb 1994.

Ponte PR, Higgins JM, James JR et al: Development needs of advance practice nurses in a managed care environment, *JONA* 23:13-19, November 1993.

Schoolfield M, Orduna A: Understanding staff nurse responses to change: utilization of a grief-change framework to facilitate innovation . . . introduction of patient-focused care, *Clinical Nurse Specialist* 8:57-62, Jan 1994.

Sherman S: A master class in radical change, *Fortune* 128:82-90, December 13, 1993.

Spiker BK: Making change stick, *Industry Week* 243:45, March 7, 1994.

Stevens CA, Gambrell S: Managing change with configuration-value management, *Indust Eng* 25:54-58, May 1993.

Taft SH, Stears JE: Organizational change toward a nursing agenda: a framework from the strengthening hospital nursing program, *JONA* 21:12-21, February 1991.

Terez T: A manager's guidelines for implementing successful operational changes, *Indust Manage* 32:18-20, July-August 1990.

Thomson P: Public sector management in a period of radical change: 1979-1992, *Public Money and Management* 12:33-41, July-September 1992.

Tiffany CR, Cheatham AB, Doornbos D et al: Planned change theory: survey of nursing periodical literature, *Nurs Manage* 25:54-59, July 1994.

CASE STUDY

You are going to start using critical pathways instead of nursing care plans on the unit. What are the driving and restraining forces related to this innovation? How would you go about implementing the five tracks for organizational planned change?

CRITICAL THINKING AND LEARNING ACTIVITIES

1. Identify a change you would like to make in your life. Using Worksheet 11-1, apply Kurt Lewin's force-field analysis. Identify the restraining forces and the driving forces. Plan strategies to weaken the restraining forces and strengthen the driving forces.

2. Identify a group to which you belong. List the norms. What are the do's and don'ts? List what you would like the norms to be? Identify culture gaps, using Worksheet 11-2.

3. Write a job description.

✍ **Worksheet 11-1**

Force Field Analysis

Identify a change you want to make: _____

Identify the driving forces and the restraining forces:

Driving forces	Restraining forces
1.	1.
2.	2.
3.	3.
4.	4.
5.	5.

Plan strategies to strengthen the driving forces and weaken the restraining forces.

Strengthen driving forces	Weaken restraining forces
1.	1.
2.	2.
3.	3.
4.	4.
5.	5.

✍ **Worksheet 11-2**

Culture Gaps

List the organizational norms, what you would like the norms to be, and identify culture gaps.

Organizational norms	Desired norms	Culture gaps
1.	1.	1.
2.	2.	2.
3.	3.	3.
4.	4.	4.
5.	5.	5.
6.	6.	6.
7.	7.	7.
8.	8.	8.
9.	9.	9.
10.	10.	10.

Bibliography
Part Two

Albrecht K, Zemke R: *Service America: doing business in the new economy*, New York, 1990, Warner.

Althaus JN, Hardyck NM, Pierce PB, Rodgers MS: *Nursing decentralization: the El Camino experience*, Wakefield, Mass, 1981, Aspen Systems.

Beckhard R, Harris RT: *Organizational transitions: managing complex change*, Redwood City, Calif, 1987, Addison-Wesley.

Belcher DW: *Compensation administration*, Englewood Cliffs, NJ, 1987, Prentice Hall.

Bennis WG, Benne KD, Chin R: *The planning of change*, ed 4, New York, 1985, Holt, Rinehart & Winston.

Blanchard K, Oucken W, Burrows H: *The one minute manager meets the monkey*, New York, 1989, William Morrow.

Brooten DA: *Managerial leadership in nursing*, Philadelphia, 1986, JB Lippincott.

Campbell JP, Campbell RJ, et al: *Productivity in organizations*, San Francisco, 1988, Jossey-Bass.

Charns MP, Schaefer MJ: *Health care organizations: a model for management*, Englewood Cliffs, NJ, 1983, Prentice Hall.

Christain WP, Hannah GT: *Effective management in human services*, Englewood Cliffs, NJ, 1983, Prentice Hall.

Dale E: *Management theory and practice*, ed 4, New York, 1978, McGraw-Hill.

Davis K, Newstrom J: *Human behavior at work: organizational behavior*, ed 7, New York, 1985, McGraw-Hill.

Davis SM, Lawrence PR: *Matrix*, Reading, Mass, 1977, Addison-Wesley.

Desl TE, & Kennedy AA: *Corporate cultures*, Reading, Mass, 1982, Addison-Wesley.

French WL: *The personnel management process*, ed 6, Boston, 1986, Houghton Mifflin.

Fuszard B: *Self-actualization for nurses*, Rockville, Md, 1984, Aspen Systems.

Green PE, Tull DS, Albaum G: *Research for marketing decisions*, Englewood Cliffs, NJ, 1988, Prentice Hall.

Hall RH: *Organizations: structure and process*, ed 3, Englewood Cliffs, NJ, 1987, Prentice Hall.

Hand L: *Nursing supervision*, Reston, Va, 1980, Appleton & Lange.

Hickman CR, Silva MA: *Creating excellence: managing corporate culture, strategy, and change in the new age*, New York, 1986, New American Library.

Jernigan DK, Young AP: *Standards, job descriptions, and performance evaluations for nursing practice*, Norwalk, Conn, 1983, Appleton & Lange.

Joos IM, Nelson R, Lyness A: *Man, health, and nursing: basic concepts and theories*, Reston, Va, 1985, Appleton & Lange.

Kaluzny AD et al: *Management of health services*, Englewood Cliffs, NJ, 1982, Prentice Hall.

Kanter RM: *The change masters*, New York, 1985, Simon & Schuster.

Kilmann RH: *Managing beyond the quick fix*, San Francisco, 1991, Jossey-Bass.

Kotler P: *Marketing for nonprofit organizations*, Englewood Cliffs, NJ, 1975, Prentice Hall.

Kotler P: *Marketing management: analysis, planning, and control*, Englewood Cliffs, NJ, 1994, Prentice Hall.

Kotter JP, Schlesinger LA, Sathe V: *Organization: text, cases, and readings on the management of organizational design and change*, ed 3, Homewood, Ill, 1991, Irwin.

Laliberty R, Christopher WI: *Enhancing productivity in health care facilities*, Owings Mills, Md, 1984, National Health.

Lancaster J, Lancaster W: *Concepts for advanced nursing practice: the nurse as a change agent*, St Louis, 1981, CV Mosby.

Langford TL: *Managing and being managed,* Englewood Cliffs, NJ, 1990, Appleton & Lange.

Lassey WR, Sashkin M: *Leadership and social change,* San Diego, 1983, University Associates.

Lawrence PR, Lorsch JW: *Developing organizations: diagnosis and action,* Reading, Mass, 1969, Addison-Wesley.

Lawrence PR, Lorsch JW: *Organization and environment,* Homewood, Ill, 1986, Irwin.

Lippitt R, Watson J, Westley B: *The dynamics of planned change,* New York, 1958, Harcourt, Brace & World.

Magula, M: *Understanding organizations,* Wakefield, Mass, 1982, Nursing Resources.

Martel L: *Mastering change,* New York, 1986, Simon & Schuster.

Mauksch IG, Miller MH: *Implementing change in nursing,* St Louis, 1981, CV Mosby.

McCarthy EJ: *Basic marketing,* ed 11, Homewood, Ill, 1992, Irwin.

McConnell CR: *The effective health care supervisor,* ed 3, Germantown, Md, 1993, Aspen Systems.

McConnell EA: *Burnout in the nursing profession,* St Louis, 1982, CV Mosby.

Mintzberg H: *Structures in fives: designing effective organizations,* ed 2, Englewood Cliffs, NJ, 1992, Prentice Hall.

Mintzberg H: *The structuring of organizations,* Englewood Cliffs, NJ, 1983, Prentice Hall.

Newman WH, Summer CE, Warren EK: *The process of management,* ed 5, Englewood Cliffs, NJ, 1981, Prentice Hall.

Morgan G: *Images of organization,* Beverly Hills, Calif, 1986, Sage.

Porter-O'Grady T, Finnigan S: *Shared governance for nursing: a creative approach for professional accountability,* Rockville, Md, 1984, Aspen Systems.

Price M, Franck P, Veith S: *Nursing management: a programmed text,* ed 2, New York, 1980, Springer.

Quinn JB: *Strategies for change: logical incrementation,* Homewood, Ill, 1980, Irwin.

Rice GH, Bishoprick DW: *Conceptual models of organization,* New York, 1971, Appleton-Century-Crofts.

Ries A, Trout J: *Positioning: the battle for your mind,* New York, 1987, McGraw-Hill.

Robey D: *Designing organizations,* ed 3, Homewood, Ill, 1990, Irwin.

Robbins SP: *Organizational behavior: concepts, controversies, and applications,* ed 6, Englewood Cliffs, NJ, 1992, Prentice Hall.

Schein EH: *Organizational culture and leadership,* ed 2, San Francisco, 1992, Jossey-Bass.

Schmied E, editor: *Organizing for care: nursing units and groups,* Wakefield, Mass, 1982, Aspen Systems.

Vistal, KW: *Nursing management: concepts and issues,* Philadelphia, 1995, JB Lippincott.

Weick KE: *The social psychology of organizing,* ed 2, Reading, Mass, 1986, Random House.

Wilkins AL: *Developing corporate character,* San Francisco, 1989, Jossey-Bass.

P A R T
Three

Staff

Nature and Purpose of Staffing

Staffing is the third managerial function. Having planned and organized, the manager must now staff to accomplish the goals of the organization. Staffing involves the selection of personnel and assignment systems and the determination of staffing schedules. There are many variables to be considered when planning for staffing. The more accurate the assessment, the higher the probability of containing costs while providing high-quality care.

Chapter

12

Selection of Personnel

Chapter Objectives

◆ Describe why retention measures are at least as important as recruitment efforts.

◆ Identify three activities related to selection of personnel.

◆ Describe affirmative action.

◆ Identify and discuss at least four cultural phenomena and their influence on the interviewing process.

Major Concepts and Definitions	
Personnel	persons employed in an agency or department
Recruitment	the process of enlisting personnel for employment
Retention	capacity to retain employees once they are hired
Affirmative action	actions taken to remedy past discriminatory practices
Cultural diversity	communication, space, social organization, time, environmental control, and biological variations among cultures

SELECTION OF PERSONNEL

Recruitment and Retention

The acquisition of qualified people in any agency is critical for the establishment, maintenance, and growth of the organization. Therefore, active recruitment is important, and the attraction of qualified applicants is the first step in selection of personnel. Modes for active recruitment include employee recommendations and word of mouth; advertisements in local newspapers, nursing organization bulletins, and nursing journals; recruitment literature, such as flyers and newsletters; posters; career days; job fairs; contacts with schools' graduating classes; placement services; open houses; nursing conventions; and frequent, low-cost, credit-carrying, continuing education courses for outsiders as well as employees (see Box 12-1).

Word of mouth can be very effective, but it can also lead to the hiring of friends and relatives of the current workforce; this practice may foster nepotism and violate equal opportunity employment requirements. The use of advertisements in professional journals, in newspapers, and on radio and television, employment agencies, and contacts with schools' graduating classes offers the prospective employer a broader field for selection and more opportunities to hire from minority groups. Hiring minority group members may require active recruitment to meet public policy.

Each institution needs someone responsible for recruitment. Recruiters should know nursing qualifications and the needs of the institution. They should be able to

Box 12-1   **MODES FOR RECRUITMENT**

Employee recommendations	Posters
Word of mouth	Career days
Advertisements	Job fairs
Flyers	Placement services
Newsletters	Open houses
Bulletins	Nursing conventions

represent the institution with candor and enthusiasm. It is important that the recruiter relate well to people. Referrals from employees should be sought and in-house applicants encouraged; however, favoritism should not be shown. To aid in the selection of the best candidate for the job, an adequate budget should be provided for necessary advertisement, and these advertisements should depict an institution that cares about employees and patients. That image should also be reflected at open houses, during conventions, and at high school and college career days.

The content is more important than the form of advertising. The recruiter should determine the needs and desires of potential applicants and demonstrate how the institution will meet those needs. New graduates are likely to be interested in thorough orientation, in-service education, staff development, and intern programs. Some nurses will be interested in tuition reimbursement and release time to work on educational degrees. Single people will be more interested in health benefits than married people whose spouses have family coverage. Older nurses will be increasingly interested in retirement plans. Refresher courses, chartered buses for people who live in suburban areas, childcare programs, part-time work, and flexible personnel policies may appeal to inactive nurses. The nurse recruiter needs to assess nurses' interests and show how the institution can address their concerns.

The recruiter should respond to inquiries immediately. Records of inquiries noting the origin (how the job applicant learned of the opening) and disposition (hired or not and length of tenure) should be compiled and evaluated. The most productive recruitment method should be maximized. Out-of-town or out-of-state applicants should be assisted with information about the community and housing.

The major sources of personnel are persons seeking their first jobs, dissatisfied employees, and the unemployed. These classifications are important, for the categories indicate types of information the nursing manager should obtain, and they influence the selection process. Recent graduates or nurses who have not practiced since graduation may have a limited idea of job opportunities. Their choice of a first job may be strongly influenced by their education, achievement level, geographical preference, salary, mate's occupation, and peer pressure. They are likely to take several jobs before settling down. This variety of jobs, along with growing family responsibilities and maturity, helps develop the nurse's capabilities.

The dissatisfied employees are often not actively seeking other employment but are likely to be receptive to news of openings and job offers. If nursing managers attribute the dissatisfaction to the misuse of the person's talents and abilities, they may explore how to employ that person more effectively within their own agency. Job dissatisfaction is not uncommon, for every job has disadvantages. Agencies that require special job skills should expect applications from nurses who are looking for a better job with fewer disadvantages.

Hiring an unemployed worker who has been released from a previous job because of an infraction or a quarrel with the previous employer demands careful assessment. The nursing manager may wish to hire nurses who were fired because they refused to falsify records or perform a task for which they were not adequately prepared. They would not want to hire a nurse who was terminated because of high absenteeism and irresponsibility, unless the nurse could adequately explain the situation and assure the nursing manager that the problem had been resolved. For instance, the prospective employee might have been caring for a dying child at that time, or having a marital crisis that has since ended in divorce.

It is unlikely that nurse applicants have been laid off from previous jobs because of slack times. If so, the nursing manager should consider the chances of the nurses' returning to their old jobs when the slack has ended. Seniority and other vested interests may influence nurses' desires to return to their previous positions.

Because of the costs of recruiting, selecting, and training employees, the decreased quality of care while orienting new workers, and the emotional drain of turnover on continuing employees, serious attention should be given to retention efforts. Exit interviews, particularly anonymous questionnaires, can help identify the reasons people resign. Posttermination questions mailed to the homes of former employees a month or two after their resignation may obtain more accurate information than does the exit interview. After a period of time has elapsed, a person may be less emotional and more objective with some distance from the job and may feel more anonymous with less fear of retaliation. In addition, attitude surveys can be used with current employees to identify sources of dissatisfaction and concern. Focus groups can be used to identify and solve problems. Once stressors are identified, strategies to reduce them can be planned. It is important to meet personnel's psychosocial needs for advancement, responsibility, achievement, and recognition. Nurses want input into decision making and control over their own lives.

Screening of Staff

Investment in well-qualified nurses can produce a high rate of return, and errors, whether they be failure to hire a promising nurse or hiring someone who fails to achieve the organization's expectations, can be expensive mistakes. In general there are three underlying philosophies in the screening process: (1) The manager should screen out applicants who do not fit the agency's image. Although this practice is common among some corporations, it is not a standard procedure for selecting health personnel. (2) The manager should try to fit the job to a promising applicant. Examples include part-time positions, split-shift hours, and opportunities for handicapped people. (3) Usually the manager should try to fit the applicant to the job. This philosophy assumes that both the person and the position are unique.

Application forms and résumés. Once the applicants have been attracted, they should submit biographical data. The application form is a quick way to collect demographic information. Data in the personal history—educational background, work experience, and other pertinent information—can be used to:

- Determine whether the applicant meets minimal hiring requirements such as minimal educational level or minimal job experience requirements
- Furnish background data useful in planning the selection interview
- Obtain names of references that may be contacted for additional information about the applicant's work experience and general character
- Collect information for personnel administration, that is, Social Security number, number of dependents, and so forth

Letters of reference.   Letters of recommendation may be requested from references listed on the application form, from previous employers, or both. However, these letters may be inaccurate and misleading because the person writing may not have had sufficient exposure to the nurses to become familiar with their capabilities, or they may not have even known the nurse. Because of rapid turnover of nursing personnel, it is possible that few current staff members worked with the previous employee, and the current manager, who joined the agency after the applicant had resigned, may have to write the letter of reference based on an inadequate personnel file. The applicant may not know the current whereabouts of previous managers. To prevent these problems, employees could ask that a letter of reference be sent to a placement bureau at the time of termination, but this measure does not necessarily solve the problem. They have no assurance that the letter writer can express themselves well or is even willing to be accurate.

All of the above indicate that letters of reference should be used cautiously. More emphasis should be placed on comments made by previous employers and co-workers, because they tend to give more critical evaluations than do subordinates and personal acquaintances. Most emphasis should be placed on characteristics consistently cited and on the general tone of the letters.

Interview.   A preemployment interview to predict job success should be conducted with the most qualified applicants. Information obtained from the application form and letters of reference should be taken into consideration during the interview. The purposes of the interview are to obtain information, to give information, and to determine if the applicant meets the requirements for the position. The interviewer judges the applicant's dependability, willingness to assume responsibility for the job, willingness and ability to work with others, interest in the job, adaptability, consistency of goals with available opportunities, and conformance of manners and appearance to job requirements. The interviewer answers questions, explains policies and procedures, and helps acquaint the applicant with the position. Finally, the interviewer must predict whether the applicant's overall performance will be satisfactory. The value of the interview is determined by the interviewer's ability to evaluate applicants and to predict accurately their future success.

The interview has definite purposes and should avoid social chitchat, although a brief warm-up period may help put the interviewee at ease. One of the main purposes is to learn about the prospective employee. Therefore it behooves the interviewer to concentrate on listening, as well as to provide necessary information and answer questions from the applicant. Managers should avoid giving clues about what pleases or displeases them, should not be argumentative, and should try to avoid premature judgment. They should also beware of the halo effect: judgment based on appearances. Although individuals wear clothing that reflects their personality, they are likely to select clothes for the interview that project the image they wish to convey.

It is advisable to train managers in the art of interviewing. Training might include methods of establishing rapport with an interviewee, interviewing techniques, therapeutic communication, and predicting applicant job performance. It is helpful to construct an interview recording form designed for the needs of the agency or for a specific position. Use of the job description to define and specify job dimensions on the form increases interviewer reliability. A personal profile of what the person hired should be, including education, experience, abilities, aptitudes, and interests, is helpful. Standardization of the interview promotes nondiscriminatory hiring practices and is particularly important when more than one person does the interviewing.

The heading of the form contains the date, name of the applicant, position desired, and the interviewer's name. The body categorizes traits required for the position. This allows the interviewer to assess the applicant more systematically. One area might be work history. Does the applicants' work history indicate that they have the ability to learn and understand the requirements of the job for which they are applying? More specifically, is there any evidence of lack of ability? Have they had past experience in performing the same or similar tasks? Are they familiar with the equipment and procedures? Have they had special project or task force assignments? Have they had job progression? Education is another area to be evaluated. Have applicants had adequate formal education? Is there evidence of on-the-job training? Have they participated in continuing education or in self-initiated skill development by reading books and journals and watching related television specials? Are they active in professional organizations?

Certainly applicants' dependability demands assessment. Is it likely that they will have a good attendance record and maintain good work habits? Or is there evidence of poor work habits or work performance? What do past attendance and safety records indicate? Of equal concern is applicants' sense of responsibility. Will they seek assistance when needed and take initiative when appropriate to get the job done? Will they see jobs through to the end? Is there evidence of past independent thought and action, or do they tend to blame others for problems? Finally, is the nurse capable of assuming leadership when required?

Are applicants cooperative and able to get along with others and work well as team members, or do they have a preference for working alone? Is there evidence of success or friction with managers, peers, and staff associates? Are they open to criticism, or do they react excessively? Are applicants involved in the community? Have they been open and candid during the interview? Job interest, poise, manners, appearance, and aspirations are other areas to investigate.*

During the interview, the interviewer explains the purpose and plan of the interview. This helps create a positive climate. The interviewer learns the most by listening rather than talking, and can encourage the job candidate to talk freely by asking open-ended questions. These are nondirective questions that help reveal feelings and attitudes. Examples of nondirective questions are the following: What qualifies you for this job? What aspects of your last job appealed to you? How were your relations with your peers?

Closed-ended questions are directive and can often be answered yes or no. They solicit less information than open-ended questions but are appropriate for objective and factual information. The following are examples of closed-ended questions: Who was your last employer? How long did you work for that agency? Did you get along with your co-workers? Do you think you are qualified for this job?

---

* These questions are adapted and modified from Osburn HG, Manese WR: *How to install and validate employee selection techniques,* Washington, DC, 1971, American Petroleum Institute, pp. 69-70.

Topic to explore	Open-ended question	Self-appraisal question	Direct question

Figure 12-1   Grid of topics to explore during interviews.

The funnel technique incorporates both open-ended and closed-ended questions. When using the funnel technique, the interviewer starts with an open-ended question such as, What subjects did you like most in school? This gets objective information and sets a nonthreatening tone. The scope of the discussion is then funneled by asking a self-appraisal question such as, Why do you think you liked those courses in particular? This elicits subjective information. The interviewer closes the discussion of a particular subject by asking direct questions to clarify the self-appraisal. A direct question might be, What classes did you take for your nursing electives?

A grid of topics to explore and the funnel technique can help the interviewer sequence questions in a logical order and decide what kind of questions to ask (see Fig. 12-1).

Initially it may be helpful to fill in the topics and potential questions. The questions may be modified during the interview. See Table 12-1.

After obtaining information from the candidate, it is appropriate for the interviewer to share information about the job, policies, the agency, and how the interviewee will be informed of the decision. The applicant is given an opportunity to ask questions. The interviewer closes the interview by telling applicants when and how they can expect to hear the decision. For example, the interviewer can say, "I will be interviewing a few more applicants this week. You can expect to hear from me by the first of next week." Or, "You should receive a letter regarding our decision within 2 weeks."

The facts collected during the interview are used as the basis for assumptions or inferences. They should be checked throughout the interview as new information is collected. It is possible to make both positive and negative assumptions from the same information. For example, if an applicant did not work for 3 months between jobs, the negative assumption could be that the person was escaping, undirected, or lazy. A positive inference could be that the applicant was clarifying goals and fulfilling personal objectives. Inferences are often more reflective of the person making them than of the applicant, thus making it particularly important to test interpretations.

Women, men, minority applicants, and persons with disabilities should be treated in the same professional manner. The same general questions and the same standards should be required for all applicants. One should follow a structured interview plan to help achieve fairness in interviewing and should treat all applicants with fairness, equality, and consistency.

Table 12-1 **Topics and Questions to be Explored During an Employment Interview**

Topic to Explore	Open-Ended Question	Self-Appraisal Question	Direct Question
Education	Why did you choose to go to that school?	What courses were most useful to you and how were they useful?	What courses did you take as electives?
Prior employment	Where have you worked?	What did you like best about your last job? What did you like least about your last job?	How long did you work there? What was your title? On what service areas did you work?
Life experiences	What life experiences have you had that help qualify you for this job?	How will raising your own children help you in this job?	How long have you spoken Spanish? How frequently do you use sign language?
Professional	What are your professional goals?	How do you plan to accomplish your goals?	What do you plan to be doing 5 years from now?

Interviewers can talk about applicants' qualifications, abilities, experiences, education, and interests; the duties and responsibilities of the job; where the job is located, travel, equipment, and facilities available; and the organization's missions, programs, and achievements.

Discriminatory behavior is improper even when it is not intended, and appearance is as important as reality. Questions not related to the job have been used in a discriminatory way and should be avoided. Because improper significance might be given to questions regarding marriage plans or family matters, one should not inquire about marital status or nonmarital arrangements; what the significant other does or earns; how the significant other feels about the applicant's work life, travel arrangements, possible relocation; medical history concerning pregnancy or any questions relating to pregnancy; or whether there are children, how many, and their ages. Use either first or last names for all candidates and persons involved in the recruitment.

Applicants with disabilities should also be asked questions relevant to the job. Whether the individual needs any reasonable accommodations or assistance during the hiring or interviewing process and the individual's ability to perform essential job functions with or without reasonable accommodations may be discussed. Avoid discussions of past or present serious illnesses or physical/ mental conditions; the nature or severity of an apparent disability; problems an individual may have had because of a disability; or how the person became disabled.

Because people are presumed innocent until proven guilty, records of arrest without convictions are meaningless. One may inquire about an applicant's conviction record for jobs where that is relevant.

When discussing the location, mention the special features: lakes, parks, and urban areas; sports, cultural, and other recreational features; and renting and buying options.

Avoid references to the applicant's personal happiness and do not suggest that one is interested in hiring a woman, minority person, or person with a disability as a statistic to improve the Affirmative Action/Equal Opportunity profile. Applicants are being considered for a position based on qualifications.

Testing.   Personality and interest testing is sometimes done but does require a trained psychologist. Ability tests are rarely used when hiring nurses. However, in-basket exercises, problem analysis, mock selection interviews, oral presentations, and debates have been used to select management personnel. Testing is useful for selecting clerical help. Tests can measure knowledge and skills possessed and estimate the rate at which the applicant can acquire the knowledge and skills required for the position. They measure clerical and mechanical aptitudes, general intelligence, and mental, perceptual, and psychomotor abilities.

EQUAL OPPORTUNITY AND AFFIRMATIVE ACTION

The employer is subject to a number of legal requirements that have been enacted to provide equal opportunity and affirmative action in the workplace. Requirements for providing equal opportunity are contained in Title VI and Title VII of the Civil Rights Act of 1964, Title IX of the Education Amendments of 1972, the Equal Pay Act of 1963, and the Age Discrimination in Employment Act of 1967. Affirmative action requirements are contained in Executive Order 11246, Section 503 of the Rehabilitation Act of 1973, and in Section 402 of the Vietnam Era Veterans Readjustment Assistance Act of 1974.

Title VI and Title VII of the Civil Rights Act of 1964, as amended by the Equal Employment Act of 1972, prohibit discrimination because of race, color, religion, sex, or national origin in any term, condition, or privilege of employment.

Title IX of the Education Amendments of 1972 prohibits discrimination on the basis of sex in any educational program or activity receiving federal financial assistance. The Equal Pay Act, as amended by the Education Amendments of 1972, requires the same pay for men and women doing substantially equal work, requiring substantially equal skill, effort, and responsibility under similar working conditions in the same establishment.

The Age Discrimination in Employment Act of 1967, as amended, prohibits age discrimination against individuals between 40 and 70 years of age.

Executive Order 11246 (as amended by EO 11375) prohibits all government contracting agencies from discriminating against any employee or applicant for employment and requires that contractors take affirmative action to ensure that applicants are employed and that employees are treated during employment without regard to their race, color, religion, sex, or national origin.

Sections 503 and 504 of the Rehabilitation Act of 1973 prohibit discrimination because of handicap in employment and in programs and activities receiving federal funds. Section 503, in addition, requires contractors to take affirmative action to employ and advance in employment qualified handicapped individuals.

Section 402 of the Vietnam Era Veterans Readjustment Assistance Act of 1974 requires contractors to take affirmative action to employ and advance in employment qualified disabled veterans and veterans of the Vietnam era.

Affirmative action in Executive Order 11246 requires the employer to make extra efforts to recruit, employ, and promote qualified members of formerly excluded groups. It is based on the premise that unless action is taken to overcome systematic exclusion and discrimination based on national origin, race, color, sex, or religion, employment practices will perpetuate the status quo indefinitely. In addition to the elimination of all existing discriminatory practices, affirmative action requires actions beyond neutral nondiscrimination.

A major portion of an affirmative action program must recognize and remove barriers and establish affirmative measures to remedy past discriminatory practices. Such measures include additional aid to prepare disadvantaged people for jobs. It is noteworthy that recent Supreme Court rulings state that such measures are not restricted to workers who have not individually been victims of discrimination.

Development of an affirmative action program includes the addition of affirmative action intent to the agency's philosophy, development of affirmative action policies and procedures, appointment of a manager responsible for the program, inclusion of affirmative action responsibilities in appropriate job descriptions, and publication of the affirmative action commitment internally to all employees and externally to sources for recruitment, to minority and women's organizations, to organizations of handicapped individuals, to appropriate veterans' service organizations, to community agencies, and to the community in general.

The affirmative action policy is disseminated internally by including it in the policy manual, annual reports, and other media, such as the agency newsletter. It can also be posted on bulletin boards. Nondiscrimination clauses are included in union agreements. Articles about the affirmative action program, its progress, and the activities of disadvantaged workers are published in agency publications. When employees are pictured in handbooks or advertising brochures, minority and nonminority men and women should be included.

Top administration should discuss the intent of the policy and individuals' responsibilities for its implementation with management personnel. Special meetings should be scheduled with all employees and the policy discussed in orientation and management training classes.

A workforce analysis of job classifications by departments is the first step toward identifying where minorities, women, and men are currently employed and discovering areas of concentration and underuse. The availability of minorities, women, and handicapped persons having requisite skills is considered when determining whether there is underuse: How many minorities, women, and handicapped persons are in the geographical area from which the institution recruits? What percentage of the total workforce in the area is minorities, women, and handicapped persons? How many are unemployed? How many can be recruited from the local community or the nation? Are there training programs available to prepare minorities, women, and handicapped people with skills the agency can use? Can the agency prepare minorities, women, and handicapped personnel? A hospital may be able to prepare nurse's aides or assistants but would need to rely on other institutions to prepare licensed practical or vocational nurses and registered nurses. Are there disadvantaged people already employed by the agency who are transferable or promotable? Programs to correct underutilization must be developed when there are fewer minorities, women, and handicapped persons in a job classification than would be expected by their availability.

Once management has completed its utilization and availability analysis, it establishes goals and timetables to improve use. To correct identifiable deficiencies, management needs goals that are measurable and attainable. Goals for minorities and women are presented separately. Those goals and the timetables for completion along with supportive data and analysis are major parts of the written affirmative action program.

Programs to achieve these goals must be developed and implemented next. This phase begins with a review of the employment process to identify barriers. Recruitment procedures and the selection process—including job requirements, job descriptions, application forms, testing, and interviewing—are examined. The upward mobility system, including training, assignments, job progressions, seniority, transfers, promotions, and disciplinary action policies, is reviewed. Wage and salary structure, benefits, conditions of employment, and union contracts are also studied. Appropriate changes are made, and an internal audit and reporting system to monitor and evaluate the affirmative action program is implemented. Records of referrals, placements, transfers, promotions, and terminations should be maintained for 3 years. Formal reports regarding attainment of goals and timetables are prepared on a regular basis. The manager of the affirmative action program reviews the reports with other managers, advises top administration of the program effectiveness, and submits recommendations for improvement of unsatisfactory performance.

Compliance status is not judged solely by whether goals have been met by the time set for achieving them. A review of the program's content and the efforts made toward realization of the goals are factors that are considered in determining its effectiveness.

It is important to keep in mind that goals are not inflexible quotas that must be met but are targets that are reasonably attainable through good faith efforts. Goals, therefore, should be realistic, measurable, and achievable by the time established.

When interviewing applicants for positions, one should remember that some employment inquiries are acceptable, whereas others are not. The purpose of the question determines its propriety. Appropriate inquiries have a direct relationship to the applicant's capacity to do the job. Inappropriate questions may receive answers that will limit the person's opportunities because of ancestry, race, color, age, religion, sex, marital or parental status, or handicap. Some information needed for payroll or personnel purposes—such as age, proof of citizenship, and number of dependents— can be obtained after the person has been hired. Questions about the applicant's religious preferences, sex, marital status, credit rating, number and ages of dependents, or marital and family plans are not appropriate. Questions that would identify the person as being over 40 or general questions about disabilities are not acceptable. Applicants may be asked to prove they are over 18 years of age and able to perform job-related functions. One can ask for an address and length of residence in a city or state but not for rental or ownership information. Questions about ability to read, write, or speak a language are acceptable, but questions about one's primary language or the way one acquired the ability to use a language are unacceptable. One's legal right to remain in the United States can be questioned, but questions about naturalization of parents or spouse are unacceptable. The applicant may be asked to list membership in clubs, organizations, societies, and associations, excluding those that would indicate the national origin, race, color, or religion of the membership. Requests for all memberships are not appropriate. General questions about military service are inappropriate.

When interviewing minority candidates, the interviewer should not pretend interest in, or knowledge of, an ethnic culture or use ethnic vernacular or a foreign language one does not speak well. It is inappropriate to talk about one's minority friends or to expect the candidate to know all other minority members. Lack of eye contact should not be judged negatively, since some cultures interpret direct eye contact as disrespectful. The interviewer should be aware that body language and voice tone give messages that provoke confidence or mistrust and suggest support or indifference.

The manager should be aware that some minority applicants may not have well-defined aspirations and career goals because their opportunities may have been limited and they may feel they have little control over their careers. Minority applicants often have frequently changed jobs in search of better pay. Therefore, steady work and work progression histories may be of little use in evaluating minority applicants who have had limited opportunities.

CULTURAL DIVERSITY

People bring with them assumptions, attitudes, and behaviors related to their cultural heritage. The recognition of and respect for cultural differences helps foster positive relationships. Leaders and managers need to have an awareness of how their own cultural background effects their performance.

Individuals within a cultural group vary widely, but the majority of individuals within a cultural group generally agree on common norms and traits. Communication is an important aspect of one's culture. It includes spoken and nonverbal expressions. Misunderstandings can result from silence, words used, tone of voice, pitch, and body movements. What a person says and does can be interpreted in a variety of ways. Unless the person's cultural heritage is understood, an interpretation could be wrong. Someone speaking loudly with animation might be misinterpreted as being aggressive, pushy, or rude. Someone speaking in a soft, low voice may be viewed as passive, afraid, or shy.

Context of speech refers to use of emotion in communications. Mexican Americans, Irish and Italians often use emotions, whereas Black Americans, Germans, and the Jewish rarely do. Kinesics is the use of gestures, stances, and eye movements when communicating. Alaskan Eskimos blink to indicate agreement. Irish and Italian Americans use gestures, stances, and eye movements to emphasize points. Persons in certain socioeconomic groups in India are to avoid eye contact with persons in lower or higher socioeconomic groups and persons of the opposite sex.

Dialect and language styles often differ among cultural groups. Some cultures convey feelings and emotions through touch. Others find touch intrusive or consider it to have sexual connotations.

There are four zones of interpersonal space: (1) intimate, (2) personal, (3) social consultative, and (4) public. Each zone has distinctive distance and intimacy techniques for verbal and nonverbal communication. The intimate zone is zero to 18 inches, is reserved for close personal relationships, and is considered taboo in some cultures.

The personal space, 18 inches to 4 feet, is where touching family and friends and some counseling interactions are permitted. The social consultative zone, 4 to 12 feet, is for casual social interactions. The public zone, beyond 12 feet, is beyond the sphere of personal involvement, and verbal communication is usually formal. The preferred space between people in the United States is 2 to 3 feet. In general, Asians do not mind closer spaces, whereas Black Americans do not want their personal space invaded.

People tend to be past, present, or future oriented. People who value the past maintain tradition and are not likely to set goals for the future. People who focus on the present tend to be unappreciative of the past and do not plan for the future. People with future orientations plan and organize for the future.

Americans tend to be individualistic and desire to control their own lives. Chinese, Mexican, Vietnamese, and Puerto Rican Americans tend to consider the family as the most important social organization. Some cultural groups, such as the Italians and Appalachians, extend their family beyond blood lines.

Environmental control relates to the ability to control nature and direct the environment. Some groups believe they can control nature; others feel controlled by it. Still others, such as many Native American nations, believe humanity should attempt to live in harmony with nature.

There are also biological variations among cultures. Features, skin color, body size, and enzyme differences are related to cultural heritage. Understanding cultural variables can help leaders and managers recruit, retain, direct, and evaluate personnel. Understanding cultural variables can help one understand oneself better, as well (Giger and Davidhizar, 1990).

AMERICANS WITH DISABILITIES ACT

Three categories of individuals with disabilities are protected by the Americans with Disabilities Act (ADA): (1) individuals who have a physical or mental impairment that substantially limits one or more major life activities; (2) individuals who have a record/history of a physical or mental impairment that substantially limits one or more major life activities; and (3) individuals who are regarded as having such an impairment whether they have the impairment or not. Disability in a major life activity includes caring for one's self, walking, breathing, hearing, seeing, speaking, and learning.

Physical impairments include but are not limited to orthopedic, visual, speech, and hearing impairments; cerebral palsy, epilepsy, muscular dystrophy, multiple sclerosis, cancer, diabetes, and HIV-positive status, tuberculosis; drug addiction; and alcoholism.

Mental impairments include but are not limited to mental retardation, organic brain syndrome, emotional or mental illness, and specific learning disabilities.

Other conditions covered by the ADA include homosexuality or bisexuality; transvestism, transsexualism, pedophilia, exhibitionism, voyeurism, gender identity disorders, compulsive gambling, kleptomania, and psychoactive substance use disorders. ADA excludes current drug users from coverage when an adverse action is taken against an individual based on such use.

Temporary conditions may be considered a disability depending on the duration and the extent to which one or more major life activities is limited. Qualified individuals with a disability must meet the essential eligibility requirements of the agency, with or without (1) reasonable modification to the agency's rules, policies, or practices; (2) removal of architectural, communication, or transportation barriers; or (3) provisions of auxiliary aids or services.

People who pose a direct threat to the health or safety of others are not qualified for protection under the ADA. Determination may not be based on generalizations or stereotypes but must be based on an individualized assessment that relies on current medical evidence or the best available objective evidence to assess (1) the nature, duration, and severity of the risk; (2) the probability that the potential injury will actually occur; and (3) whether reasonable modification of policies, practices, or procedures will mitigate or eliminate the risk. Modifications that fundamentally alter the nature of the program, service, or activities are not required.

An agency should have procedures by which people who identify potential difficulties with meeting essential performance standards can receive appropriate assistance and guidance. When a person believes that he or she cannot meet one or more of the standards without accommodations or modifications, the agency must determine on an individual basis whether or not the necessary accommodations or modifications can be made. Reasonable accommodations are defined by the ADA to include (1) making existing facilities readily accessible to and usable by individuals with disabilities; and (2) job restructuring, part-time or modified work schedules, acquisition or modification of equipment or devices, appropriate adjustment or modification of examinations, training materials, or policies, the provision of qualified readers or interpreters, and other similar accommodations for individuals with disabilities. Each agency should rely on its legal resources to make informed decisions.

BIBLIOGRAPHY

Burdett JO: Recruitment: more than a side show, *Canadian Manager* 17:8-12, September-October 1992.

de Savorgnani AA, Haring RC, Galloway S: Recruiting and retaining registered nurses in home healthcare, *JONA* 23:42-46, June 1993.

Dubnicki C, Sloan S: Excellence in nursing management: competency-based selection and development, *JONA* 21:40-45, June 1991.

Eagle J, Fortnum D, Price P et al: Developing a rationale and recruitment plan for a nurse researcher, *Canadian Journal of Nursing Administration* 3:5-10, May-June 1990.

Fish J: How to choose the right applicant, *Br J Nurs* 1:352-355, July 23-August 13, 1992.

Fleischmann ST: Effective ways to conduct recruiting and hiring, *Employment Relations Today* 10:485-489, Winter 1991/1992.

Giger JN, Davidhizar R: Transcultural nursing assessment: a method for advancing nursing practice, *Int Nurs Rev* 37:199-202, 1990.

Heslin KA, Faux SA: The staff nurse employment interview selection process: judgement and decision errors and how to avoid them part 1, *Canadian Journal of Nursing Administration* 4:25-29, November-December 1991.

Hughes KK, Marcantonio RJ: Recruitment, retention, and compensation of agency and hospital nurses, *JONA* 23:46-52, October 1991.

Jolma DJ: Relationship between nursing work load and turnover, *Nurs Econ* 8:110-114, March-April 1990.

Jones CB: Staff nurse turnover costs: a conceptual model part 1, *JONA* 20:18-23, April 1990.

Leidy K: Effective screening and orientation of independent contract nurses, *Journal of Continuing Education in Nursing* 23:64-68, March-April 1992.

Loveridge CE: Contingency theory: explaining staff nurse retention, *JONA* 18:22-25, June 1988.

Mackey CL: Creative retention and recruitment, *Nurs Manage* 19:25-27, February 1988.

Mann EE: A human capital approach to ICU nurse retention, *JONA* 19:8-16, October 1989.

Mann EE, Jefferson KJ: Retaining staff: using turnover indices and surveys, *JONA* 18:17-23, July-August 1988.

Marquis B: Attrition: the effectiveness of retention activities, *JONA* 18:25-28, March 1988.

Marriner A: The selection of personnel, *Superv* Nurse 7:18-22, January 1976.

Martin EG, Harris AM, Kirk RKN et al: Retention strategies that work, *Nurs Manage* 20:721-728, June 1989.

Mercer MW: Screening for the right candidates, *Human Resources Professional* 6:9-13, Fall 1993.

Neathawk R, Dubuque SE, Kronk CA: Nurses' evaluation of recruitment and retention, *Nurs Manage* 19:38-45, December 1988.

Schofer KKK: The promotion decision: a key step in successful clinical ladders, *Recruitment and Retention Report* 4:1-3, November 1991.

Smith LL: Coping with disability: nurse administrators' obligations under the Americans with Disabilities Act, *JONA* 22:29-31, March 1992.

Southern Council on Collegiate Education for Nursing: The Americans with Disabilities Act: implications for nursing education, *MAIN Dimensions* 4:1-2,4, February 1993.

Strasen L: Supporting the middle manager, *JONA* 19:6-7, April 1989.

Taunton RL, Krampitz SD, Woods CQ: Manager impact on retention of hospital staff, *JONA* 19:15-19, April 1989.

Taylor C: How to make the right choice: a new model for the selection interview, *J Adv Nurs* 18:312-320, February 1993.

Tibbles LR: The structured interview: an effective strategy for hiring, *JONA* 23:42-46, October 1993.

Wall LL: Plan development for a nurse recruitment-retention program, *JONA* 18:20-26, February 1988.

Williams CR, Labig CE, Stome TH: Recruitment sources and posthire outcomes for job applicants and new hires: a test of two hypotheses, *J Appl Psychol* 78:163-174, April 1993.

Winland-Brown JE, Pohl C: Administrators' attitudes toward hiring disabled nurses, *JONA* 20:24-27, April 1990.

CASE STUDY

You are responsible for hiring staff for your unit. You have one staff nurse position available. You have four applicants. They have all graduated from the same school of nursing with the same level of education, and they have all had similar clinical experiences. Three are white and one is black. What criteria will you use to make your decision? What is the affirmative action policy at your institution? What is the diversity mix on your unit? What is the cultural background of the clients you serve? What will your decision be and why?

CRITICAL THINKING AND LEARNING ACTIVITIES

1. In preparation for hiring a staff nurse for the unit, use Worksheet 12-1 to prepare a grid of topics to explore, including open-ended questions, self-appraisal questions, and direct questions to get at what you consider important topics to explore.

2. Write an advertisement for the staff nurse position on your unit. Decide what modes you are going to use to recruit nurses for your unit.

3. Form diads in class and interview each other for specific positions.

✍ Worksheet 12-1

Interview Grid

Prepare a grid of topics to explore, including open-ended, self-appraisal, and direct questions.

Topics	Open-ended questions	Self-appraisal questions	Direct questions

Chapter

13

Staff Development

Chapter Objectives

♦ Describe the importance of orientation.

♦ List at least six ways to accomplish staff development.

♦ Describe career mapping.

Major Concepts and Definitions	
Orientation	familiarization with and adaptation to an environment
Staff development	education of the employees
Preceptor	teacher or instructor
Mentor	a wise and faithful counselor
Career mapping	strategic plan for one's career

ORIENTATION

Having chosen from the available applicants, the manager introduces the nurse to the new job, agency policies, facilities, and co-workers. Orientation is important, and the manager who does not take the time to assist a new employee is making a serious mistake. Communicating regulations and exactly what is expected of the nurse diminishes uncertainty, relieves anxiety, and prevents unnecessary misunderstandings. One's security usually increases when someone is considerate enough to help one adjust to a new situation. The manner in which nurses are treated during their first day at a new job may be critical to their future job satisfaction and performance.

Orientation to the institution typically includes a tour of the facilities; a description of the organizational structure; a discussion of different departmental functions; a presentation of the philosophy, goals, and standards; an interpretation of administrative policies and procedures; and possibly an explanation of hospital relationships with the community. Next the nurse will need an orientation to the nursing service, including interdepartmental relationships, departmental organization, administrative controls, philosophy, goals, policies, procedures, and job descriptions.

After the general orientation, new nurses may be assigned to an experienced nurse for orientation to their specific job. New nurses will need a tour of the unit so that they know the location of supplies, equipment, and policy and procedure books. Information about how the unit is run, specific methods of practice, and communication systems is important. Introductions to other personnel can help the new person feel welcome.

Frequent visits to see that the nurse is comfortable and that the orientation is progressing satisfactorily are helpful. Documentation of the orientation process is useful. The documentation may be a simple checklist that itemizes information such as the organizational structure, specific policies, fire and disaster plans, tour of the facilities, and procedures, with space for a signature. It can be retained in the personnel file.

Nurse internship programs are common to assist newly graduated nurses in making the adjustment from the student role to a staff nurse position. The instructor and head nurse usually work together to identify teaching-learning needs, plan rotation schedules, and evaluate the intern's performance. Classes are held on a regular basis for orientation, role adjustment, problem solving, and information about pathophysiology. There is a concentration on the mastery of technical skills. Some programs also present leadership instruction. Nurse internship programs help new graduates build self-confidence, lower frustration levels, increase nursing care planning, improve patient care, improve job satisfaction, and reduce turnover.

Near the end of the probationary period, it is advisable to have a systematic evaluation. The nurse should know what characteristics will be evaluated. Two independent judgments, such as those of the manager and a head nurse, may be secured and used to check reliability of the evaluation. The results of the evaluation are indicative of the success of the selection process.

STAFF DEVELOPMENT

Staff development goes beyond orientation. It is a continuing liberal education of the whole person to develop his or her potential fully. It deals with aesthetic senses as well as technical and professional education and may include activities such as orientation, internships, in-service education, courses, conferences, seminars, journal or book clubs, programmed learning, and independent study.

Nurse managers play an important role in the support of staff development and have a responsibility to review the goals for the staff development program and to provide a budget for those activities. They participate in needs identification and analyze how education effects change in nursing services. In addition, they must be careful to differentiate staff development needs from administrative needs. If staff nurses know how to do a procedure properly but do not because the necessary supplies and equipment are not available to them, the need is administrative rather than educational. Nursing managers are legally liable for the quality of nursing services. Their ability to document staff development is strong supportive evidence for the manager. Conversely, the reception of staff development will be largely related to the reward system developed. Positive reinforcement through recognition, such as oral praise on the unit or acknowledgment of accomplishments in a newsletter, is useful. Staff development can also be related to retention, pay raises, advancement to other positions, or termination.

Preceptorship

Preceptorships may be used to help recruit, retain, orient, and develop staff. They may be used before students graduate to orient them to the agency and to recruit them for hire. If students have worked at an agency before graduation and are familiar with it, they can make sounder decisions about where to work, are not as likely to be unprepared for the work situation, and, consequently, are likely to be retained longer. The preceptorship also gives agency personnel an opportunity to evaluate students and determine if they are suitable candidates for employment.

During the preceptorship, faculty facilitate, monitor, and evaluate student learning. Faculty direct students to resources, offer suggestions regarding patient care problems, and lead discussions at conferences. The faculty member is responsible for student learning and encourages students to apply class content.

The preceptor is responsible for the quality of patient care and facilitates the student's learning. Preceptors are liaisons between students and the agency. They help students learn skills and how to organize their work. They provide real-life experiences for students before graduation to help reduce the difficulties of transition from school to work.

The professional nurturance of a preceptorship can be likened to the "good old boy" network or godfathers who look after godsons. It allows students to use and increase their knowledge and skills so they can assume increasing responsibilities. They gain experience with a variety of patients and different levels of staff. They have opportunities to discuss and adjust to professional-bureaucratic conflicts. Preceptorships are a potential recruitment tool for the agency and can increase the job satisfaction of nurses. Preceptors may even learn from the students and are likely to find the preceptor role challenging and stimulating.

There are also disadvantages to preceptorships. They add to staff nurse responsibilities and require time. Sometimes busy nurses have little time to spend with students. It becomes difficult for faculty to evaluate students because they have little direct observation of the students' work. The use of preceptors requires considerable planning and coordination. Role descriptions should clarify who chooses learning experiences for the student, who supervises the student, and who evaluates the student. Practical evaluation tools of the student, preceptor, and faculty should be developed and used. Educational and service administrative support are needed.

The faculty member serves as a preceptor of preceptors. A workshop to prepare preceptors is desirable. It is appropriate to discuss and clarify role descriptions, skill inventory lists for students, and guidelines for preceptor evaluation of students. Information about teaching methods, counseling, and evaluation is useful. Finding a time and place for the workshop and getting release time for the preceptors may create problems. Awarding continuing education credits for the workshop and preceptor experience may be considered as a way to reward preceptors.

The preceptor model can also be used by the staff development department and nurses after a graduate has been hired. The staff development faculty may present formal content in orientation and development programs that is reinforced by preceptors on the units.

Mentorship

Preceptors are role models who may become mentors. Mentors give their time, energy, and material support to teach, guide, assist, counsel, and inspire a younger nurse. It is a nurturing relationship that cannot be forced. Close, trusted counselors, usually in their forties or fifties, acquaint younger nurses, usually in their twenties or thirties, with the values, customs, and resources of the profession. The mentor is a confidante who personalizes role modeling and serves as a sounding board for decisions. The mentor is a resource person who supports the development of the young person through influence and promotion.

There are phases to the mentoring process (see Box 13-1). At first, during the invitational stage, mentors must be willing to use their time and energy to nurture someone who is goal directed, willing to learn, and respectfully trusting of the mentor. The younger professionals have a career goal, a vision of what they want to become; the mentors are people who have reached that goal and are willing to share the secrets of their success. Then there is a period of questioning, when the young person has self-doubt and fears of being unable to meet the goals. The mentor helps clarify those

PHASES OF THE MENTORING PROCESS

Invitational: ● Mentor uses time and energy to nuture a younger professional who is goal directed, willing to learn, and respectfully trusting of the mentor.

Questioning: ● Mentee experiences self-doubt and questioning of goals.
● Mentor helps clarify goals and provides guidance.

Transitional: ● Mentor helps student personalize learning and become aware of own strengths and uniqueness.
● Mentee is now prepared to be a mentor.

goals through self-discrimination. Next mentors share information about power and politics, tell how they became successful, and serve as a sounding board. The transitional phase is the final phase, when mentors help students personalize learning and become aware of their own strengths and uniqueness. Younger nurses are then prepared to be mentors and to tell others how they became what they are.

Mentorship should provide an opportunity to share information, review work, provide feedback, explore issues, plan strategies, and solve problems. It helps socialize novices into professional norms, values, and standards. Career advancement and success are promoted, thus increasing self-confidence, self-esteem, and greater personal satisfaction.

CAREER MAPPING

Career mapping is a strategic plan for one's career. It provides direction for formal education, experience, continuing education, professional associations, and networking. The individual nurse needs to choose an area of specialization. There are many opportunities for nurses: hospitals, ambulatory care, long-term care, community health, industrial nursing, school nursing, government, and so on. The many specialties and subspecialties include the medical, surgical, obstetrical, pediatric, psychiatric, and intensive cardiac care. Functional areas include practice, teaching, research, and consultation.

Nurses need to assess their own values and define success for themselves. Job security, sense of accomplishment, and opportunities for professional advancement are often considered important. Other issues to consider are work hours, salary, fringe benefits, retirement plans, organizational and geographical climate, and location.

Nurses also need to assess their skills. What do they do well, do poorly, want to do, not want to do, or have the potential to develop?

Once one has (1) assessed interests and skills, one should (2) determine goals, (3) develop a map, and (4) pursue strategies to maintain the map. It is appropriate to make a list of interests and skills and to set 1-, 5-, and 10-year plans. The time frame can be illustrated in a career map with a 10-year time frame across the top of the paper. Then one can write in years of specific experience under "Dates" and types of education under "Experiences." One might focus on continuing education classes for a time or work on an advanced degree during certain periods.

Ongoing maintenance of the map will reflect advancement efforts: writing, personal presentations, networking, and professional development. The curriculum vitae (CV) and the résumé are used interchangeably to present oneself in writing. The CV is a listing of educational, professional, and scholarly accomplishments most commonly used in academic settings. The résumé is a concise history of education and experiences in a few pages. The vitae should have an attractive format and contain such information as professional goal, education, work experience, professional memberships, continuing education, research, publications, and presentations. If there have been no accomplishments in a category to date it is best to omit that category from the vitae. Place of education, degree, and year degree was granted should be listed. Name of agency, city, state, and years of employment should be listed for occupational experiences. Professional memberships and dates of membership are listed under professional memberships. Offices and committee membership and related dates can be added. Name of presentation, location, and date of attendance may be listed under continuing education. Résumés are updated periodically, especially when one is applying for a job. It is helpful to keep information files listing continuing education, organizational memberships, offices, committees, research, publications, and presentations so that accurate information is available for updating the résumé. A cover letter should accompany a résumé to introduce the sender and explain the purpose for sending the résumé: interest in a position.

One must present oneself in person for an interview. *One-on-one interviews* are common. The applicant is typically asked, What are your goals? What are your strengths and weaknesses? Why do you want to work here? What do you have to offer this agency? In *serial interviews,* the applicant sees one person after another. Looking attractive, having a positive attitude, remaining consistent, and treating each interviewer as if that person alone will make the decision are appropriate. Serial interviews are increasingly common as one applies for jobs higher in the hierarchy. The interviewers are interested in the interrelationship with their specific area of responsibility. One's communication skills are tested during *group interviews,* when the applicant is interviewed by several people at once. *Stress interviews* are sometimes used to test an applicants' reactions to stress. They may leave a very negative feeling about the job; the applicant should try to remember such a test is not a personal attack. After the initial screening, the most serious candidates may be asked back for a *reinterview.*

It is helpful to network with colleagues inside and outside the organization. Identify individuals who have influence over your career, who can serve as mentors, who can give you career guidance, and who can serve as references. Join professional organizations where you can meet colleagues with similar interests. Volunteer for committee work. Attend conventions and meetings. Have business cards made up and swap them with colleagues. Keep in touch with your colleagues, ask for what you need, give feedback, and follow up with contacts (Vestal, 1987).

One progresses in professional development by systematically reviewing professional journals, collecting and filing articles and materials topically, developing a professional library, achieving professional certification, chairing a committee to develop leadership skills, presenting an in-service, and fostering a support group.

BIBLIOGRAPHY

Bethel PL: RN orientation: cost and achievement analysis, *Nurs Econ* 10:336-341, September-October 1992.

Brown RL: Mentoring program builds million dollar agencies, *Managers Magazine* 65:10-18, May 1990.

Brunt BA: Role of continuing educators in encouraging use of clinical practice guidelines, *Journal of Continuing Education in Nursing* 25:8-10, January-February 1994.

Cunningham JB, Eberle T: Characteristics of the mentoring experience: a qualitative study, *Personnel Review* 22:54-56, 1993.

Driggers DL, Nussbaum JS, Haddock KS: Role modeling: an educational strategy to promote effective cancer pain management, *Oncology Nursing Forum* 20:959-963, July 1993.

Ellis C: Incorporating the affective domain into staff development programs, *Journal of Nursing Staff Development* 9:127-130, May-June 1993.

Finnick M, Crosby F, Ventura MR: Staff development challenge: assuring nurses' competency in quality assessment and improvement, *Journal of Nursing Staff Development* 9:136-140, May-June 1993.

Fitzgerald W: Training versus development, *Training and Development* 46:81-84, May 1992.

Halbert TL, Underwood JE, Chambers LW et al: Population based health promotion: a new agenda for public health nurses, *Canadian Journal of Public Health* 84:243-245, July-August 1993.

Horn PB, Kopser KG, Carpenter AD: A systematic evaluation of a poster presentation . . . alternative methods within staff development, *Journal of Continuing Education in Nursing* 24:232-233, September-October 1993.

James LA: Orientation through self-study, *Journal of Nursing Staff Development* 9:85-87, March-April 1993.

Kallenbach AM, Lantz M: Preceptorship and skill validation programs, *Journal of Post Anesthesia Nursing* 8:316-321, October 1993.

Kihlgren M, Kuremyr D, Norberg A et al: Nurse-patient interaction after training in integrity promoting care at a long-term ward: analysis of video-recorded morning care sessions, *International Journal of Nursing Studies* 30:1-13, February 1993.

Leonard DJ: Workplace education: adult education in a hospital nursing staff development department, *Journal of Nursing Staff Development* 9:68-73, March-April 1993.

Lewis ML, Govoni A, Camp Y et al: Competency based nursing in a rehabilitation setting, *Rehabilitation Nursing* 18:221-225, July-August 1993.

Macari GH: Self-study packets: an in-service strategy for today's emergency department, *Journal of Emergency Nursing* 19:156-157, April 1993.

Ozcan YA, Shukla RK: The effect of a competency based targeted staff development program on nursing productivity, *Journal of Nursing Staff Development* 9:78-84, March-April 1993.

Ponte PR, Higgins JM, James JR et al: Development needs of advance practice nurses in a managed care environment, *JONA* 23:13-19, November 1993.

Rooda L, Gay G: Staff development for culturally sensitive nursing care, *Journal of Staff Development* 9:262-265, November-December 1993.

Speers AT: Games in nursing staff development, *Journal of Nursing Staff Development* 9:274-277, November-December 1993.

Tibbles LR, Smith AE, Manzi SC: Train the trainer for hospital wide safety training, *Journal of Nursing Staff Development* 9:166-169, November-December 1993.

Twardon C, Gartner MK, Cherry C: A competency achievement orientation program: professional development of the home health nurse, *JONA* 23:20-25, July-August 1993.

Williams J, Baker G, Clark B et al: Collaborative preceptor training: a creative approach in tough times, *Journal of Continuing Education in Nursing* 24:153-157, July-August 1993.

Williams A, Poroch D, McIntosh W: Fun projects: increasing awareness of nursing research in hospitals, *Australian Journal of Advanced Nursing* 11:14-18, September-November 1993.

Wilson JA, Elman NS: Organizational benefits of mentoring, *Academy of Management Executive* 4:88-94, November 1990.

Zanzi A, Arthur MB, Shamir B: The relationships between career concerns and political tactics in organizations, *Journal of Organizational Behavior* 12:219-233, May 1991.

CASE STUDY

A new graduate is starting on your unit next week. Using Worksheet 13-1, make a list of what the employee needs to be oriented to and identify who should tell the employee about what. Would you assign the new graduate to a preceptor, and if so what part would the preceptor play in the orientation? What is your role as patient care coordinator? What might the inservice department of the hospital do? Identify some of the new graduate's learning needs and identify means for facilitating the nurse's lifelong learning needs.

CRITICAL THINKING AND LEARNING ACTIVITIES

1. Update your résumé. Start or maintain a file of your accomplishments.

2. Using Worksheet 13-2, list your interests and skills.

3. Draw your career map.

4. Design your business card.

Orientation

Identify what the new employee needs to know or be oriented to and who should orient the employee to each topic.

Orientation topic	Orienter

✍ **Worksheet 13-2**

Interests and Skills

List your interests and skills as a basis for planning your future.

Interests	Skills
1.	1.
2.	2.
3.	3.
4.	4.
5.	5.
6.	6.
7.	7.
8.	8.
9.	9.
10.	10.

Chapter

14

Assignment Systems for Staffing

Chapter Objectives

◆ Identify at least five patient care delivery modes or assignment systems.

◆ Compare and contrast at least three patient care delivery modes or assignment systems.

◆ Differentiate between managed care and case management.

Major Concepts and Definitions

Case method	each patient is assigned to a nurse for total patient care
Functional nursing	hierarchical division of labor
Team nursing	registered nurses supervise auxiliary nursing staff
Modular nursing	district nursing
Primary nursing	registered nurses give total patient care to a few patients
Managed care	unit-based care system that uses critical paths
Case management	management and coordination of the care a patient receives in all settings throughout an episode of illness
Collaborative practice	cooperative interdisciplinary practice
Differentiated practice	distinction between professional and technical nursing
Partners in practice	interdisciplinary team

ASSIGNMENT SYSTEMS FOR STAFFING

Changes in assignment systems are a response to changing needs. In the 1920s, the case method and private duty nursing were popular. By 1950, functional nursing was predominant in response to the shortage of nurses. During that decade, team nursing was introduced to maximize use of the knowledge and skills of professional nurses and to supervise auxiliary workers. The late 1960s and 1970s witnessed a shift back to care of the patient by a professional nurse through primary nursing. Managed competition emerged as an economic strategy guiding health care reform during the 1990s. It stimulated partners in practice, which is an interdisciplinary team. Case management and managed care became popular during the 1980s. Each system has advantages and disadvantages (see Box 14-1).

Case Method

In the case method each patient is assigned to a nurse for total patient care while that nurse is on duty. The patient has a different nurse each shift and no guarantee of having the same nurses the next day. The patient care coordinator, with no obligation to assign nurses to the same patient, supervises and evaluates all of the care given on the unit. Popular during the 1920s along with private duty nursing, the case method emphasized following physicians' orders.

Box 14-1

PROS AND CONS OF VARIOUS ASSIGNMENT SYSTEMS

Assignment System	Pros	Cons
Care method	Total patient care	Different nurse, different shifts, different days
Functional nursing	Efficiency	Nurses do managerial work Nurses' aides do patient care
Team nursing	Team effort Frees patient care coordinator to manage the unit Nursing care conferences help problem solve and develop staff Nursing care plan	Time to coordinate delegated work
Modular nursing	Useful where there are few RNs RNs plan care	Paraprofessionals do technical aspects of care
Primary nursing	RNs give total patient care Primary nurse has 24 hour a day responsibility Associate nurse works with patient while the primary nurse is off duty Accountability in place Continuity of care is facilitated Reduces number of errors from relay of orders Fewer patient complaints Shorter hospitalization	Confines nurse's talents to a limited number of patients Associate nurse may change care plan without discussing with primary nurse
Managed care	Unit-based Can be used with any nursing care delivery system Standard critical paths	Questionable continuity of care
Case management	Focuses on entire episode of illness Emphasizes achievement of outcomes Incorporates managed care Care is coordinated by a case manager Second-generation primary nursing Critical paths Variation analysis Intershift reports Health care team meetings Quality assurance Interdisciplinary approach	Effort to coordinate

Functional Nursing

In the 1950s, when few registered and only some practical nurses were available, much patient care was given by nurses' aides. In functional nursing, hierarchical structure predominates. The medication nurse, treatment nurse, and bedside nurse are all products of this system. The functional method implements classic scientific management, which emphasizes efficiency, division of labor, and rigid controls. Procedural descriptions are used to describe the standard of care, and psychological needs typically are slighted. Registered nurses keep busy with managerial and nonnursing duties, and nurses' aides deliver the majority of patient care.

Although efficient, the functional assignment method does not encourage patient and staff satisfaction. Regimentation of tasks may bore nurses because they no longer have the satisfaction of seeing the effects of their total patient care. On the other hand, the functional system may work satisfactorily during critical staffing shortages. Routinized patient care for patients with similar needs may meet those needs more consistently than other systems, and some staff members may be satisfied by doing repetitive jobs well.

Team Nursing

After World War II, registered nurses were still scarce, although the number of auxiliary personnel had increased. Team nursing was introduced during the 1950s to improve nursing services by using the knowledge and skills of professional nurses and to supervise the increasing numbers of auxiliary nursing staff. The result was an improvement in patient and staff satisfaction. Team nursing is based on a philosophy that supports the achievement of goals through group action. Each team member is encouraged to make suggestions and share ideas. When team members see their suggestions implemented, their job satisfaction increases, and they are motivated to give even better care.

The team is led by a professional or technical nurse who plans, interprets, coordinates, supervises, and evaluates the nursing care. Team leaders assign team members to patients by matching patient needs with staff's knowledge and skills. They also do the work other members of the team are not qualified to perform. They set goals and priorities for patient care; centralizes information through the use of a Kardex; direct the planning of care by directing care conferences and developing care plans; fix responsibility for the work; provide for coverage during absences, such as breaks, meals, and conferences; and coordinate and evaluate team activities. The team members report to the team leader, who reports to the patient care coordinator. This is a form of decentralization that frees the patient care coordinator to manage the unit.

One of the main features of team nursing is the nursing care conference. Its primary purpose is the development and revision of nursing care plans by providing an opportunity to identify and solve problems. Precision in the identification of problems is increased through information sharing. The belief that the total group has more information about a topic than any one person enhances the staff's appreciation of group work. A resulting consensus increases the commitment to the decisions made. Identification of the problem and determination of goals early in the conference necessarily precede planning intervention. During the conference, one care plan can be developed or the care plans for a case load can be updated.

Team conferences also provide the opportunity to identify and work through staff educational needs. Nurses can review standards of care by comparing the actual patient's condition to the textbook example. They can review procedures and learn specialized nursing care and the operation of infrequently used equipment. By studying critical incidents, they may prevent problems from recurring and identify the contributing components of excellent care. Team conferences also provide an opportunity to discuss and resolve interpersonal problems and the chance to prevent future ones. Consequently, team spirit is fostered.

The team leader is responsible for planning and conducting the team conference, which should be limited in time and scope. Meeting for 15 to 30 minutes at the same time each day helps the conference become a part of the daily routine. A time that least interferes with other activities and a place away from the hub of activity are preferable. The team leader must arrange for coverage of the unit during the conference, because relief from patient care responsibilities is essential to prevent interruptions. Staff should be informed of the time, place, and purpose of the conference, so that they can plan their other work around the conference and be well prepared on arrival. Interest can be stimulated by allowing the staff to decide which patient they wish to discuss at the next conference and by having one of the team members record patient problems and solutions during the conference.

Preparation of the meeting area is also a responsibility of the team leader. Temperature, ventilation, lighting, and chair arrangements should be controlled. Refreshments may be appropriate. The team leader introduces the topic and starts the meeting on time to motivate latecomers to be more prompt. A brief review of the patient's condition is appropriate. The team leader monitors the group process, records problems and solutions on the nursing care plan or delegates that task, does appropriate teaching, and summarizes the major points. The nursing care plan is then available to the staff. The team leader serves as a role model by referring to the care plan while receiving and giving reports, making out assignments, and administering nursing care.

The nursing care plan is another main feature of team nursing. A care plan identifying present and potential problems and long- and short-term objectives should be developed for each patient. The care plan should be realistic, to prevent morale problems that result from setting unattainable objectives. Care plans should be individualized, reflecting the interrelatedness of psychosocial and physiological needs and involving patient and family participation. Problems, mutually acceptable goals, objectives, actions, and responses are identified. The care is evaluated according to how well the objectives are met.

Team nursing contributes to the satisfaction of patient and staff needs. Each patient is treated as a unique individual. Staff can identify their contributions and the correlation between their work and patient outcomes. The closer interaction of staff contributes to esprit de corps.

Because each staff member does many tasks for a limited number of patients instead of a single task for a large number of patients, there is an increased likelihood of errors and a need to spend more time monitoring for them. It also takes time to coordinate delegated work. Although team leaders probably have the least contact with the patients, they are responsible for assessment, planning, and communicating with the physician. Continuity of care is not a given, because patients are not assigned to the same staff all of the time and large assignments make individualized patient care difficult. Changing team membership makes it difficult for the team leader to know team members well enough to match their talents with patient needs. Team nursing is similar to functional nursing when the team leader administers medications and treatments other team members are not qualified to give. Team conferences are often omitted because they are difficult to fit into busy days, and care plans (if done) usually note functional duties relative to the physician's orders. Care plans rarely depict the patient as a total person and consequently are not comprehensive. Medication precautions, fluid intake requirements, dietary and environmental adaptations, protective measures, psychological support, teaching, rehabilitation, and referrals are seldom mentioned. In reality the key features of team nursing—nursing care conferences and nursing care plans—often receive inadequate attention, and resulting care is routinized.

Modular, or District, Nursing

Modular, or district, nursing is a modification of team and primary nursing. It is sometimes used when there are not enough registered nurses to practice primary nursing. Each registered nurse, assisted by paraprofessionals, delivers as much care as possible to a group of patients. The registered nurse plans the care, delivers as much of it as possible, and directs the paraprofessionals for the more technical aspects of care. The registered nurse's role is closer to that of a coordinator and information processor than that of a charge nurse.

Modular nursing decreases the sense of isolation and unrealistic expectations often associated with primary nursing. When nurses are consistently assigned to the same module, continuity and quality of care can increase. More time may be spent in direct care. Fiscal savings are possible. Morale can also improve when staff know they are making a difference (Bennett and Hylton, 1990).

Some physical changes may be necessary to implement modular or district nursing. For example, a medication cart may be placed in the hall instead of using a medication room. Kardexes may be kept on the medication cart. Charts may be moved to the patient's room. Patient Kardexes and staff identification badges may be color-coded.

Primary Nursing

During the late 1960s and early 1970s, primary nursing was instituted in some hospitals by professional nurses who were unhappy with fragmented care and lack of direct patient contact. Based on the philosophy that patients, instead of tasks, should be the focus of professional nurses, primary nursing features a registered nurse who gives total patient care to four to six patients. The RN remains responsible for the care of those patients 24 hours a day throughout the patient's hospitalization. The associate nurse cares for the patient by using the care plan developed by the primary nurse while the primary nurse is off duty. The associate nurse is expected to contact the primary nurse regarding changes in the care plan. The number of patients assigned to one nurse varies according to length of hospitalization, complexity of care, number of medical and paramedical personnel involved with the patient's care, availability of support systems, and the shift worked. Day-shift nurses are assigned the greatest number of patients; evening nurses have some; and night nurses are primarily auxiliary nurses because of their reduced contact with patients and families.

The primary nurse does the admission interview and develops the nursing care plan, including teaching and discharge planning, which is shared with the associate nurse. Primary nurses have autonomy and authority for the care of their patients. Consequently, accountability is placed and continuity of care is facilitated. Primary nursing decreases the number of people in the chain of command and reduces the number of errors that can result from a relay of orders. Other advantages include mobile use of auxiliary workers and increased satisfaction by both nurse and patient. Nurses can identify patient outcomes as a result of their work. Patients have the security of knowing the nurse is available and has to cope with fewer people than in other assignment systems. Research suggests that patients have fewer complications and a shorter hospitalization when cared for by a primary nurse.

Unfortunately, primary nursing confines a nurse's talents to a limited number of patients. Other patients cannot benefit, and if a patient has a nurse who is not capable, the patient may be worse off than if cared for by numerous people, some of whom might meet the patient's needs. Another problem occurs when the associate nurse changes the care plan without discussing the reasons with the primary nurse. Thus it is critical that the primary nurse communicate verbal and written plans to the associate nurse. The success of primary nursing seems to depend on the quality of the nursing staff and administrative support.

Managed Care

Managed care is a unit-based care system that can be used with any nursing care delivery system in any clinical setting. It uses standard critical paths with nursing care plans, analyzes the positive and negative variations from the critical paths, and uses them in change-of-shift reports. A critical path is a one-page version of a case management plan that shows the key incidents that occur at predictable times to achieve the length of stay permitted by a diagnostic-related group category. Critical paths are not revised for individual patients, but variations are documented. Activities, consultations, diet, discharge planning, medications, teaching, tests, and treatments are noted. The critical path is used to plan and monitor the care. It can be kept in a nursing Kardex and accompanies the patient to various services.

Case Management

Case management focuses on an entire episode of illness, including all settings in which the client receives care. It emphasizes achievement of outcomes in designated time frames with limited resources. Typically, it incorporates managed care. Care is coordinated by a case manager. Case management is sometimes called second-generation primary nursing.

Case management involves critical paths, variation analysis, intershift reports, case consultation, health care team meetings, and quality assurance. Critical paths visualize outcomes within a time frame. Variation analysis notes positive or negative changes from the critical path, the cause, and the corrective action taken. This information is reported in intershift reports. Case consultation may be indicated when the client's condition differs from the critical path as noted in the intershift report. Case consultation is conducted about once a week for a few minutes immediately after intershift report to deal with variations. It can also be conducted informally whenever a staff member identifies a variation and consults others. The problem solvers focus on the variation and the desired outcomes, brainstorm ideas to achieve desired outcomes, and use open communication to evaluate a plan. A summary can be used to close the session.

Health care team meetings provide an interdisciplinary approach to problem solving. The case manager needs to identify no more than three priority goals and decide what team members should be present after considering the patient, family, physician, social service, various therapists, and others involved. The case manager should set the time and place for the meeting, make the arrangements, and post the date, time, place, and people to attend in the Kardex. The case manager calls the meeting to order, states the goals, initiates discussion, documents the plans, and sets time limits for follow through. The variance between what is expected and what happened is assessed for quality assurance.

Collaborative Practice

Collaborative practice can include interdisciplinary teams, nurse-physician interaction in joint practice, or nurse-physician collaboration in care giving. Collaboration is cooperative and assertive. The interaction between nurses and physicians or other health team members in collaborative practice should enable the knowledge and skills of the professions to influence the quality of patient care provided synergestically.

The American Nurses' Association and the American Medical Association established the National Joint Practice Committee (NJPC) in 1972 with funding from the W.K. Kellogg Foundation. The report supported collaborative practice and suggested that increased collaboration results in improved quality of care and patient and nurse satisfaction, and a decreased need for physician supervision of nurses. Primary nursing, nurse decision making, integrated patient record, a joint practice committee, and a joint record review were found to enhance nurse-physician collaboration.

Differentiated Practice

Differentiated practice generally refers to the difference between professional and technical nursing. Complexity of decision making, timeline of care, and structure of the setting are its main distinctive features. Professional nurses have received a baccalaureate or graduate degree. They give direct care to patients with complex interactions of nursing diagnosis and relate to their families from preadmission to postdischarge in a variety of more or less structured settings. The technical nurse has received an associate degree and gives nursing care to patients with common conditions and to their families in structured settings.

The original Integrated Competencies of Nurses (ICON) model addressed entry into practice roles by developing a differentiated practice model. The baccalaureate-prepared nurses assessed, planned, and evaluated. The associate degree-prepared nurses implemented care. One professional and two or three associate nurses cared for 10 to 15 patients during the day. ICON 11 responded to the shortage of nurses by "grandfathering" all RNs into the professional role. Licensed practical nurses (LPNs) then filled the technical role (Tonges, 1989).

Mathey's Primary Practice Partners model responds to the nursing shortage by recommending former military corpsmen, emergency medical technicians (EMTs), and registered certified technicians (RCTs) with special technical training to be nurse extenders. These and other job categories may expand differentiated practice models.

LEVEL OF STAFF

The level of staff available greatly influences the assignment systems used. When there are a few registered nurses and a few practical nurses, many aides are quickly oriented and used. This is an expensive and relatively dangerous mix, because aides do not have the educational background to do most of what needs to be done or to recognize what needs to be reported. After the aides have done all they can, there is still much work to be done. Consequently, there is considerable downtime. This staffing mix lends itself best to functional nursing.

Team nursing is appropriate when there are some registered nurses, even more practical nurses, and fewer aides. The registered nurses plan and direct the care, pass medications, and do the more complicated treatments. Although this provides better physical care, the staff is still not adequately educated to understand the pathophysiological basis of symptoms, to plan nursing intervention, and to detect changes in the status of the patient at an early stage so they may promptly report pertinent information to the physician. There is also a dearth of patient education and response to psychosocial needs.

Modular nursing is appropriate when more registered nurses are available, and primary nursing works best with a staff of only registered nurses. Research regarding exclusively RN staffs indicates an increase in staff, patient, and physician satisfaction. There is an increase in professional orientation, personal liking of colleagues, and cooperation with others. Collegial relationships are more common, and there is more mobility on units because nurses can cover for each other. There is greater competence in skills, creative interventions, personalized care, and continuity of care.

All-registered nurse staffing is economical. It has been found to save money through decreased turnover, sick leave, unpaid absences, float hours, and overtime. Registered nurses can give better care in fewer hours. Patients have fewer complications, shorter hospitalizations, and lower readmission rates. Hospitals also generate more revenue when patients have shorter stays with a concentration of treatments. Unfortunately, frequent shortages of nurses make all-RN staffs unlikely.

Pure applications of case method, functional method, team nursing, modular nursing, and primary nursing are possible, but they seldom exist in pristine form. Rather, it is common to find elements from more than one assignment system combined and used at the same time. Managed care can be used with any nursing care delivery mode and can incorporate differentiated practice.

BIBLIOGRAPHY

Abbott J: Making the commitment to managed care, *Nurs Manage* 24:36-37, August 1993.

Abts D, Hofer M, Leafgreen PK: Redefining care delivery: a modular system, *Nurs Manage* 25:40-46, February 1994.

Ahrens T: Nurse clinician model of managed care, *AACN Clin Issues Crit Care Nurs* 3:761-768, November 1992.

Ambutas S: A comparison of two patient classification systems for an MICU, *Nurs Manage* 19:64A-64H, September 1988.

Anderson CL, Hughes E: Implementing modular nursing in a long-term care facility, *JONA* 23:29-35, June 1993.

Barger SE: The nursing center: a model for rural nursing practice, *Nurs Health Care* 12:290-295, June 1991.

Barger S, Rosenfield P: Models in community health care: findings from a national study of community nursing centers, *Nurs Health Care* 14:426-431, October 1993.

Barnsteiner JH, Mohan A, Milberger P: Implementing managed care in a pediatric setting, *AACN Clin Issues Crit Care Nurs* 3:777-787, November 1992.

Boston CM: Nurse assistive programs, *JONA* 20:5-6, January 1990.

Brett JJ, Tonges MC: Restructured patient care delivery: evaluation of the proact model, *Nurs Econ* 8:36-44, January-February 1990.

Buerhaus PI: Economics of managed competition and consequences to nursing part 1, *Nurs Econ* 12:10-17, January-February 1994.

Cesta TG: The link between continuous quality improvement and case management, *JONA* 23:55-61, June 1993.

Edelstein EL, Cesta TG: Nursing case management: an innovative model of care for hospitalized patients with diabetes, *Diabetes Educator* 19:517-521, November-December 1993.

Erkel EA: The impact of case management in preventive services, *JONA* 23:27-32, January 1993.

Feldman C, Olberding L, Shortridge L et al: Decision making in case management of home healthcare clients, *JONA* 23:33-38, January 1993.

Fielo SB, Crowe RL: A nursing center in Brooklyn, *Nurs Health Care* 13:488-493, November 1992.

Gardner M: Nursing case management: a model for care delivery, *AANA Journal* 19:156, April 1992.

Hamptom DC: Implementing a managed care framework through care maps, *JONA* 23:21-27, May 1993.

Hayes PM: Team building: bringing RNs and NAs together, *Nurs Manage* 25:52-54, May 1994.

Hicks L, Stallmeyer JM, Coleman JR: Nursing challenges in managed care, *Nurs Econ* 10:265-276, July-August 1992.

Hinshaw AS, Scofield R, Atwood JR: Staff, patient, and cost outcomes of all-registered nurse staffing, *JONA* 11:30-36, November-December 1981.

Huber DG, Blegen MA, McCloskey JC: Use of nursing assistants: staff nurse opinions, *Nurs Manage* 25:64-68, May 1994.

Hyams-Franklin E, Rowe-Gilliespie P, Harper A et al: Primary team nursing: the 90s model, *Nurs Manage* 24:50-52, June 1993.

Krieger JW, Connell FA, LoGerfo JP: Medicaid prenatal care: a comparison of use and outcomes in fee for service and managed care, *Am J Public Health* 82:185-190, February 1992.

Madden JM, Ponte PR: Advanced practice roles in the managed care environment, *JONA* 24:56-62, January 1994.

Mahn VA: Clinical case management: a service line approach, *Nurs Manage* 24:48-50, September 1993.

Malloch KM, Milton DA, Jobes MO: A model for differentiated nursing practice, *JONA* 20:20-26, February 1990.

Manthey M: Primary practice partners (a nurse extender system), *Nurs Manage* 19:58-59, March 1988.

Miller AM: Health care reform: clarifying the concepts, *J Community Health Nurs* 10:199-211, 1993.

Neidlinger SH, Bostrom J, Stricker A et al: Incorporating nursing assistive personnel into a nursing professional practice model, *JONA* 23:29-37, March 1993.

Newman M, Lamb GS, Michaels C: Nurse case management, *Nurs Health Care* 12:404-408, October 1991.

Parker M, Quinn J, Viehl M et al: Case management in rural areas: definition, clients, financing, staffing, and service delivery issues, *Nurs Econ* 8:103-109, March-April 1990.

Phillips CY, Carson JA, Huggins CM et al: Care manager/nurse manager: a blending of roles, *Nurs Manage* 24:26-28, October 1993.

Ponte PR, Higgins JM, James JR et al: Development needs of advance practice nurses in a managed care environment, *JONA* 23:13-19, November 1993.

Powers PH, Dickey CA, Ford A: Evaluating an RN/co-worker model, *JONA* 20:11-15, March 1990.

Schull DE, Tosch P, Wood M: Clinical nurse specialists as collaborative care managers, *Nurs Manage* 23:30-33, March 1992.

Shamian J, Frunchak V, Miller G, Georges P et al: Role responsibilities of head nurses in primary nursing and team nursing units, *JONA* 18:7, May 1988.

Stein LJ, Watts DT, Howell T: Sounding board: the doctor-nurse game revisited, *N Engl J Med* 322:546-549, February 1990.

Uzark K, LeRoy S, Callow L et al: The pediatric nurse practitioner as case manager in the delivery of services to children with heart disease, *J Pediatr Health Care* 8:74-78, March-April 1994.

Wadas TM: Case management and caring behavior, *Nurs Manage* 24:40-46, September 1993.

CASE STUDY

You are responsible for the budget on your unit. You have a registered nurse vacancy, which you may fill with one registered nurse or two unlicensed personnel. What will you do and why?

CRITICAL THINKING AND LEARNING ACTIVITIES

1. Identify the patient care delivery mode for at least one health care setting with which you are familiar. Use Worksheet 14-1 to help you identify the basic characteristics of the patient care delivery modes discussed in this chapter.

2. Form diads to compare and contrast three patient care delivery modes.

3. Form small groups and discuss the similarities and differences between managed care and case management.

✍ Worksheet 14-1

Patient Care Delivery Modes

List characteristics of the following patient care delivery modes:

Case method
1.
2.
3.
4.
5.

Functional nursing
1.
2.
3.
4.
5.

Team nursing
1.
2.
3.
4.
5.

Modular nursing
1.
2.
3.
4.
5.

Primary nursing
1.
2.
3.
4.
5.

Managed care
1.
2.
3.
4.
5.

Case management
1.
2.
3.
4.
5.

Chapter
15

Staffing Schedules for Productivity

Chapter Objectives

◆ List at least six policy issues related to staffing schedules.

◆ Describe the pros and cons of centralized and decentralized scheduling.

◆ Identify at least three different staffing patterns and discuss the pros and cons of each.

◆ Describe how to calculate the number of full-time staff needed for vacation, holiday, and absentee coverage per year.

Major Concepts and Definitions	
Staffing schedules	work schedules for personnel
Centralized scheduling	scheduling done in one location
Decentralized scheduling	scheduling done in local areas
Self-scheduling	staff coordinating their own work schedules
Rotating work shifts	alternating work hours among days, evenings, and nights
Permanent shifts	personnel working the same hours repeatedly
Block scheduling	using the same schedule repeatedly
Variable staffing	determining the number and mix of staff based on patient needs
Patient classification systems	calculating staffing needs based on patient acuity
Staffing formulas	calculations used to determine staffing needs

STAFFING SCHEDULES

Staffing schedules are largely influenced by staffing policies. To determine staffing policies, one must consider the following questions:

What is the best organization for staffing—centralized or decentralized to clinical areas or nursing units?

Who is responsible for the original scheduling or daily adjustments?

Where are nursing hours posted and an accurate copy kept?

For what period will schedules be prepared—1, 2, 4, or 6 weeks?

How far in advance will personnel know their work schedule?

Will there be an adjustment in staffing based on the identification of patient needs?

Will there be shift rotation?

If there is shift rotation, how often—daily, weekly, monthly?

How much time should elapse between rotated shifts?

What day starts a calendar week—Sunday or Monday?

Will there be 2 days off each week or an average of 2 days a week?

How often are weekends off guaranteed?

What days does a weekend comprise—Friday, Saturday, Sunday?

Will days off be split or consecutive?

What are the maximum and minimum work spans?

How many holiday and vacation days are allowed?

How far in advance of scheduling should employees request time off?

How will holiday time off be determined?

Will part-time help be used?

If so, what is the most economical ratio between full- and part-time personnel?

Will part-time help be allowed to specify when they can and cannot work?

Will part-time help be required to work weekends? If so, how often?

Centralized Scheduling

Two major advantages of centralized scheduling are fairness to employees through consistent, objective, and impartial application of policies and opportunities for cost containment through better use of resources. Centralized scheduling also relieves head nurses from time-consuming duties, freeing them for other activities. Centralized scheduling is not without its critics, however. Lack of individualized treatment of employees is a chief complaint, and centralized scheduling has brought to the surface previously unrecognized organizational and managerial problems.

Organizational and managerial problems can be reduced when (1) the philosophy and goals of the agency are identified; (2) the goals, objectives, and organizational structure are defined; (3) scheduling policies are stated; (4) standards of nursing care practices are set; (5) acuity of care is determined as it relates to staffing needs; (6) patient needs, personnel policies such as vacation and personal leave, and staff development are taken into account in personnel schedules; and (7) quality of care is measured.

Resistance to centralized scheduling may be reduced when head nurses prepare and control their own budgets, understand and approve the scheduling policies, and have open communication with the scheduler. Line and staff accountability need to be carefully defined to prevent confusion over responsibility and authority when staff personnel make decisions where line managers are accountable. Line authority is accountable for decisions, and staff provides support to help line make decisions.

The staff functions of the scheduler include scheduling employees according to staffing policies, implementing procedures for position control and reallocation of staff, maintaining records for line managers, gathering information and preparing reports to help line authority prepare personnel budgets, and maintaining communications with other appropriate departments, such as personnel and payroll.

Line responsibilities of managers include developing a master staffing pattern; establishing procedures for adjustment of staff; clarifying requirements for each job description and staff position; hiring, developing, promoting, disciplining, and firing employees when appropriate; and defining and controlling the personnel budget.

Computers can be used for centralized scheduling. Before implementing a computer system, an analysis of policies and procedures is done and baseline data collected. Agency policies regarding the nature of the schedule—straight, alternating, or rotating shifts; frequency of alternating or rotating shifts; work stretch; weekends-off sequence; and use of part-time help—are constants in the information process system. Variables such as census, acute conditions of patients, special requests, special assignments, vacations, and holidays can be fed into the computer.

Advantages of centralized computer scheduling include cost-effectiveness through the reduction of clerical staff and better use of professional nurses by decreasing the time spent in non-patient-care activities; unbiased, consistent scheduling; equitable application of agency policies; an easy-to-read work schedule developed in advance so employees know what their schedules are and can plan their personal lives accordingly; and availability of data for monitoring the effect of staff size and composition, quality of care, and cost.

Decentralized Staffing

When managers are given authority and assume responsibility, they can staff their own units through decentralized staffing. Personnel feel that they get more personalized attention with decentralized staffing. Staffing is easier and less complicated when done for a small area instead of for the whole agency. Each manager learns the responsibility and challenges of staffing. With a philosophy of sharing and mutual trust, managers can work together to solve chronic staffing problems. Because of their knowledge and experience, managers can form a support system and offer each other informed advice. Managers and charge nurses are freed from staffing responsibilities and have more time for other tasks.

Unfortunately, some staff members may receive individualized treatment at the expense of others, and work schedules can be used as a punishment-reward system. Staffing, which is very time-consuming, takes managers away from other duties or forces them to do the scheduling while off duty. Decentralized staffing may utilize resources less efficiently and consequently make cost containment more difficult (see Box 15-1).

Self-Scheduling

Self-scheduling is a system that is coordinated by staff nurses. It is a process by which nurses and other staff collectively develop and implement work schedules, taking policies and variables affecting staffing into consideration. A process might allow about 2 weeks for staff to indicate the days, shifts, weekends, holidays, and vacation days that they want. Then about 2 weeks is needed for negotiations to finalize a schedule that accommodates both the staff and the unit's needs. Staff may negotiate before and after work and during break and lunch times. They may also write notes to each other and wait for responses.

Self-scheduling can help create a climate where professional nursing can be practiced. It saves the manager considerable scheduling time and changes the role of the manager from supervisor to coach. It increases the amount of time staff spends on

Box 15-1 **ADVANTAGES AND DISADVANTAGES OF VARIOUS SCHEDULING METHODS**

SCHEDULING METHOD	PROS	CONS
Self-scheduling	Coordinated by staff nurses Saves manager scheduling time Helps develop accountability Increased perception of autonomy Increased job satisfaction Improved team spirit Improved morale Decreased absenteeism Reduced turnover Effective for recruitment and retention	Increases amount of time staff spends on scheduling
Rotating work shifts	Can rotate teams	Rotate among shifts Increases stress Affects health Affects quality of work Disrupts development of work groups High turnover
Permanent shifts	Can participate in social activities Job satisfaction Commitment to the organization Fewer health problems Less tardiness Less absenteeism Less turnover	Most people want day shift New graduates predominately staff evenings and nights Difficulty evaluating evening and night staff Nurses may not appreciate the work load or problems of other shifts
Block or cyclical scheduling	Same schedule repeatedly Nurses not so exhausted Sick time reduced Personnel know schedule in advance Personnel can schedule social events Decreased time spent on scheduling Staff treated fairly Helps establish stable work groups Decreases floating Promotes team spirit Promotes continuity of care	Rigidity
Variable staffing	Use census to determine number and mix of staff Little need to call in unscheduled staff	

scheduling, increases their ability to negotiate with each other, and helps develop a more accountable and professional staff.

Self-scheduling has been associated with increased perception of autonomy, increased job satisfaction, increased cooperative atmosphere, improved team spirit, improved morale, decreased absenteeism, and reduced turnover. It has also been effective in recruitment and retention (Ringl and Dotson, 1989).

Alternating or Rotating Work Shifts

Although straight shifts are used by some institutions or for some personnel within institutions, rotating work shifts are common for staff nurses. The frequency of alternating between days and evenings, or days and nights, or rotating through all three shifts varies among institutions. Some nurses may work all three shifts within 7 days.

Alternating and rotating work shifts create stress for staff nurses. Environmental cues, such as sunrise and sunset, fluctuate in a predictable cycle. Instruments that designate hours, minutes, and seconds correspond to the natural daily cycle and allow knowledge of one's location in that cycle. Social and work routines synchronize with the internal circadian rhythms as the body rhythms are timed to coincide with the usual activities. Thus, when environmental conditions are changed by altering work hours, sleep time, hour for rising, meal times, and social and recreational activities, the body must make accommodations for the environmental changes. Body rhythms need time to adjust to the discrepancy between the person's activity cycle and the new demands of the environment. The ability of the body functions to adjust varies considerably among individuals. It may take 2 to 3 days to 2 weeks for a person to adjust to a different sleep-wake cycle.

Alternating and rotating work shifts affect the health of nurses and the quality of their work. The rapid shift of work schedules causes stress. Nurses complain of restlessness and nervousness while trying to sleep, wakefulness or sleepiness at inappropriate times, anorexia, digestive disturbance, disruption in bowel habits, fatigue, slower reaction time, lower job performance, and error proneness. There are changes in the patterning of temperature, blood pressure, and urine excretory cycles, and a possible lowered resistance to disease. Resultant increase in medication errors, equipment failures, and errors in problem solving are probable.

To guarantee that nurses work their share of weekends, holidays, and unpopular evening and night hours, alternating and rotating assignments currently focus on the time patterns of an individual nurse rather than on well-integrated work groups. The rotation of personnel on an individual basis is disruptive to the development of work groups.

The Federal Aviation Agency's (FAA) rotation of teams of airport personnel may be used as a model by nursing services. The FAA rotates entire teams consisting of four or five controllers plus trainees and a leader, chosen because of their qualifications, amount of experience, and anticipated compatibility. Their schedules are planned a year in advance so that team members can plan their personal lives with confidence. Emergencies and vacations are handled within the team. Absenteeism affects the workload of the peers with whom one must continue to work; therefore, team identification reduces absenteeism because of team pressure. Controllers have a low turnover rate.

In hospitals, rotation of teams instead of individuals could contribute to team development. If a group of personnel works together consistently, they can help each other through the dependence of the orientation phase of group development and the conflict experienced during the organizational phase, when the role negotiations of who will be responsible for what occurs. The staff has a chance to become an interdependent, cohesive group with good communication and effective problem-solving abilities. Unfortunately, there is usually a high turnover of nursing personnel, which complicates team development. Perhaps more attention to team development would reduce turnover.

Permanent Shifts

Permanent shifts relieve nurses from stress and health-related problems associated with alternating and rotating shifts. They also provide social, educational, and psychological advantages. When nurses are able to choose the shift that best suits their personal life, they can participate in social activities (such as hobbies, sports, and community, professional, or church organizations) even when they require regular attendance. They may be able to continue their education by planning courses around their work schedule. Child-care arrangements can be stable. Nurses may develop a sense of belonging to a shift and feel and work better because the shift suits them. In studies conducted with Montreal nurses, those working permanent shifts had higher averages on psychological scales such as mental health, job satisfaction, social involvement, and commitment to the organization. They had fewer health problems and less tardiness, absenteeism, and turnover.

Although the day shift is not always the preferred shift, it is likely to be. Consequently, assignment to preferred shift may need to be done on a seniority-priority basis. This usually results in a predominance of new graduates staffing the evening and night shifts. Managers may have difficulty evaluating the evening and night shift personnel unless they make some observations during those shifts; therefore, it may be easier for evening and night supervisors to evaluate permanent staff on those shifts. One disadvantage of permanent shifts is that nurses may not develop an appreciation for the workload or problems of other shifts.

Block, or Cyclical, Scheduling

Block, or cyclical, scheduling uses the same schedule repeatedly. With a 6-day forward rotation, personnel are scheduled to work 6 successive days followed by at least 2 days off. The schedule repeats itself every 6 weeks.

Personnel can be scheduled with every other weekend off and 1 day during the week so that there are no more than 4 consecutive days of work. Several blocks are possible. Because nurses are not exhausted by working too many consecutive days, sick leave can be reduced. By having one team member at a time vacation and by rotating holidays among the workers, vacations and holidays can be scheduled to avoid changes in the block. However, some nurses fear that 1 day off at a time is not adequate to feel rested. But nurses who currently do not work more than 4 consecutive days report that 1 day is adequate to refresh themselves.

There are several advantages to established rotations. Personnel know their schedules in advance and consequently can plan their personal lives. Absences because of social events decrease because staff can plan their social activities around their work schedules. There is a decrease in preoccupation with staffing, time for scheduling, time for maintenance of schedule, and conflict over preferred days off. Staff is treated more fairly by equitable distribution of popular and unpopular days on duty. The scheduling of appropriate number and category mix of personnel is simplified. Once the appropriate mix is determined, it is repeated. This helps establish stable work groups and decreases floating, thus promoting team spirit and continuity of care. A decrease in flexibility of staffing, however, may be perceived as a disadvantage.

Variable Staffing

Variable staffing is a method that uses patient needs to determine the number and mix of staff. Time measures are done for direct and indirect patient care. A patient classification system is developed, and tables are designed to determine the number of nursing hours required, depending on the number of patients in each category. This provides the information to determine staff needs by skill levels. Nursing pools, floats, and part-time help can be used to supplement the regular staff to accomplish the variable staffing. With a study of previous staffing needs, redistribution of peak routine work, and slight overstaffing in some areas to create float personnel for last-moment needs, there may be little need to call in unscheduled staff.

Eight-Hour Shift, Five-Day Workweek

The 5-day, 40-hour workweek became popular during the late 1940s. It was a radical change from the 10-hour day, 5-day workweek that contained split shifts and few holidays. It has been a predominant pattern since then. The shifts are usually 7 AM to 3:30 PM, 3 PM to 11:30 PM, and 11 PM to 7:30 AM, allowing for a half-hour lunch break and a half-hour overlap time between shifts to provide for continuity of care.

Ten-Hour Day, Four-Day Workweek

The Intensive Coronary Care Unit at Saint Elizabeth Community Health Center in Lincoln, Nebraska, has implemented the 10-hour day, 4-day workweek with an every-other-weekend-off staffing pattern. The shifts are 7 AM to 5:30 PM, 1 PM to 11:30 PM, and 9 PM to 7:30 AM. A cyclical schedule allows at least 14 hours off between shifts and a 4-day weekend every 6 weeks for those who rotate. The workweek begins on Sunday, and the weekend is Saturday and Sunday for all shifts. The main problem is fatigue, but it was not found to be as serious a problem as anticipated. The long weekends and extra days off are attractions (Bauer, 1971).

Ten-Hour Day Plus Five- or Six-Hour Shift

Roger Williams General Hospital in Providence, Rhode Island, has implemented two 10-hour shifts and one 5-hour shift. The shifts are 7 AM to 5:00 PM, 5 PM to 10 PM, and 9 PM to 7 AM. A 2-week cyclical schedule posts 2 days on, 2 days off, 3 on, 2 off, 2 on, and 3 off with two teams working complementary schedules. The younger nurses seem to have a more positive attitude toward the 10-hour shift and cite the social opportunities as a major benefit. However, the 10-hour system did contribute to greater fatigue, poorer communication between physicians and nurses, and discontinuity of patient care (Colt et al., 1974).

Nursing service at Sacred Heart Hospital in Eau Claire, Wisconsin, was able to capitalize on a pool of inactive registered nurses by developing a 6-hour evening shift and a 10-hour day shift. Shifts are 7 AM to 5 PM, 5 PM to 11 PM, and 11 PM to 7 AM. Problems encountered were overtime, which may have been partially due to adjustment, and absences of ill nurses from 10-hour shifts—a difficult deficit to fill, and one that burdened other staff members and lowered morale (Minor, 1971).

Ten-Hour Shift, Seven-Day Workweek

Evergreen General Hospital in Kirkland, Washington, has implemented a 7-70 plan that includes a 10-hour shift 7 days a week, followed by 7 consecutive days off. Two teams alternate weeks from Tuesday through Monday. There is no rotation of shifts. Each team contains permanent day, evening, and night shifts. The shifts are 6:45 AM to 5:15 PM, 12:45 PM to 11:15 PM, and 9:15 PM to 7:45 AM. Initially there was no extra pay for holiday or vacation time, because that was compensated for in the pay for 80 hours when only 70 hours were worked. Later, vacation time was instituted, dependent on length of employment and ranging from 70 hours annually for 1 to 3 years of employment to 140 hours per year for 11 or more years of employment.

Advantages of the 10-hour day, 7-day workweek include increased continuity of care, more consistency of care between weekdays and weekends, improved communications, better understanding of the patients' needs resulting from longer time with patients, more consistent patient teaching, more flexibility for meeting patient needs instead of hospital regimens, and improved job satisfaction because of advanced knowledge of work schedule and prolonged rest periods that facilitated a more normal home life and more control over one's personal affairs. Sick leave and resignations decreased. However, nurses were tired at the end of the 7-day workweek (Hutchins and Cleveland, 1978).

Twelve-Hour Shift, Seven-Day Workweek

The 12-hour shift, starting at 7 or 7:30 AM and ending at 7 or 7:30 PM, has been adopted by some institutions. The better use of nursing personnel lowers staffing requirements; this consequently lowers the cost per patient day. Nurses find they get to know their patients better because they have more time to study charts and can visit patients more frequently. They have more time to get new admissions settled before the change of shift and feel that they can give better patient care because they are not so rushed. They find that there are fewer communication gaps and better continuity of care. Consequently, there are improved nurse-patient relations, job satisfaction, and morale.

Working relations are improved. Personnel work with the same group of people, so team development is possible. There is less friction and no 3-to-11 shift to blame for problems. Less daily reporting results in less confusion about physicians' orders and changes in procedures and routines. Less time is required for staffing, thus freeing supervisors and head nurses for other duties.

Total time off is increased with an increased usefulness of time. Travel time is reduced. There is less personal expense for babysitting, gas, and meals. Nurses find they have more time to relax and enjoy their days off and are able to return to work refreshed. Flexibility for personal schedules improves staff morale.

Overtime pay has been of some concern. The 1966 Amendments to the Fair Labor Standards Act permit agencies to calculate overtime pay on a 14-consecutive-day work period. Consequently, overtime pay is only required for more than 80 hours in a 2-week period.

Some nurses complain that the extra time they have for learning and research becomes boring. Mental exhaustion and tension increase by the end of the work-week. Increases in minor accidents and medication errors have been reported. Others, however, have reported no such increases as a result of the cumulative fatigue. Nurses also complain that their home and social lives suffer the week they work.

The wide variety of staffing practices suggests there is no right or wrong staffing schedule. Rather, there is much variability to consider when designing the best staffing schedule for a given situation.

Baylor Plan

Baylor University Medical Center in Dallas, Texas, started a 2-day alternative plan. Nurses have the option to work two 12-hour days on the weekends and be paid for 36 hours for day shifts, or 40 hours for night shifts, or to work five 8-hour shifts Monday through Friday. This plan requires a larger nursing staff but has filled weekend positions and reduced turnover. Some hospitals have implemented the Baylor plan, indicating that the extra pay on weekends compensates for vacations, holidays, and sick time.

Some hospitals have nurses work 12-hour shifts when they work weekends. This way fewer people have to work weekends and, consequently, staff can have weekends off more frequently.

Variations

Medical College of Virginia Hospitals in Richmond has combined two 8-hour shifts and two 12-hour shifts per week for a total of 40 hours in a 4-day week (Alivizatos, 1981).

Intensive care nurses at Baptist Medical Center-Montclair in Birmingham, Alabama, have worked seven consecutive 8-hour nights from 10:30 PM to 7 PM, followed by seven nights off. They opted to be paid for 7½ hours for the 16 hours in excess of 40 per week rather than to accrue time off. The system was so popular it was expanded to other units.

When staff nurses designed their own staffing pattern at Valley Medical Center in Fresno, California, they designed a 3-day workweek with two 13-hour days, one

14-hour day, and 4 days off. It has decreased absenteeism and turnover and increased staff morale.

At Woman's Hospital of Texas in Houston, personnel can work the 5-day, 40-hour week, the two 16-hour weekend shifts for 40 hours' pay, or the three 12-hour shifts with at least one of those days on the weekend. The staff scheduling is done at the unit level. If nurses wish to work the three 12-hour day shift, they must have a buddy complete the 24-hour coverage.

Shared jobs where two part-time nurses fill one full-time position; half-shifts where two nurses each work 4 hours to fill one 8-hour shift; shifts at nontraditional times such as 9:00 AM to 5:00 PM or 10 AM to 6:00 PM; and 8 or fewer staggered hours scheduled during the busiest times are also options.

VARIABLES AFFECTING STAFFING

Although institutional and nursing service philosophy and objectives guide staffing, various patient, staff, and environmental factors also affect staffing patterns. The types of patients, their expectations, fluctuations in admissions, length of stay, and complexity of care complicate staffing (see Box 15-2). Personnel policies, educational and experiential levels of staff, job descriptions, the mix of work titles or leveling, hour and rotation policies, absenteeism, and the competitive market also affect staffing. Environmental factors, such as the floor plan of the unit and hospital, number of patient beds, availability of supplies and equipment, the organizational structure, and support services from other departments and agencies, are also considered when planning staffing patterns.

Budget submission is done periodically by submitting a summarization of the revenue and expense sections of the budget for review. A narrative justification is used to negotiate changes in the budget.

Managers are responsible for implementation of the budget to meet the staffing needs of the unit including weekends, holidays, vacations, and sick leave coverage through busy and slow periods.

Staffing Studies

Three major types of staffing studies are used to predict the number, level, and mix of personnel required for staffing. Nursing care needed may be predicted from patient classification systems by assigning patients to categories according to diagnosis, acuity of care, or amount of self-sufficiency. Number, level, and mix of staff needed can be determined by noting the number of patients in each category. Then a cost-effective nursing personnel budget based on the needs of patients and the qualifications of nursing personnel can be determined. Patient classification systems can be combined with nursing care plans, and costs to individual patients can be determined. Systems that charge patients for the care they receive can be designed.

Time standards can be determined for nursing procedures by listing and analyzing the procedures required by each patient. The time required for each patient and the sum for all patients on a unit can then be calculated. Formulas deduced from statistical analysis of work sampling data can be used to predict the number of nursing care hours needed.

Box 15-2   **VARIABLES THAT AFFECT STAFFING**

Workload budgets indicate the amount of work produced by a unit in terms of units of service, which are used to calculate expense budgets.

Activity reports measure statistics about current activity centering on the number of units of service given compared with the capacity.

Average daily census is the average number of patients cared for per day for a period of time.

Average length of stay is the average number of days that patients stay in the agency.

Adjusted units of service allows budgeting based on expected workload units of service adjusted for the expected mix of patients.

Care hours calculation determines the average required care hours per patient per 24 hours for each classification level and the sum or the total hours of care needed for all patients.

Personnel expense budget is the budget for all personnel assigned to a unit.

Fixed staff are employees who do not vary with the patient volume.

Variable staff are responsive to the projected number of care hours needed.

Establishing positions should involve the manager's discretion for use of full-time and part-time personnel to total the number of full-time equivalents needed to meet the care needs.

Labor costs are calculated by calculating the dollar basis of the straight-time salary, differentials, overtime, raises, and fringe benefits for each employee used by the unit.

Expense budget (other than personnel) is a combination of the direct unit expenses plus the indirect overhead expenses.

Revenue budget is the unit's income.

Adapted from Finkler SA, Kovner CT: *Financial management for nurse managers and executives,* Philadelphia, 1993, WB Saunders, pp 315-347.

PATIENT CLASSIFICATION SYSTEMS

The three basic styles of patient classification systems are (1) descriptive, (2) checklist, and (3) time of relative value unit standard. In the *descriptive style,* the nurse classifies the patient in the category that most closely describes the care received. The tool used is a narrative on a concise acuity table. Category 1 may be self-care and category 4 complete care, including feeding, frequent skin care, complete bath, complete bed rest, and frequent positioning. The patient does not have to receive all of the care received in a category to be classified in that category. The nurse chooses the category that best describes the patient. The major problem with this style is interrater reliability, caused by the subjectivity of the interpretation of the patient's degree of care. The descriptive style is a quick-check guide, but the poor interrater reliability leads to a wide range of requested nurse-to-patient ratios. Many administrators have moved away from this subjective style of patient classification.

The *checklist style acuity table* divides descriptions of care routines into activity categories, such as eating and bathing. Activity levels are described in each category.

Levels in the eating category might be self-care, help setting up, feed, and frequent feedings. Each activity is assigned an activity level point score, such as one for routine or self-care and 4 for comprehensive care. The nurse checks the activity level for each patient in each category and totals the points for each patient to determine the level of care. This is usually done at each shift or daily. It, too, is a subjective system.

Time standard or relative value unit (RVU) systems assign a value unit (usually a measure of time) to various activities of patient care. Those activities are usually clustered according to categories, such as diet, bathing, and mobility. There is considerable variation in the complexity of these systems (Lewis and Carini, 1984).

To develop patient classification systems, acuity definitions must be established and validated through work sampling. Warstler (1972) identifies five categories for patient classification: category I, self-care requiring from 1 to 2 hours per day; category II, minimal care requiring from 3 to 4 hours; category III, intermediate care requiring from 5 to 6 hours; category IV, modified intensive care requiring from 7 to 8 hours; and category V, intensive care requiring from 10 to 14 hours.

Regnery (1977) developed a four-level patient care classification system for public health nursing service that describes the characteristics of the family situation, psychological component, therapeutic competence, knowledge of health conditions, health attitudes, principles of general hygiene, environmental milieu, and community resources for each level. Level I is for clients who require a high degree of nursing skill, level II includes families that need regular public health nursing service, level III is for people requiring occasional service, and level IV is for clients and families requiring limited public health nursing service. Other four-level patient classification systems include category 1, minimal nursing care; category 2, moderate nursing care; category 3, considerable direct nursing care; and category 4, intensive nursing care. Another four-category system labels the labels self-, partial, complete, and intensive care.

Three-level categories have been labeled minimal, moderate, and maximal; minimal, intermediate, and intensive; and essential, progressive, and comprehensive. Nurses at the Visiting Nurse Association of Cleveland classify therapeutic visits as essential nursing care. The progressive patient care category is for the client who is achieving independence in situations requiring continuing evaluation. Clients requiring a high degree of nursing knowledge and skill are placed in the comprehensive nursing care category.

Time Standards

When figuring time standards for nursing care, one should consider both direct and indirect care. Direct care involves the patient and includes feeding, bathing, treating, and giving medications. Indirect care involves all activities that are not direct care, such as preparation of and cleaning up after medications and treatments, clinical work, reporting, communications, and coffee and lunch breaks.

Once the number and kind of care activities required by each patient are identified and the length of time it takes to do the activities calculated, one can add up the time required by all patients on a unit and divide by the number of productive work hours on a shift to determine the number of personnel needed. The mix of nursing personnel can be predicted by categorizing the care needed by the qualifications needed to give it, adding the time in each category, dividing by productive hours on a shift, and obtaining the number of specific types of personnel required to meet the patients' needs. Once this is accomplished, patients can be charged by the level of care required.

Staffing Formulas

When determining the number of staff to hire, one must consider hours needing coverage, vacations, holidays, absenteeism, and staff development time. If nurses work 5 days a week and coverage is needed for 7 days, it takes 1.4 nurses to have one nurse on duty 7 days and 2.8 to have two nurses on duty for 7 days. This is calculated by multiplying the number needed on duty by days of the week needing coverage and dividing by the number of days each employee works per week to determine the number of personnel needed for coverage. For example:

Number Needed		Days of Week		Number of Days Each Workweek		Number of People Required
1	×	7	÷	5	=	1.4
2	×	7	÷	5	=	2.8
3	×	7	÷	5	=	4.2
4	×	7	÷	5	=	5.6
5	×	7	÷	5	=	7.0

This figure does not allow for vacations, holidays, absenteeism, or staff development time.

To calculate vacation coverage, multiply the number of vacation days per year by the number of people at that skill level. Dividing the total number of vacation days per skill level by the total days worked per year per person determines the number of people needed for vacation coverage. For example:

$$\text{Number of vacation days per year} \times \text{Number of full-time people at that skill level} = \text{Total vacation days by skill level}$$

$$\text{Total vacation days by skill level} \div \text{Total days worked per person per year} = \text{Number of full-time people needed for vacation relief coverage}$$

To determine holiday coverage, multiply total number of personnel required (7-day coverage per skill level) by the number of holidays to determine the number of holiday days to be staffed. Then divide the total holiday relief days by the total days worked per year per person to obtain the number of personnel required per skill level for holiday coverage per year.

$$\text{Number of personnel} \times \text{Number of holidays} = \text{Number of holidays needing coverage}$$

$$\text{Number of holiday relief days} \div \text{Number of days worked per year per person} = \text{Number of personnel required for holiday coverage per year}$$

The percentage of absenteeism is used to calculate absentee relief coverage.

$$\text{Weeks/year} \times \text{Days worked/week} \times \text{\% of absenteeism} = \text{Absentee days/person/year}$$

$$\text{Personnel requirements (7days/week)} \times \text{Absenteeism days/person/year} = \text{Absentee coverage for staffing}$$

$$\text{Absentee coverage required} \div \text{Total days worked/person/year} = \text{Full-time personnel required for absentee coverage per year}$$

Personnel required for staff development relief per year can also be calculated.

$$\text{Number of hours required or recommended for staff development per year per person} \times \text{Number of staff} = \text{Number of hours per year for staff development needing relief coverage}$$

$$\text{Number of staff development hours needing coverage} \div \text{Hours worked/day} \div \text{Total days worked/person} = \text{Full-time personnel required for staff development coverage}$$

A staffing slide rule can be developed to save time when computing the number of budgeted positions needed to meet staffing standards by preparing a table that identifies the number of persons needed on duty, number of persons needed to cover days off, and number of persons needed to cover additional days off for vacation, holiday, sick, and personal leaves. For example:

Number Needed on Duty	Number Needed to Cover Days Off	15.6 Extra Days + 6%	18.2 Extra Days + 7%	20.8 Extra Days + 8%	23.4 Extra Days + 9%
1	1.4	1.46	1.47	1.48	1.49
2	2.8	2.92	2.94	2.96	2.98
3	4.2	4.38	4.41	4.44	4.47
4	5.6	5.84	5.88	5.92	5.96
5	7.0	7.30	7.35	7.40	7.45

Staffing to Meet Fluctuating Needs

Full-time staff.   Full-time staff may be hired to meet the average staffing needs of an institution. The most common adjustment for an increased workload is to transfer staff from a less busy area to the overloaded area. This is economical for the agency but disrupts the unity of work groups, causes the transferred nurse to feel insecure, and contributes to job dissatisfaction and turnover. Some units require specialized knowledge and skill that not every nurse has. Cross-training is helpful.

In the companion floor system, two units relieve each other. Staff nurses are oriented to the second unit and know that if they are transferred it will be to the companion unit. Thus staff aggravation is minimized, flexibility is possible, and quality of care is maintained.

At best, a complementary, or float, staff is full-time staff nurses who are oriented to many areas and like the challenge of different types of patients and settings. Unfortunately, most nurses prefer stability. Consequently, the float staff is likely to be part-time staff or new personnel waiting for a permanent assignment.

Having full-time staff work double shifts and overtime is another option. The nurse is already oriented to the area, and continuity of care is facilitated. There are also disadvantages, however. Institutional costs increase. The nurses may become tired, errors are likely to increase with fatigue, and overtime may interfere with the nurses' personal lives.

Part-time staff.   Flexible working hours can be an incentive for inactive nurses to start part-time employment and can thus reduce staffing shortages. Most nurses are women who have to combine their nursing role with many others, such as wife, mother, and homemaker. A part-time job can broaden the woman's horizons beyond her home, increase her income, give her ego satisfaction, and help her maintain her nursing skills. It is not uncommon for nurses to want to work part-time while continuing their education. Part-time nurses tend to work more than their share of unpopular hours, and some prefer evening and night duty exclusively. When part-time nurses' other responsibilities decrease, they are likely candidates for full-time work.

There are, of course, disadvantages to the use of part-time nurses. Educational and administrative expenses are higher proportionately for part-time than for full-time help. For example, it is likely to cost as much to orient a part-time as a full-time nurse, thus costing more per hours worked. Maintaining continuity of care is complicated, because two or more part-time people may fill budgeted full-time positions. There are also disadvantages for the employee. The part-time nurse may not receive benefits such as paid sick or vacation days and is not likely to be considered for promotion. Sometimes benefits are prorated for part-time workers.

Temporary help is another option. Some institutions hire temporary help for the summer to give relief for vacations. The University of Virginia Hospital in Charlottesville has used temporary bed and bath teams to reduce weekend staffing shortages (Rinker et al., 1975). Rochester Methodist Hospital in Rochester, Minnesota, has used a "premium day" approach to reduce the weekend staffing shortage. Staff nurses get an extra day off (a premium day) if they work one additional weekend within a 4-week schedule (Fisher and Thomas, 1974). Some nurses may be willing to work on an on-call basis the year around.

External temporary help agencies are available in some areas. The use of such agencies can greatly reduce the amount of time middle management must spend on staffing. The supervisor merely calls the external agency and requests so many nurses, and the agency makes the necessary contacts. The agency has a registry of available nurses who are allowed to have highly flexible, self-determined schedules. This allows some nurses to work who could not otherwise and consequently helps those nurses maintain their skills. It is then more likely for those nurses to return to nursing practice on a full-time basis than if they had remained inactive. Their availability may boost morale, and they may introduce new ideas and stimulate creativity among the regular staff.

Unfortunately, there are also disadvantages to temporary help agencies. The matching of the nurses' credentials and qualifications with assignments and orientation to assignments are severe problems. Although some temporary help agencies do keep orientation information and procedure manuals for their client institutions on file, their use may still be optional. It is likely to take considerable time for the regular staff to orient the temporary help, errors are likely to increase, and continuity of care is jeopardized. The temporary nurses get preferred schedules, leaving the regular staff with more of the less-attractive hours. Consequently, morale may be lowered.

A central placement service run by the state board of nursing or the state nurses' association could be useful for matching nurses' qualifications and interests with vacancies and anticipated vacancies throughout the state.

There are many variables to be considered when planning staffing schedules. The more accurately those variables are assessed, the better one is able to contain costs while providing high-quality care.

Rightsizing/downsizing. Declining inpatient activity and changing patient care patterns have caused some institutions to rightsize, or downsize. Proactive rightsizing measures may eliminate or minimize the need for downsizing. Rightsizing is a comprehensive and systematic process that studies ineffective, costly programs and generates ideas for replacing them with revenue-generating programs. Units that should be investigated include those where the occupancy rate is below 60%, where care-giver worked hours per patient have increased by several percentage points in a year, where fixed staffing levels have increased by a small percentage of the full-time equivalents, where productivity goals are not met, where costs exceed revenues, and where the units have been out of service (Bruce and Patterson, 1987).

Finding new work for present departments can delay the need for downsizing. Examples are contracting out continuing education and laundry services and attracting work through expanded or new services such as geriatrics. Slow times can be used for inservice personnel to increase competence, cross-training personnel to work in more than one area, carry out special projects, and update policies and procedures. Reducing overtime, encouraging use of holidays, vacation time, and leaves of absences without pay, reducing temporary help, and deferring hiring can decrease the budgetary deficit (Borg and Jensen, 1985).

Use of attrition, temporary early retirement, and conversion of full-time to part-time positions may be considered before termination. When it becomes necessary to implement layoffs, there are many issues to consider: Will they be based on seniority, job skills, job classification, or a combination of those factors? It is beneficial to involve managers from the patient care coordinator position up in deciding the criteria for layoffs. If seniority is used, is there a bumping policy? Bumping through transfers, demotions, and layoffs makes layoffs much more complicated and time-consuming, and involves about five times more people than originally targeted. People who know their positions are in jeopardy may experience more stress than those who have actually been bumped. Nurses may be angry and frustrated that they are transferred outside their specialty area. They may not be suited to their new positions and may file grievances that are time-consuming and costly to both staff and management. Many nurses would rather be laid off and be eligible for unemployment compensation than work where they do not feel qualified. Orientation and training for the new positions also cost time and money. Nurses may be too angry to orient people who will replace them. Those who are staying may worry about being responsible for inexperienced nurses placed on their units. Those who retrain may leave the institution as soon as they find another position in their area of interest. Many qualified people may leave voluntarily but discuss their unhappy experiences in the community.

There are also communication issues. Many people prefer to be informed about the layoff by personal communication rather than in writing. It is common to have a public meeting with immediate written follow-up. Many want information about why cuts are needed, the extent of the cuts, and the potential effects. They may want to be informed as soon as possible so they can make necessary arrangements.

Attention must be given to morale building through increased communication and input into decision making. A central communication office may be helpful by allowing personnel to call or stop in for clarification or information. A meeting may be scheduled to explain rules, present facts, and answer questions in an attempt to reduce anxiety. Discussion of the organization's bumping policy and procedures is particularly appropriate. Recall policy should also be discussed so that retained and laid-off personnel know their rights and responsibilities concerning future vacancies. Support groups can be formed to allow for venting anger and sharing feelings. Stress management workshops are appropriate.

A placement committee may be formed to match affected personnel to openings, or a review process implemented to respond to objections. Job skill evaluation and job counseling may be offered to affected personnel. Clear-cut procedures for matching personnel skills and openings are essential. Training opportunities to prepare for new jobs should be provided, and prospective employees should be informed of the organization's layoff policies before they are hired (Meehan and Price, 1988). Public relation efforts for community image will need attention.

Productivity.   Productivity is the product or work produced through a specific amount of resources, measured as outputs divided by inputs. For example, productivity can be measured as required staff hours divided by provided staff hours multiplied by 100. Improvements in productivity involve more work or product produced for less overall cost. Productivity can be increased by decreasing the staff hours provided while holding the required staff hours constant or increasing them. It is often measured through the patient classification system: average daily census, number of patient days per month, number of patients treated, and number of procedures performed are productivity measures.

Many actions can be taken to increase outputs while maintaining or reducing inputs. Recognizing the need to do better, involving staff, seeking staff ideas and recommendations, creating challenges, management interest in staff achievements and concerns, and praise and reward for good performance can help. Evaluating the problems, resources, and realities in the organization; using work flow analysis and work simplification procedures; and improving use of time by helping personnel keep and analyze time diaries, and decreasing waiting time can make a difference. There are many ways to improve productivity: set a climate for productivity by asking personnel what would help them be more productive and implementing their ideas. Set targets for increasing outputs. Have personnel set personal objectives and measure performance against them. Seek new approaches to old problems and improve products and services. Staff development, attention to process, ethics, and aesthetics enhance productivity through attention to doing the right things the right way (Swansburg, 1995).

BIBLIOGRAPHY

Alivizatos MS: A new concept in scheduling for nurses, *Superv Nurse* 12:20-22, February 1981.

Bauer J: Clinical staffing with a 10-hour day, 4-day workweek, JONA 1:12-14, November-December 1971.

Bennett MK, Hyton JB: Modular nursing: partners in professional practice, *Nurs Manage* 21:20-24, March, 1990.

Borg JH, Jensen DL: Managing layoffs: a comprehensive approach, *Nurs Manage* 16:31-37, August 1985.

Bruce A, Patterson D: Resizing hospital nursing organizations, an alternative to downsizing, *Nurs Manage* 18:33-35, August 1985.

Capozzi S, Glahn S: A 24-hour shift option in level one trauma ORs, *Nurs Manage* 21:96y-96z, May 1990.

Colt AM, Corley TF: What nurses think of the 10-hour shift, *Hospitals* 48:134-142, February 1974.

DeGroot HA: Patient classification system evaluation 2. System selection and implementation, *JONA* 19:24-30, July-August 1989.

Fisher DW, Thomas E: A "premium day" approach to weekend nurse staffing, *JONA* 4:59-60, September-October 1974.

Giovannetti P, Johnson JM: A new generation patient classification system, *JONA* 20:33-40, May 1990.

Hung R: Improving productivity and quality through workforce scheduling, *Indust Manage* 34:4-6, November-December 1992.

Hutchins C, Cleveland R: For staff nurses and patients—the 7-70 plan, *Am J Nurs* 78:230-233, February 1978.

Johnson JM: Quantifying an ambulatory care patient classification instrument, *JONA* 19:36-42, November 1989.

Kirk R: Using workload analysis and acuity systems to facilitate quality and productivity, *JONA* 20:21-30, March 1990.

Lewis EN, Carini PV: *Nurse staffing and patient classification: strategies for success,* Rockville, Md, 1984, Aspen.

Meehan M, Price C: Managing layoffs with minimum loss of productivity, *Nurs Adm Q* 13:26-32, Fall 1988.

Minor MA: Ten- and 6-hour nursing shifts solve staffing problem, *Hosp Prog* 52:62-66, July 1971.

Murphy CA, Watts L, Cavouras CA: The PRN plan: professional reimbursement for nurses, *Nurs Manage* 20:64q,645,64v-64x, October 1989.

Regnery G: Patient care needs: an index for community health staffing, *Nurs Adm Q* 2:79-89, Fall 1977.

Ringl KK, Dotson L: Self-scheduling for professional nurses, *Nurs Manage* 20:42-44, February 1989.

Rinker KL, Norris CL, Jordan MF: "Bed and bath teams": one solution to the weekend staffing shortage, *JONA* 4:34-35, May 1975.

Shukla RK: Effect of an admission monitoring and scheduling system on productivity and employee satisfaction, *Hospital and Health Services Administration* 35:429-441, Fall 1990.

Stenske JE, Birdi DL, Gilles DA et al: Resource teams: their structure and use, *JONA* 18:34-38, April 1988.

Strasen L: Implementing salary cost per unit of service productivity standards, *JONA* 20:6-10, March 1990.

Tonges MC: Redesigning hospital nursing practice: the professionally advanced care team (proact) model *I JONA* 19:31-38, July-August 1989.

Young SW, Daehn LM, Busch CM: Managing nursing staff productivity through reallocation of nursing resources, *Nurs Adm Q* 14:24-30, Spring 1990.

Warstler ME: Some management techniques for nursing service administration, *JONA* 2:25-34, November-December 1972.

CASE STUDY

Using the case study in the appendix, determine an assignment system to be used on one of the units at Lake View Hospital. Determine how the scheduling will be done and how shifts and workweeks will be defined (8-, 10-, 12-hour days on a permanent or rotating basis). Determine the number and level of staff needed. Discuss the rationale for and advantages and disadvantages of your decisions with your classmates.

CRITICAL THINKING AND LEARNING ACTIVITIES

Form a small group with two or three classmates and do the following activities:

1. List at least six policy issues related to staffing schedules.

2. Describe the pros and cons of centralized and decentralized scheduling, using Worksheet 15-1.

3. Identify at least three different staffing patterns and discuss the pros and cons of each, using Worksheet 15-2.

✍ Worksheet 15-1

Centralized and Decentralized Scheduling

Identify the pros and cons of centralized and decentralized scheduling.

	Centralized	Decentralized
Pros	1. 2. 3. 4. 5.	1. 2. 3. 4. 5.
Cons	1. 2. 3. 4. 5.	1. 2. 3. 4. 5.

✍ Worksheet 15-2

Staffing Patterns

Identify at least three staffing patterns and the pros and cons of each.

Staffing Patterns	Pros	Cons
1. _____	a.	a.
	b.	b.
	c.	c.
	d.	d.
	e.	e.
2. _____	a.	a.
	b.	b.
	c.	c.
	d.	d.
	e.	e.
3. _____	a.	a.
	b.	b.
	c.	c.
	d.	d.
	e.	e.

Bibliography
Part Three

Althaus JN, Hardyck NM, Pierce PB, et al: *Nursing decentralization: the El Camino experience,* Rockville, Md, 1981, Aspen.

Berger MS, Elhart D, Firsick SC, et al, editors: *Management for nurses,* ed 2, St Louis, 1980, Mosby.

Boyle JS, Andrews MM: *Transcultural concepts in nursing care,* Glenview, Ill, 1989, Scott, Foresman.

Bradford LP: *Making meetings work: a guide for leaders and group members,* La Jolla, Calif, 1976, University Associates.

Cohen EL, Cesta TG: *Nursing care management: from concept to evaluation,* St Louis, 1993, Mosby-Year Book.

Deines E: *Staffing for DRGs: a unit-specific approach for nurse managers,* Chapel Hill, NC, 1983, Ganong.

Fraser LP: *Contemporary staffing techniques in nursing,* ed 6, Norwalk, Conn, 1986, Appleton & Lange.

French WL: *The personnel management process,* ed 5, Boston, 1982, Houghton Mifflin.

Glover SM: *Recruitment and retention,* Baltimore, 1989, Williams & Wilkins.

Jelinek RC, Munson F, Smith RL: *SUM (service unit management): an organizational approach to improved patient care,* Battle Creek, Mich, 1971, Kellogg Foundation.

Kelly KJ: *Nursing staff development: current competence, future focus,* Philadelphia, 1992, JB Lippincott.

Lewis EN, Carini PV: *Nurse staffing and patient classification: strategies for success,* Rockville, Md, 1984, Aspen.

Marram G, Flynn K, Abaravich W, et al: *Cost-effectiveness of primary and team nursing,* Wakefield, Mass, 1976, Aspen.

Marram GD, Schlegel MW, Bevis EO: *Primary nursing: a model for individualized care,* St Louis, 1974, Mosby.

Mayer GG, Bailey K: *The middle manager in primary nursing,* New York, 1982, Springer.

McClure ML, Poulin MA, Sovie MD et al: *Magnet hospitals: attraction and retention of professional nurses,* Kansas City, Mo, 1983, American Academy of Nursing.

Meyer D: *GRASP Too: applications and adaptations of the GRASP nursing workload management system,* Morganton, NC, 1981, MCS.

Newcomb DP, Swansburg RC: *The team plan,* New York, 1971, Putnam's.

Popiel ES: *Nursing and the process of continuing education,* ed 2, St Louis, 1977, Mosby.

Price JL: *The study of turnover,* Ames, Ia, 1977, Iowa State University Press.

Prince J, Mueller CW: *Absenteeism and turnover of hospital employees,* Greenwich, Conn, 1986, JAI Press.

Schindler-Rainman E, Lippitt R, Cole J: *Taking your meetings out of the doldrums,* La Jolla, Calif, 1988, Pfeiffer.

Stewart CJ, Cash WB: *Interviewing: principles and practices,* ed 4, Dubuque, Ia, 1985, WC Brown.

Swansburg RC: *Team nursing: a programmed learning experience,* New York, 1989, Putnam's.

Swansburg RC: *Nursing staff development: a component of human resource development.* Boston, 1995, Jones and Bartlett.

Tobin HM, Hull PK, Wise PSY, et al: *The process of staff development,* ed 2, St Louis, 1979, Mosby.

Vistal KW: *Nursing management: Concepts and issues.* Philadelphia, 1995, JB Lippincott.

Vogt JF, Cox JL, Velthouse BA, et al: *Retaining professional nurses: a planned process,* St Louis, 1983, Mosby.

Zurlage C, editor: *The nurse as personnel manager,* Chicago, 1982, S-N Publications.

PART
Four

Direct

Nature and Purpose of Directing

After managers have planned, organized, and staffed, they must direct personnel and activities to accomplish the goals of the organization. Knowledge of one's leadership style, managerial philosophy, sources of power and authority, and political strategies is important. To get the work done by others, the manager must deal with conflict and motivate and discipline staff; all of these tasks require good communication skills and assertive behavior.

Chapter

16

Theories of Leadership

Chapter Objectives

◆ Identify the two dimensions of leadership behavior and at least three activities in each dimension.

◆ List the three aspects of a situation that structure the leader's role as identified by Fiedler in contingency theory.

◆ Identify the variable from which Hersey and Blanchard's situational leadership theory predicts the most appropriate leadership style.

◆ Describe the differences between transactional and transformational leadership.

◆ Identify at least three of the strategies for taking charge as identified by Bennis and Nanus.

◆ Outline the five basic practices and two specific behaviors for each practice as identified by Kouzes and Posner in *The Leadership Challenge.*

Major Concepts and Definitions	
Lead	to show, mark the way, guide the course
Transaction	the negotiation of business
Transformation	a change in the nature of someone or something
Charisma	an inspirational quality that some leaders possess
Situational	appropriate to the needs of different situations
Contingency	the uncertainty of an event's occurrence

THEORIES OF LEADERSHIP

Theories of leadership are numerous. The following survey covers the alternatives, beginning with the oldest notion and advancing to ideas currently in vogue. By familiarizing themselves with them, nurses can select and adapt the most suitable approach for dealing with different situations. As a role model, the nursing leader can reduce the autocratic atmosphere and, hence, some of the role conflicts.

Great Man Theory

The great man theory argues that a few people are born with the necessary characteristics to be great. Leaders are well rounded and simultaneously display both instrumental and supportive leadership behavior. Instrumental activities include planning, organizing, and controlling the activities of subordinates to accomplish the organization's goals. Obtaining and allocating resources such as people, equipment, materials, funds, and space are particularly important. Supportive leadership is socially oriented and allows for participation and consultation from subordinates for decisions that affect them. People who use both instrumental and supportive leadership behaviors are considered "great men" and supposedly are effective leaders in any situation. Many find this theory unattractive because of its premise that leaders are born and not made, which suggests that leadership cannot be developed.

Charismatic Theory

People may be leaders because they are charismatic, but relatively little is known about this intangible characteristic. What constitutes charisma? Most agree that it is an inspirational quality possessed by some people that makes others feel better in their presence. The charismatic leader inspires others by obtaining emotional commitment from followers and by arousing strong feelings of loyalty and enthusiasm. Under charismatic leadership, one may overcome obstacles not thought possible. However, because charisma is so elusive, some may sense it while others do not.

Yukl (1989) has reported findings from House's, Bass's, and Conger and Kanungo's research about charisma. House found that followers of charismatic leaders trust the leader's beliefs; have similar beliefs; exhibit affection for, obedience to, and unquestioning acceptance of the leader; and are emotionally involved in and believe they can contribute to the mission. House found that charismatic leaders had a strong conviction in their own beliefs, high self-confidence, and a need for power. They are likely to set an example by their behavior, communicate high expectations to followers and express confidence in them, and arouse motives for the group's mission.

Conger and Kanungo's research approached charisma as an attributional phenomenon. They found that charisma is more likely attributed to a leader who advocates a vision discrepant from the status quo, emerges during a crisis, accurately assesses the situation, communicates self-confidence, uses personal power, makes self-sacrifices, and uses unconventional strategies.

Bass proposed that charismatic leaders perceive themselves as having supernatural purpose and destiny and that followers may idolize and worship them as spiritual figures or superhumans. This blind obedience can lead to bad outcomes such as group suicide. Transformational leaders use charisma for good.

Trait Theory

Until the mid-1940s, the trait theory was the basis for most leadership research. Early work in this area maintained that traits are inherited, but later theories suggested that traits could be obtained through learning and experience. Researchers identified the leadership traits as energy, drive, enthusiasm, ambition, aggressiveness, decisiveness, self-assurance, self-confidence, friendliness, affection, honesty, fairness, loyalty, dependability, technical mastery, and teaching skill. Asking themselves what traits leaders possessed, various researchers arrived at different conclusions, but identified some common leadership traits:

1. Leaders need to be more intelligent than the group they lead. However, a highly intelligent person may not find leadership responsibilities challenging enough, may prefer to work with abstract ideas and research, and may have difficulty relating to the group.
2. Leaders must possess initiative, the ability to perceive and start courses of action not considered by others.
3. Creativity is an asset. Having originality—the ability to think of new solutions to problems and ideas of new ways to be productive—is helpful.
4. Emotional maturity with integrity—a sense of purpose and direction, persistence, dependability, and objectivity—is another important trait. Mature leaders do what they say they will and are consistent in their actions. They often work long hours, apply themselves intensely, and spread enthusiasm to followers. Energy, drive, and good health are necessary to endure the long hours, overcome obstacles, and sustain continuous achievement. Self-assurance is self-confidence. It is hoped that leaders perceive themselves as effective problem solvers who can successfully handle the difficulties that confront them.
5. Communication skills are important. The leader needs to understand others and speak and write clearly.
6. Persuasion often is used by leaders to gain the consent of followers. The leader may make suggestions, supply supportive data, ask penetrating questions, make compromises, and request action to persuade others.

7. Leaders need to be perceptive enough to distinguish their allies from their opponents and to place their subordinates in suitable positions.
8. Leaders participate in social activities. They can socialize with all kinds of people and adapt to various groups. Approachable, friendly, and helpful, they gain the confidence and loyalty of others in such a way that makes people willing to cooperate.

The trait theory expanded knowledge about leadership, but it was not without its flaws. Few, if any, traits are identified in all trait theory research. They are not mutually exclusive, and there is considerable overlap between categories or definitions of the characteristics. It is not clear which traits are most important, which traits are needed to acquire leadership, and which traits are needed to maintain it. Trait theory does not view personality as an integrated whole, does not deal with subordinates, and avoids environmental influences and situational factors.

Ohio State Leadership Studies researchers compiled a list of about 1800 examples of leadership behavior that factored out two dimensions: consideration and initiating structure. Consideration involves behaving in a friendly and supportive way, looking out for others' welfare, showing concern, treating others as equals, taking time to listen, consulting others on important matters, being willing to accept suggestions, and doing personal favors.

Initiating structure is the way the leader structures roles to attain the goals. It includes assigning tasks, defining procedures, setting deadlines, maintaining standards, suggesting new approaches, and coordinating activities.

Researchers at the University of Michigan focused on identification of relationships among leader behavior, group process, and group performance. They found that three types of leadership behavior marked the difference between effective and ineffective leaders: (1) task-oriented behavior, (2) relationship-oriented behavior, and (3) participative leadership. Task-oriented behavior includes planning, scheduling, and coordinating activities. Relationship-oriented behavior includes acting friendly and considerate, showing trust and confidence, expressing appreciation, and providing recognition. Participative leadership uses group meetings to enlist associate participation in decision making, improve communications, promote cooperation, and facilitate conflict resolution.

Situational Theory

Situational theories became popular during the 1950s. These theories suggest that the traits required of a leader differ according to varying situations. Among the variables that determine the effectiveness of leadership style are factors such as the personality of the leader; the performance requirements of both the leader and followers; the attitudes, needs, and expectations of the leader and followers; the degree of interpersonal contact possible; time pressures; physical environment; organizational structure; the nature of the organization; the state of the organization's development; and the influence of the leader outside the group. A person may be a leader in one situation and a follower in another or a leader at one time and a follower at others, because the type of leadership needed depends on the situation.

**Box
16-1**   **GROUP-ATMOSPHERE SCALE**

Describe the atmosphere of your group by checking the following items:

	8	7	6	5	4	3	2	1	
1. Friendly	:	:	:	:	:	:	:	:	Unfriendly
2. Accepting	:	:	:	:	:	:	:	:	Rejecting
3. Satisfying	:	:	:	:	:	:	:	:	Frustrating
4. Enthusiastic	:	:	:	:	:	:	:	:	Unenthusiastic
5. Productive	:	:	:	:	:	:	:	:	Nonproductive
6. Warm	:	:	:	:	:	:	:	:	Cold
7. Cooperative	:	:	:	:	:	:	:	:	Uncooperative
8. Supportive	:	:	:	:	:	:	:	:	Hostile
9. Interesting	:	:	:	:	:	:	:	:	Boring
10. Successful	:	:	:	:	:	:	:	:	Unsuccessful

From Fiedler FE: *A theory of leadership effectiveness*, New York, 1967, McGraw-Hill, p. 269.

Contingency Theory

During the 1960s, Fred Fiedler introduced the contingency model of leadership. Refuting the ideal leadership style theory, he argued that a leadership style will be effective or ineffective, dependent on the situation. He identified three aspects of a situation that structure the leader's role: (1) leader-member relations, (2) task structure, and (3) position power.

Leader-member relations involve the amount of confidence and loyalty the followers have in their leader. Leadership is assessed by a group-atmosphere scale. Fiedler also used a sociometric index of the least-preferred co-worker (LPC) score (Box 16-1). Followers were asked to think of everyone they have ever worked with and to rate the least-preferred co-worker on an eight-point bipolar adjective scale, which includes adjectives such as friendly and cooperative. A high score describes the person in favorable terms, and a low score is a negative rating. Although the LPC scores are difficult to interpret and it is hard to say what they measure, Fiedler suggests that high scorers are relationship oriented and low scorers are mostly task oriented.

Task structure is high if it is easy to define and measure a task. The structure is low if it is difficult to define the task and to measure progress toward its completion. Fiedler used four criteria to determine the degree of task structure: (1) goal clarity: goal understood by followers; (2) extent to which a decision can be verified: know who is responsible for what; (3) multiplicity of goal paths: number of solutions; and (4) specificity of solution: number of correct answers. Technical nursing, which focuses on

Table 16-1   Summary of Fiedler Investigations of Leadership

	Group Situation			Leadership Style Correlating with Productivity
Condition	Leader-Member Relations	Task Structure	Position Power	
1	Good	Structured	Strong	Directive
2	Good	Structured	Weak	Directive
3	Good	Unstructured	Strong	Directive
4	Good	Unstructured	Weak	Permissive
5	Moderately poor	Structured	Strong	Permissive
6	Moderately poor	Structured	Weak	No data
7	Moderately poor	Unstructured	Strong	No relationship found
8	Moderately poor	Unstructured	Weak	Directive

From Donnelly JH Jr, Gibson JL, Ivancevich JM: *Fundamentals of management functions, behavior, models,* Dallas, 1981, Business Publications. © 1981 by Business Publications, Inc.

procedures, may have a high task structure, but situations involving human relations and value judgments may have numerous solutions with no specific correct answer and consequently have low task structure.

Position power refers to the authority inherent in a position, the power to use rewards and punishment, and the organization's support of one's decisions. Directors of nursing, managers, and sometimes patient care coordinators have high position power with the right to hire and fire, promote, and adjust salaries. People with low position power may be elected, function in an acting position, or be subject to removal by peers or subordinates. Elected committee chairpersons have low position power. Team leaders and staff nurses usually have low position power. Given the critical conditions, Fiedler argues that one can predict the most productive leadership style (Table 16-1).

If a task is structured but the leader is disliked and therefore needs to be diplomatic, or if the task is ambiguous and the leader is liked and therefore seeks the cooperation of the workers, the considerate, accepting leadership style probably will be most productive. When a disliked leader faces ambiguous tasks, a directive style is more productive. The most productive leadership style is contingent on the situational variables.

Empirical evidence does not supply conclusive evidence for the contingency model. It is difficult to say what the psychologically distant manager and psychologically closer manager measures are really recording. Correlations were used for predicted direction even when they were not statistically significant. The model is primarily academic in that it has not been used in management development for improving group performance and organizational effectiveness, and Fiedler's complex, three-dimensional contingency model has contributed to leadership theories.

Path-Goal Theory

Robert J. House derived the path-goal theory from the expectancy theory. The expectancy theory argues that people act as they do because they expect their behavior to produce satisfactory results. In the path-goal relationship, the leader facilitates task accomplishment by minimizing obstructions to the goals and by rewarding followers for completing their tasks. The leader helps staff associates assess needs, explores alternatives, helps associates make the most beneficial decisions, rewards personnel for task achievement, and provides additional opportunities for satisfying goal accomplishment.

House noted that studies done during the 1950s revealed that leaders who structured activities for staff associates generally had more productive work groups and got higher performance evaluations from superiors. Structure includes planning, organizing, directing, and controlling through activities such as clarifying expectations of staff associates, scheduling work, making assignments, determining procedures, and setting standards. Structured activity can increase motivation by reducing role ambiguity and allowing for externally imposed controls. In contrast, considerate leaders had more satisfied workers. They created an atmosphere of friendliness, warmth, and support by tending to the personal welfare of their subordinates. Leader consideration seems particularly important for routine jobs. People who perform a variety of tasks may find their jobs more satisfying and have less need for social support.

House recognized that individual differences will affect the staff associates' perception of leader behavior. For instance, experienced staff associates may prefer a task-oriented style, whereas less mature, less experienced, and consequently less secure individuals may prefer a considerate leader. Staff associates with a high need for achievement probably will prefer a task-oriented leader, but people with a high need for affiliation will prefer a considerate leader. The path-goal theory introduced staff associates as a variable.

Situational Leadership Theory

The situational leadership theory predicts the most appropriate leadership style from the level of maturity of the followers. Paul Hersey and Kenneth H. Blanchard illustrate this theory in a four-quadrant model (Fig. 16-1). A horizontal continuum registers low emphasis on the accomplishment of tasks on the left side of the model to a high emphasis on task behavior on the right side. The vertical continuum depicts low emphasis on interpersonal relationships at the bottom of the model to high emphasis on relationships at the top. The lower left quadrant, therefore, represents a laissez-faire type of leadership style with little concern for production or relationships. The lower right quadrant represents an autocratic leadership style with considerable concern for production but little concern for relationships. The upper right quadrant designates a high concern for both tasks and relationships. The left upper quadrant represents a leadership style that stresses relationships but shows little concern for tasks.

The maturity level of the group or individual is depicted on a continuum from high maturity on the left to low maturity on the right under the four quadrants. The

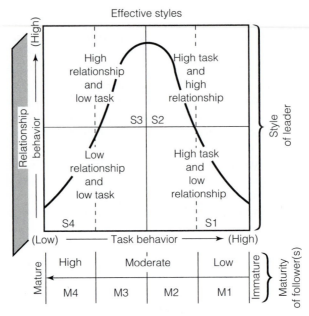

Figure 16-1 Situational leadership theory. (From Hersey P, Blanchard KH: *Management of organizational behavior: utilizing human resources,* ed 3, Englewood Cliffs, NJ, 1977, Prentice Hall, p. 194. © 1977. Reprinted by permission of Prentice Hall, Englewood Cliffs, New Jersey.)

maturity levels are superimposed on the quadrants with dashed lines. The best leadership style for given levels of maturity is shown by a curvilinear line in the four quadrants. To determine the most appropriate leadership style, one must assess the maturity level of the individual or group, plot it on the maturity continuum, and project a line at a right angle from that point until it intersects with the curvilinear line. The quadrant in which the intersection occurs depicts the most appropriate leadership style. With increased maturity, less structure and emotional support are needed. In contrast, high-task and low-relationship style is considered best for below-average maturity. The leadership styles in quadrants 2 and 3 are recommended for the average group or individual.

This model is consistent with Argyris's immaturity-maturity continuum, which indicates that as people mature, they progress from a passive to an active state and from dependence to independence. With maturity they pass from a need for structure and little relationship through a decreasing need for structure and increasing need for relationship to little need for either. The progression is not always smooth. Stress may cause members of the group to regress, and leaders must adjust their behavior accordingly. The situational leadership theory therefore emphasizes the importance of the maturity level of the group, and the leader needs to adapt leadership styles accordingly.

Transformational Leadership

Transactional leaders organize groups around their personal goals and believe that others are also motivated by personal goals. They are likely to use coercion and

**Box
16-2**   **VIEWS OF TRANSFORMATIONAL LEADERSHIP**

Bass (1985)	Bennis and Nanus (1985)	Kouzes and Posner (1987)	Bass and Avolio (1993)	Hitt (1993)

Character-istics of transfor-mational leadership:
• Charisma
• Inspirational leadership
• Individualized consideration
• Intellectual stimulation
	Strategies for taking charge:
	
	• Attention through vision
	• Meaning through communi-cation
	• Trust through positioning
	• Deployment of self
		Basic leadership practices:
		
		• Challenging the process
		• Inspiring a shared vision
		• Enabling others to act
		• Modeling the way
		• Encouraging the heart
			Character-istics of transfor-mational leaders:
			• Idealized influence
			• Inspirational motivation
			• Intellectual stimulation
			• Individual-ized con-sideration
				Types of knowl-edge needed by leaders and core functions of leaders:
				• Types of knowledge
				  Knowing oneself
				  Knowing the job
				  Knowing the organization
				  Knowing the business
				  Knowing the world
				• Core functions
				  Valuing
				  Visioning
				  Coaching
				  Empowering
				  Team building
				  Promotes quality

rewards. Transformational leaders motivate others through values, vision, and empowerment. Box 16-2 summarizes the key points of several views of transformational leadership.

Bass (1985) has described transformational leaders in terms of charisma, inspirational leadership, individualized consideration, and intellectual stimulation.

Bennis and Nanus (1985) indicate that leaders do the right things, whereas managers do things right. Leaders focus on effectiveness, managers deal with efficiency. Bennis and Nanus identified four strategies for taking charge: (1) attention through vision, (2) meaning through communication, (3) trust through positioning, and (4) deployment of self. The leader's vision needs to be clear, attractive, and attainable. Communication through stories, allegories, fables, parables, analogies, and so on helps give meaning to the vision. The leader's position must be clear because associates are more likely to be trusting when they know the leader's view of the organization. Open communications, honesty, and consistency are important to building trust. Leaders are continuous learners and use the organization as a learning environment. They deploy themselves as they foster a learning environment.

Kouzes and Posner (1987) identified five basic practices and ten specific behaviors that leadership involves: (1) challenging the process by searching for opportunities and experimenting and taking risks, (2) inspiring a shared vision by envisioning the future and enlisting others, (3) enabling others to act by fostering collaboration and strengthening others, (4) modeling the way by setting an example and planning small wins, and (5) encouraging the heart by recognizing individual contributions and celebrating accomplishments.

Bass and Avolio (1993) indicate that transformational leaders change the organization by realigning the organization's culture with the new vision and revision of assumptions, values, and norms. They identify four components that characterize transformational leaders: (1) idealized influence, (2) inspirational motivation, (3) intellectual stimulation, and (4) individualized consideration. They believe that organizations should maintain a base of effective transactional qualities while moving in the direction of transformational qualities.

Hitt (1993) defines leadership as affecting people so that they will strive willingly toward group goals. He identified five types of knowledge needed by a leader: (1) knowing oneself, (2) knowing the job, (3) knowing the organization, (4) knowing the business, and (5) knowing the world. He also identified six core functions of leaders: (1) valuing, (2) visioning, (3) coaching, (4) empowering, (5) team building, and (6) promoting quality. He listed the attributes essential for leadership as identity, independence, authenticity, responsibility, courage, and integrity.

Integrative Leadership Model

From a review of leadership theories, obviously there is no one best leadership style. Leaders are rarely totally people or task oriented. Leader, followers, situation—all influence leadership effectiveness. Consequently, an integration of leadership theories seems appropriate. Leaders need to be aware of their own behavior and influence on others, individual differences of followers, group characteristics, motivation, task structures, environmental factors, and situational variables, and adjust their leadership style accordingly. Leadership behavior needs to be adaptive.

BIBLIOGRAPHY

Andrews M: Importance of nursing leadership in implementing change, *Br J Nurs* 2:437-439, April 22-May 12, 1993.
Austin NK: Supervising without spying, *Incentive* 167:13, October 1993.
Baker AM: An emerging leadership paradigm, *Nurs Health Care* 12:204-207, April 1991.
Balutis AP: Leadership in a time of change, *Public Manager* 21:21-23, Fall 1992.
Bass BM: From transactional to transformational leadership: learning to share the vision, *Organ Dyn* 18:19-31, Winter 1990.
Bass BM, Avolio BJ: Transformational leadership and organizational culture, *Publ Adm Q* 17:112-121, Spring 1993.
Bennis WG: The four competencies of leadership, *Train Dev J* 38:4-9, August 1984.
Blanchard K: Situational view of leadership, *Executive Excellence* 8:22-23, June 1991.
Boumans MPG, Landeweerd JA: Leadership in the nursing unit: relationships with nurses' well-being, *J Adv Nurs* 18:767-775, May 1993.
Capowski G: Anatomy of a leader: where are the leaders of tomorrow? *Manage Rev* 83:10-17, March 1994.

Carr C: Empowered organizations, empowering leaders, *Training and Development* 48:39-44, March 1994.

Covey SR: Top and bottom lines, *Executive Excellence* 10:3-4, October 1993.

Davidhizar R: Leading with charisma, *J Adv Nurs* 18:675-679, April 1993.

Deeprose D: Team leader or unit boss: which do you want to be? *Superv Manage* 37:3, July 1992.

Dunham J, Klafehn KA: Transformational leadership and the nurse executive, *JONA* 20:28-33, April 1990.

Fincke MK: Orchestrating team building for harmonious leadership, *Accident and Emergency Nursing* 1:229-233, October 1993.

Gilmore TN: Effective leadership during organizational transitions, *Nurs Econ* 8:135-141, May-June 1990.

Havens DS: Nursing involvement in hospital governance 1990 and 1995, *Nurs Econ* 10:331-335, September-October 1992.

Hay J: Creating community: the task of leadership, *Leadership and Organization Development Journal* 14:12-17, 1993.

Hern-Underwood M, Kenner CA: Leadership behaviors of pediatric nurse managers, *Pediatr Nurs* 17:587-589, November-December 1991.

Hersey P, Blanchard KH, LaMonica EL: A situational approach to supervision: leadership theory and supervising nurse, *Superv Nurse* 7:17-22, May 1976.

Hitt WD: The model leader: a fully functioning person, *Leadership and Organization Development Journal* 14:4-11, 1993.

House RJ: A path goal of leader effectiveness, *Adm Sci Q* 16:321-338, September 1971.

House RJ: Mitchell TR: Path-goal theory of leadership, *J Contemp Bus* 3:81-97, Fall 1974.

Irurita V: Transforming mediocrity to excellence: a challenge for nurse leaders, *Australian Journal of Advanced Nursing* 9:15-25, June-August 1992.

Kiechel W: The leader as servant, *Fortune* 125:121-122, May 4, 1992.

Manthey M: Trends: shifting patterns of authority, *Nurs Manage* 21:14-15, October 1990.

Manthey M: Leadership: a shifting paradigm, *Nurs Educ* 17:5, 14 September-October 1992.

McDaniel C, Wolf GA: Transformational leadership in nursing service: a test of theory, *JONA* 22:60-65, February 1992.

Miller FA: Leadership strategies for professional development, *Journal of National Black Nurses' Association* 5:54-60, 1992.

Pinkerton SE: St. Michael Hospital: a shared governance model, *Nurs Adm Q* 13:35-47, 1989.

Ryan SA: A new decade of leadership: from vision to reality, *Nurs Clin North Am* 25:597-604, September 1990.

Sheafor M: Productive work groups in complex hospital units: proposed contributions of the nurse executive, *JONA* 21:25-30, May 1991.

Simms LM: The professional practice of nursing administration: integrated nursing practice, *JONA* 21:37-46, May 1991.

Stivers C: Why can't a woman be less like a man? Women's leadership dilemma, *JONA* 21:47-51, May 1991.

Wolf GA, Boland S, Aukerman M: A transformational model for the practice of professional nursing: the model part 1, *JONA* 24:51-57, April 1994.

Zurlinden J, Bongard B, Magafas M: Situational leadership: a management system to increase staff satisfaction, *Orthop Nurs* 9:47-52, March-April 1990.

CASE STUDY

You are a new patient care coordinator. The previous one was very autocratic. How will you begin changing from the autocratic atmosphere to a participative style?

CRITICAL THINKING AND LEARNING ACTIVITIES

1. Using Worksheet 16-1, write your philosophy of leadership and discuss it with a classmate.

2. Using Table 16-1 (p. 272), describe the atmosphere where you work or study.

3. Using Figure 16-1 (p. 274), consider your maturity level, where you fit on the four-quadrant model, and what type of leadership you want and need.

✍ **Worksheet 16-1**

Philosophy of Leadership

Write your philosophy of leadership, using the questions below to guide you:

• What characteristics/traits does an effective leader possess?

• What specific behaviors does an effective leader exhibit?

• What activities are appropriate to a leader?

Chapter

17

Development of Management Thought

Chapter Objectives

◆ Identify at least two theorists in each of the management eras: scientific management, classic organization, human relations, and behavioral science.

◆ Identify at least five of the concepts stressed in each management era.

◆ Compare Maslow's, Herzberg's, and McGregor's theories.

◆ Describe each of Likert's four types of management systems.

Major Concepts and Definitions	
Management	act of planning, organizing, staffing, directing, and controlling
Scientific management	focused on the best way to do a task
Classic organization	focused on planning, organizing, and controlling of the organization as a whole
Human relations	focused on the effect individuals have on the success of the organization
Behavioral science	focused on scientific validation

DEVELOPMENT OF MANAGEMENT THOUGHT

A familiarity with the development of management thought can be useful to nursing leaders in creating their own management styles. No single management theory is sufficient in itself to guide the nursing leader's every action. But through an eclectic approach, drawing from the best and most applicable theories in each situation, nurse administrators can create individual management styles to meet their particular needs.

Scientific Management

Theories of management do not remain static. Since the introduction of the earliest principles of scientific management nearly a century ago, management thought has been marked by constant change.

Taylor.   Frederick W. Taylor (1856-1915) is generally recognized as the father of scientific management. Through the use of stopwatch studies, he applied the principles of observation, measurement, and scientific comparison to determine the most efficient way to accomplish a task. Taylor conducted time-and-motion studies to time workers, analyze their movements, and set work standards. He usually found that the same result could be obtained in less time with fewer or shorter motions. When the most efficient way to complete a task was determined, workers were trained to follow that method. The most productive workers were hired, and even when they were paid an incentive wage, labor costs per unit were reduced.

Taylor, an engineer in steel manufacture, applied his pioneering experience in scientific management to the service of Bethlehem Steel in 1898 and later became an independent business consultant. Identifying the responsibilities of management and separating them from the functions of the workers, Taylor threw aside rule-of-thumb judgments and developed a systematic approach to determine the most efficient means of production. He considered management's function to be planning. Working conditions and methods had to be standardized to maximize production. It was management's responsibility to select and train workers rather than allow them to choose their own jobs and methods and train themselves. An incentive plan whereby workers were paid according to their rates of production was introduced to minimize worker dissent and reduce resistance to improved methods, increase production, and produce higher profits. Taylor's scientific management reduced wasted efforts, set standards for performance, encouraged specialization, and stressed the selection of qualified workers who could be developed for a particular job. His *Shop Management* (1911) and *The Principles of Scientific Management* (1912) spread his ideas throughout Europe and America.

Gilbreth. Frank B. Gilbreth (1868-1924) and Lillian M. Gilbreth (1878-1972) also did pioneering work in time-and-motion studies. They emphasized the benefits of job simplification and the establishment of work standards as well as the effects of the incentive wage plans and fatigue on work performance. As an apprentice bricklayer, Frank Gilbreth was instructed differently by each workman on how to lay bricks. To add to his confusion, the men used one set of motions to teach him, another for a slow pace, and still another for a fast pace. Wondering what methods would be most efficient, the young bricklayer started studying the workers' motions. Gilbreth reduced the number of motions required to lay a brick from 18 to 4 by developing a new way to stack bricks; developed an adjustable stand to eliminate excessive stooping, bending, and walking back and forth; and prescribed a mortar consistency that prevented excessive tapping on the brick with a trowel. His system of "speed work" eliminated haste and also increased work output by cutting out unnecessary motions. Workers could be paid higher wages because they accomplished more in a shorter time.

The Gilbreths were among the first to use motion-picture films to analyze workers' motions. Because early cameras did not work at a steady speed, Gilbreth developed a microchronometer, a clock with a large hand measuring 1/2000 of a minute. The clock was photographed with the task and used to study motion patterns. A small, blinking electric bulb was attached to the worker's hand so speed and direction of movement could be studied. For his study of hand motions, Gilbreth developed 17 classifications for hand movements, such as "find," "select," "grasp," "position," and "rest," which he labeled "therbligs" (*Gilbreth* spelled backward with the *th* transposed). The Gilbreths also developed the flow diagram and the process chart to record their observations. The work process was diagramed to indicate operations, delays, inspection, transportation, and storage, and the process was then studied to shorten, combine, or eliminate steps. The Gilbreths recommended written instructions to prevent misunderstandings and started a merit-rating system for workers.

Lillian Gilbreth is known as the first lady of management. Her doctoral dissertation, *The Psychology of Management* (1914), was published with the author listed as L.M. Gilbreth, thus obscuring the fact that she was a woman. It was one of the first contributions toward understanding human factors in industry. Her work on the effects of fatigue complemented her husband's efforts. The Gilbreths and their twelve children are the subjects of the popular book *Cheaper by the Dozen*.

Gantt. Henry L. Gantt (1861-1919), a disciple of Taylor, also was concerned with problems of efficiency. He contributed to scientific management by refining previous work rather than introducing new concepts. The Gantt chart, a forerunner of the PERT chart, depicts the relationship of the work planned or completed on one axis to the amount of time needed or used on the other. Gantt also developed a task and bonus remuneration plan whereby workers received a guaranteed day's wage plus a bonus for production above the standard to stimulate higher performance. Gantt recommended that workers be selected scientifically and provided with detailed instructions for their tasks. He argued for a more humanitarian approach by management, placing emphasis on service rather than profit objectives, recognizing useful nonmonetary incentives such as job security, and encouraging staff development.

Emerson. Appearing before the Interstate Commerce Commission in 1910, Harrington Emerson (1853-1936) testified that the railroads could save $1 million a day by using principles of scientific management. Emerson, one of the first management consultants, originated the term *efficiency engineering*. With emphasis on conservation and the organization's goals and objectives, he defined 12 principles of efficiency. Five are related to interpersonal relations and seven to systems in management: (1) goals and ideas should be clear and well defined, the primary objective being to produce the best product as quickly as possible at minimal expense; (2) changes should be evaluated—management should not ignore "common sense" by assuming that bigness is necessarily better; (3) "competent counsel" is essential; (4) management can strengthen "discipline," or adherence to the rules, by (5) justice, or equal enforcement on all; (6) records, including adequate, reliable, and immediate information about the expenses of equipment and personnel, should be available as a basis for decisions; (7) dispatching or production scheduling is recommended; (8) standardized schedules, (9) standardized conditions, and (10) standardized operations can be facilitated through the use of (11) written instructions; (12) "efficiency rewards" should be given for successful completion of tasks. Emerson moved beyond scientific management toward classic organizational theory.

Cook. Morris Cook (1872-1960) applied scientific management to university settings and municipal management. Studying the cost of input efforts and the resulting outputs of teaching and research, he found that management practices in education were lacking. Committee management was inefficient, inbreeding was common, and departmental autonomy undermined university coordination. Cook recommended a student hour as the standard by which to measure the efficiency of professional time. He also recommended extensive use of assistants so that more expensive faculty time could be used for more sophisticated tasks. Cook felt that professors should spend their time teaching and conducting research rather than working on committees and should leave administration to specialists. He advocated establishment of professional salaries on the basis of merit rather than longevity, discontinuance of tenure, and retirement of unfit teachers.

As director of public works in Philadelphia, Cook initiated efficient methods for personnel selection, inventory recording, equipment replacement, financial planning, subcontracting, standardization, public relations, and complaint handling. After his work there, he founded his own consulting firm.

Classic Organization

Classic administration-organization thinking began to receive attention in 1930. Deductive rather than inductive, it viewed the organization as a whole rather than focusing solely on production. Managerial activities were classified as planning, organizing, and controlling. The concepts of scalar levels, span of control, authority, responsibility, accountability, line-staff relationships, decentralization, and departmentalization became prevalent.

Fayol.   Henri Fayol (1841-1925), known as the "father of the management process school," was a French industrialist concerned with the management of production shops. Fayol studied the functions of managers and concluded that management is universal. All managers, regardless of the type of organization or their level in the organization, have essentially the same tasks: planning, organizing, issuing orders, coordinating, and controlling.

Fayol derived some general principles of administration from his observations. A believer in the division of work, he argued that specialization increases efficiency. Fayol recommended centralization through the use of a scalar chain or levels of authority, responsibility accompanied by authority, and unity of command and direction so that each employee receives orders from only one superior. He believed that although individual interests should be subordinated to agency interest, workers should be allowed to think through and implement plans and should be adequately remunerated for their services. Fayol encouraged development of group harmony through equal treatment and stability of tenure of personnel. A firm believer in order, he advocated "a place for everything and everything in its place." He also urged that management be taught in the colleges.

Weber.   Max Weber (1864-1920), a German sociologist, earned the title of "father of organization theory" by his conceptualization of bureaucracy with emphasis on rules instead of individuals and on competence over favoritism as the most efficient basis for organization. He conceptualized a structure of authority that would facilitate the accomplishment of the organizational objectives. The three bases of authority, according to Weber, are (1) traditional authority, which is accepted because it seems things have always been that way, such as the rule of a king in a monarchy; (2) charisma, typified by Abraham Lincoln and Otto von Bismarck; and (3) rational legal authority, which is considered rational in formal organizations because the person has demonstrated the knowledge, skill, and ability to fulfill the position. Weber recognized that if subordinates do not believe a person qualified for the position, they may not accept that person's authority.

Favoring a rational, legal basis for authority, he suggested the avoidance of traditional and charismatic leadership through systematic selection of personnel. Administrators are chosen for their competence; their authority is clearly defined; they are given legal means for exercising their authority; and continuity of administration is provided. In Weber's bureaucracy, administrators are appointed, not elected. They are career officials who work for fixed salaries and do not own what they administer. Like other personnel, they are subject to strict rules that are applied impersonally and uniformly. All personnel are selected for competence; the division of labor, authority, and responsibility is clearly defined; and positions are organized into a hierarchy.

Mooney.   Working independently of Fayol and Weber, James Mooney (1884-1957) formed similar ideas. Mooney believed management to be the technique of directing people and organization the technique of relating functions. Organization is management's responsibility. Mooney enumerated four universal principles of organization: (1) coordination and synchronization of activities for the accomplishment of a goal can be accomplished in part through (2) functional effects, the performance of one's job description, and (3) scalar process organizes (4) authority into a hierarchy. Consequently, people get their right to command from their position in the organization.

Urwick.   Lyndall Urwick (1891-1939) integrated the ideas of Henri Fayol and James Mooney with those of Frederick Taylor. His conceptual framework blended scientific management and classic organization theory into the beginnings of classic management theory. He described the managerial process as planning, coordinating, and controlling, and he popularized such concepts as the balance of authority with responsibility, span of control, unity of command, use of general and special staffs, the proper utilization of personnel, delegation, and departmentalization.

Human Relations

The human relations movement began in the 1940s with attention focused on the effect individuals have on the success or failure of an organization. Classic organization and management theory concentrates on the physical environment and fails to analyze the human element; human relations theory stresses the social environment. The chief concerns of the human relations movement are individuals, group process, interpersonal relations, leadership, and communication. Instead of concentrating on the organization's structure, managers encourage workers to develop their potential and help them meet their needs for recognition, accomplishment, and sense of belonging.

Barnard.   Chester Barnard (1886-1961) studied the functions of the executive while he was a manager for the New Jersey Bell Telephone System. Barnard saw the manager's responsibility as defining objectives, acquiring resources, and coordinating activities. Stressing the importance of cooperation between management and labor, he noted that the degree of cooperation depends on nonfinancial inducements, which informal organization can help provide. Formal channels of communication must be known and should be as short as possible. Barnard said authority depends on acceptance by the followers, and he stressed the role of informal organizations for aiding communication, meeting individuals' needs, and maintaining cohesiveness. Because small units are the building blocks for complex organizations, the worker contributes to the large organization as well as the basic work unit. Barnard's work, which was done at the end of the classic period before human relations were emphasized, influenced the development of a behavioral focus.

Follett. In the 1920s, Mary Parker Follett (1868-1933) stressed the importance of coordinating the psychological and sociological aspects of management. Perceiving the organization as a social system and management as a social process, she considered subordination offensive. Follett distinguished between power with others and power over others and indicated that legitimate power is produced by a circular behavior whereby superiors and subordinates mutually influence one another. The law of the situation dictates that a person does not take orders from another person but from the situation. For instance, nurses will work through their lunch break during an emergency. The problem with this idea is that it is difficult for workers to know the total situation. Follett advocated that managers study the total situation to achieve unity, because she believed that control would be obtained through cooperation among all of the elements, people, and materials. Her work was a link between the classic and human relations eras.

The Hawthorne Studies. The Hawthorne studies, though criticized for poor research methods, stimulated considerable interest in human problems on the job. Conducted at the Chicago Hawthorne plant of Western Electric by researchers from Harvard University under the direction of the psychologist Elton Mayo (1880-1949) and reported by the sociologist Fritz Rothlesberger, the studies investigated the effects of changes in illumination on productivity. Lighting was changed for the experimental group but remained constant for the control group. As the illumination was increased for the experimental group, the production of both groups increased. When it was decreased for the experimental group, production continued to increase for both groups until the level of illumination reached moonlight, at which point there was a significant decrease in output. The researchers concluded that lighting had little effect on production. The effects of the number and length of work breaks, refreshments, length of workdays and workweeks, temperature, and humidity were observed on five volunteers with little or no effects shown. A group piecework incentive plan was studied. The researchers anticipated that fast workers would pressure slow workers to increase their output. However, they found that group norms were set and workers were pressured not to be rate-busters by overproducing or chiselers by underproducing. Workers slacked off when it became apparent that they could meet the rate for the day. Work norms obviously had more influence than wage incentive plans. The Hawthorne studies gave the human relations movement its thrust.

Lewin. In the early 1930s, Kurt Lewin (1890-1947), a Jewish psychologist, fled from Germany to the United States, where he revived the study of group dynamics. Lewin maintained that groups have personalities of their own: composites of the members' personalities. He showed that group forces can overcome individual interests. He confirmed the importance of group control over output and coined the terms *life space, space of free movement,* and *field forces* to describe group pressures on individuals.

Lewin advocated democratic supervision. His research indicated that democratic groups in which participants solve their own problems and have the opportunity to consult with the leader are most effective. Autocratic leadership, on the other hand, tends to promote hostility and aggression or apathy and to decrease initiative. Conducting experiments during World War II to change people's eating habits to consumption of more organ meats, he found that only 3% of the women who attended lectures (autocratic method) changed their behavior, but 32% of the women who participated in a discussion after the lecture (democratic method) started eating more organ meats. Lewin was one of the first to apply Gestalt psychology to the study of individual personality.

Moreno. Jacob L. Moreno (1892-1974) developed sociometry to analyze group behavior. Claiming that people are either attracted, repulsed, or feel indifferent toward others, he developed the sociogram to chart pairings and rankings of preferences for others. This process of classification can be used to calculate which workers are capable of harmonious interpersonal relationships. With this knowledge, work groups can be organized with a predicted minimum of disruptive tendencies, for maximal efficiency, and for promotion of high morale. Moreno also contributed to psychodrama (individual therapy), sociodrama (related to social and cultural roles), and role-playing techniques for the analysis of interpersonal relations.

Behavioral Science

During the 1950s, advocates of the behavioral sciences became concerned that much scientific, classic, and neoclassic or human relations management had been accepted without scientific validation. Behavioral science emphasized the use of scientific procedures to study the psychological, sociological, and anthropological aspects of human behavior in organizations. Behavioral scientists indicated that management is not strictly a technical process, that it cannot be haphazard, and that it should not be executed through authority. Rather, they stressed the importance of maintaining a positive attitude toward people, training managers, fitting supervisory action to the situation, meeting employees' needs, promoting employees' sense of achievement, and obtaining commitment through participation in planning and decision making.

Maslow. Abraham Maslow (1908-1970) initiated the human behavioral school in 1943 with his development of a hierarchy-of-needs theory. He outlined a hierarchical structure for human needs classified into five categories: (1) physiological, (2) safety, (3) love, (4) esteem, and (5) self-actualization. The physiological needs are the most important and the most necessary for survival. They include the need for oxygen, water, food, sleep, sex, and activity. Safety includes freedom from danger, threat, and deprivation, such as physical harm, economic distress, ill health, and unnecessary, unexpected occurrences. Love needs are composed of affectionate relations with others, acceptance by one's peers, recognition as a group member, and companionship. Esteem comprises self-respect, positive self-evaluation, and regard by others. Self-actualization is composed of self-fulfillment and achievement of one's full capacity. In Maslow's hierarchy, physical needs must be met before other needs become prepotent, and so on, and the satisfaction of self-actualization needs is possible only after all other needs are met. Once a need is satisfied it is no longer a motivator, and the next need becomes prepotent. As a need begins to be satisfied, it decreases in importance as a motivator in relation to other needs, some of which are never completely satisfied and never completely cease to motivate.

Maslow's work has been very influential in management and has stimulated subsequent research. Although Maslow's outline is correct in general, human needs

Although there is considerable communication, both upward and downward, it has limited accuracy and is accepted with some caution. Managers are quite familiar with the problems faced by their staff associates. Broad policy is set at the top with delegation; goals are set after discussion; and there is decision making throughout the organization. Control functions are delegated to lower levels where reward and self-guidance are used. Sometimes an informal organization resists the formal goals.

Participative management, the fourth system, is associated with the most effective performance. Managers have complete confidence in their staff associates. Staff associates' ideas are always sought, and they feel completely free to discuss their jobs with the manager. Goals are set at all levels. There is a great deal of communication—upward, downward, and sideways—that is accurate and received with an open mind. Managers are very well informed about the problems faced by their staff associates, and the decision making is well integrated throughout the organization with full involvement of staff associates. Because goals are established through group action, there is little or no resistance to them. There is not an informal organization resisting the goals of the formal organization, because the goals of both are the same. Control is widely shared through the use of self-guidance and problem solving.

Likert is a strong proponent of participative management and supportive relationships. His linking-pin concept is based on studies about the differences between good and poor managers as measured by their level of productivity. Good managers were found to have more influence on their own managers than did poor managers, and their managerial procedures were better received by their staff associates. Consequently, Likert suggests that managers form groups for supportive relationships and that those groups be linked by overlapping groups of managers. This facilitates three-way communications—upward, downward, and sideways. When middle managers have the opportunity for interaction with their manager, workers can have input, and there is a chance for the individual's and the organization's goals to become similar (Fig. 17-3).

Blake and Mouton. Robert Blake (1918-) and Jane Mouton (1930-) maintain that the two critical dimensions of leadership are (1) concern for people and (2) concern for

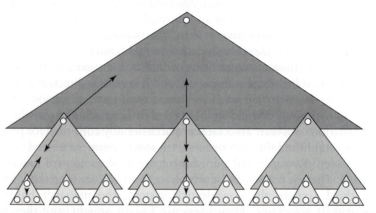

Figure 17-3 Linking-pin concept. Arrows indicate linking-pin function. (From Likert R, Likert JG: *New ways of managing conflict,* New York, 1976, McGraw-Hill, p 184.)

production, which they depict on a 9×9 or 81-square managerial Grid® (Fig. 17-4). The two dimensions are independent, so a manager can be high on both, low on both, or high on one and low on the other. The vertical axis represents the manager's concern for people, and the horizontal axis represents concern for production. Each axis is on a 1-to-9 scale from a minimal concern for people or production to a maximal concern. The five basic styles are located at each corner and in the middle.

The task manager at 9,1 has the highest regard for production and the lowest concern for people. This manager stresses operating efficiency through controls and views people as tools of production. Workers are paid to do what they are told without questioning.

As reflected on the Grid, 1,1 management is impoverished. The manager has a lack of concern for both production and people. This style may be found in some managers who feel they have been repeatedly denied promotion or otherwise mistreated and who have consequently compensated through a low level of involvement with their jobs. The organization-man management at 5,5 represents a moderate concern for

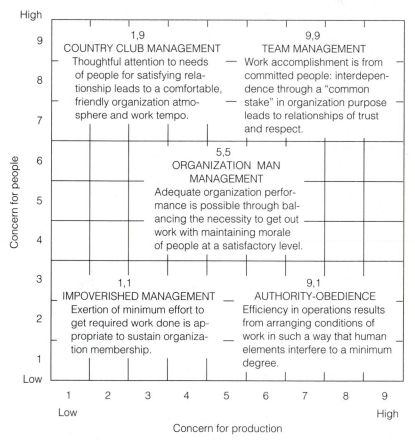

Figure 17-4   Managerial grid. (From Blake RR, Mouton JS: *The new managerial grid,* Houston, 1978, Gulf Publishing, p 11. Reproduced by permission.)

both people and production but not necessarily at the same time. The manager's emphasis shifts. The country club manager, 1,9, is thoughtful and friendly but has little concern for production.

Blake and Mouton consider team management, 9,9, the optimal managerial style. These managers integrate their concern for people and production. Problems are confronted directly, and mutual trust, respect, and interdependence are fostered.

Fiedler.   During the 1960s, Fred Fiedler (1922-) introduced the contingency model of leadership effectiveness. He identified three important dimensions of a situation for his contingency model: (1) leader-member relations, (2) task structure, and (3) position power. Leader-member relations are related to the amount of confidence and loyalty followers have in their leader. Task structure is related to the number of correct solutions to a problem. Position power depends on the amount of organizational support available to the leader.

Hersey and Blanchard.   Paul Hersey (1930-) and Kenneth H. Blanchard (1939-) extended the work of Blake, Mouton, and Fiedler by considering the maturity of the followers in more detail. As the maturity of one's followers increases, the leadership style requires less structure and emotional support. Groups with below-average maturity function best under leaders with high task-low relationship orientations. Groups with average maturity function best under leaders with high task-high relationship or high relationship-low task orientations. The most effective leadership style depends on the maturity of the group.

Drucker.   In his prolific writings about management, Peter Drucker (1909-) maintains that the only way for management to justify its existence is through economic results. However, he recognizes noneconomic consequences of managerial decisions, such as job satisfaction, as by-products of the focus on economic performance. He identifies three areas of management: managing (1) a business, (2) managers, and (3) workers. Activity, decision, and relations analyses are recommended to determine the structure and organization needed. Drucker has studied the advantages and disadvantages of decentralization, supports decentralization, and says managers should create markets and products rather than being passive.

Drucker introduced management by objectives as a way to manage managers. Relying on self-control instead of control from above, managers are directed by objectives of performance rather than by their manager. For management by objectives, the manager develops the framework, and the staff associate supplies the goals, which are agreed on by both. The staff associate gives progress reports to the manager. Objectives are developed for every level of management in the hierarchy and each unit in the organization. The manager checks objectives for compatibility with other units and contribution to the objectives at the next level of the hierarchy. Drucker maintains that it is more productive for workers to set their own norms and measure their own performance than for minimal standards to be set.

For managing the worker, Drucker recommends that jobs be designed to fit the worker, that workers be given more control over their jobs, and that the worker be considered the most vital resource in the agency.

Odiorne.   George S. Odiorne (1920-1992), director of the Bureau of Industrial Relations of the University of Michigan, was previously assistant director of personnel for General Mills, Inc., where he pioneered the installation of a management-by-objectives system. He advocates effective management through personal and agency goals and has written about the executive's responsibilities for implementing a management-by-objectives system. He also recommends training by objectives as an economic strategy for management training.

Implications for Nursing Administration

Surveying the development of management thought, one can see that there has been a trend from autocratic to democratic management and from a focus on efficiency to a greater regard for the well-being of personnel. Although the focus has changed, elements from each era maintain their validity and can be used by the nurse administrator. For example, Taylor's time studies and the Gilbreths' motion studies in the scientific era are illustrations of how the nurse can study complexity of care to predict staffing needs and study efficiency of nursing care. An adaption of Gantt's chart can be used to visualize the time element of planning and controlling, and the nurse administrator is well advised to heed Emerson's early notion of the importance of objectives in agencies. Nursing education could become more efficient by implementing some of Cook's recommendations.

Nurse administrators should be aware of their managerial tasks as defined by Fayol: planning, organizing, directing, coordinating, and controlling. His definition of management can help clarify the manager's role, and his principles of management can help direct one's actions. Assistance with the organizing function can be obtained from Weber's conceptualization of bureaucracy and authority and Urwick's popularization of such concepts as balancing authority with responsibility, unity of direction, unity of command, and span of control.

To a large extent the social environment results from organization and management. The work of Barnard, Follett, Mayo, and Lewin during the human relations era should remind the nurse administrator of the importance of developing workers to their potential and meeting their needs for recognition, accomplishment, and sense of belonging. It is hoped that nurse administrators will consider the results of Kurt Lewin's research about autocratic and democratic leadership when determining their own style. They can use Moreno's sociometry to study the group behavior of workers.

Much has been learned about management from the behavioral science studies. The nurse can apply Maslow's hierarchy-of-needs theory to the care of individual patients, to functions of individual workers, or to groups of people. The importance of achievement, recognition, responsibility, and advancement as motivators and satisfiers is stressed in Herzberg's two-factor theory. McGregor, Argyris, Likert, Blake, and Mouton's research all support the benefits of positive attitudes toward people, development of workers, satisfaction of their needs, and commitment through participation. Fiedler indicates that a leadership style may or may not be effective depending on the situation. Nurse administrators can use his work to assess their work situation to determine the most effective style or choose the work situation according to what fits their style best. The leader can also incorporate Drucker's and Odiorne's work on management by objectives for the planning, directing, and controlling phases of the management process.

By studying the development of management thought, nurse administrators can define their management role, develop their philosophy of management, learn tools and techniques for implementation of their responsibilities, and gain an increased understanding of how to work with others to accomplish goals.

BIBLIOGRAPHY

Anderson B: Voyage to shared governance, *Nurs Manage* 23:65-67, November 1992.

Basile F: What kind of manager are you? *Journal of Property Management* 55:48-49, May-June 1990.

Blanchard K, Wakin E: Managing: different styles for different people; give people feedback, not criticism, *Today's Office* 26:20-23, August 1991.

Consolvo CA: Financial management for nurse managers—the bottom line or renewal, *Journal of Continuing Education in Nursing* 22:245-247, November-December 1991.

Crawford DI: The glass ceiling in nursing management, *Nurs Econ* 11:335-341, November-December 1993.

Davidhizar R: Participative management: the power of positive manipulation, *Today's OR Nurse* 11:18-21, November 1989.

Davis PA: Unit-based shared governance, *JONA* 22:46-50, December 1992.

Dienemann J, Shaffer C: Nurse manager characteristics and skills: curriculum implication, *Nurs Connec* 6:15-23, Summer 1993.

Fulmer RM: Nine management development challenges for the 1990s, *Journal of Management Development* 11:4-9, 1992.

Hannah BA: The essence of leadership: facing the challenge of being the new manager, *Journal of Post Anesthesia Nursing* 8:43-47, February 1993.

Hempstead N: Nurse management and leadership today, *Nurs Stand* 6:37-39, May 6-12, 1992.

Jackson B: Mentorship in nurse management, *Nurs Stand* 5:36-39, June 19-25, 1991.

Johnson P: Business ethics is an inside job, *Journal of Management Development* 11:44-48, 1992.

Jung FD: Teaching registered nurses how to supervise nursing assistants, *JONA* 21:32-36, April 1991.

Katz R: Cluster management, *AACN Clin Issues Crit Care Nurs* 3:743-748, Nov 1992.

Kidwell J: Nursing management in an endoscopy setting, *Gastroenterol Nurs* 15:23-32, Aug 1992.

Knippen JT, Green TB: Coaching, *Management Accounting* 71:36-38, May 1990.

Manion J: Chaos or transformation? Managing innovation, *JONA* 23:41-48, May 1993.

Marriner A: Theories of leadership, *Nurs Leadership* 1:13-17, Dec 1978.

Marriner A: Development of management thought, *JONA* 9:21-31, Sept 1979.

Marriner A: Management moves, *Nurs Success Today* 3:8-13,, Aug 1986.

Merrett L: Developing nurses into managers, *Nurs Stand* 5:32-36, May 1-7, 1991.

Mills J: The nurse manager as mentor, *Pediatr Nurs* 17:493, Sept-Oct 1991.

Minnen TG, Berger E, Ames A et al: Sustaining work redesign innovations through shared governance, *JONA* 23:35-40, July-Aug 1993.

Muller PA: Leadership versus management: a matter of focus, *Journal of Post Anesthesia Nursing* 6:361-363, Oct 1991.

Patz JM, Biordi DL, Holm K: Middle nurse effectiveness . . . human management skill, *JONA* 21:15-24, Jan 1991.

Phifer L: Managerial leaders and their influence in nursing, *Pediatr Nurs* 16:322, May-June 1990.

Shaw S: Nurses in management: new challenges, new opportunities, *Int Nurs Rev* 36:179-184, Nov-Dec 1989.

Sonnenberg FK: A strategic approach to employee motivation, *Journal of Business Strategy* 12:41-43, May-June 1991.

Starke FA, Rempel E: Dealing with practical problems in nursing management, *Canadian Journal of Nursing Administration* 5:27-31, Nov-Dec 1992.

Suters ET: Inspirational management, *Executive Excellence* 8:15-16, Feb 1991.

Tyrrell RA: Visioning: an important management tool, *Nurs Econ* 12:93-95, March-April 1994.

Zipple AM, Selden D, Spaniol L et al: Leading for the future: essential characteristics of successful psychosocial rehabilitation program managers, *Psychosoc Rehibil J* 16:85-94, April 1994.

CASE STUDY

You have just accepted the nursing leadership role in a long-term care facility. Identify the management process and list the activities you will need to do to plan, organize, staff, direct, and evaluate.

CRITICAL THINKING AND LEARNING ACTIVITIES

1. List five major desires. In which categories of Maslow's hierarchy of needs do they belong? Do your needs fluctuate from time to time?

2. Make a list of what was happening when you felt job satisfaction and another list of what was happening when you felt job dissatisfaction. Compare and contrast the lists. Do they support Herzberg's motivation hygiene theory?

3. Consider the characteristics of Theory X and Theory Y managers. Which would you rather work with? Which do you want to be? What can you do to become the type of manager you want to be?

Chapter

18

Power and Politics

Chapter Objectives

- ◆ Identify at least five sources of power.
- ◆ Describe ways to communicate with legislators.
- ◆ Describe the process by which a bill becomes a law.
- ◆ Describe principled negotiations.
- ◆ Compare hard and soft negotiation tactics.

CHAPTER 18   POWER AND POLITICS • **299**

Major Concepts and Definitions

Power	one's capacity to influence others
Reward	something given in recompense for a good deed
Coercive	restraining, constraining, or curbing in nature
Legitimate	logically correct
Referent	a type of power based on identification with a leader and what that leader symbolizes
Expert	skillful, having knowledge and training
Authority	legitimate power determined by structure
Politics	authoritative allocation of scarce resources
Negotiation	bargaining process

POWER, AUTHORITY, AND POLITICS

Power and authority are closely related and often confused. Power is one's capacity to influence others, whereas authority is the right to direct others. One's power may be greater or less than the authority of the position. Authority is obtained through position power, but several other sources of power exist (see Box 18-1). Politics uses legitimate power.

Sources of Power

Reward.   Much of a manager's power comes from the ability to reward others for complying. When the staff associate perceives that managers have the ability to provide something valued, the manager has reward power. Sources of reward power include money, desired assignments, provision of personal space, or the acknowledgment of accomplishments. Rewards contribute to an independent system.

Coercive power.   Coercive power is the opposite of reward power and is based on fear of punishment if one fails to conform. Undesired assignments, embarrassment in front of others, withheld pay increases, and termination are sources of coercive power that contribute to a dependent system.

 Box 18-1   SOURCES OF POWER

Reward	Referent
Coercive	Expert
Legitimate	Informal

Legitimate power.   Their official positions in the organizational hierarchy give managers legitimate power. Legitimate power gives the manager the right to influence and the staff associate an obligation to accept that influence. The director of nursing has more legitimate power than the manager, who in turn has more legitimate power than the head nurse. Cultural values that give a person the right to prescribe appropriate behavior for another (such as parents for children), social structures involving a hierarchy of authority, and election processes to legitimize a person's right to an office are bases for legitimate power.

Referent power.   Referent power is based on identification with a leader and what that leader symbolizes. The leader is admired and exerts influence because the followers desire to be like the leader.

Expert power.   People gain expert power through knowledge, skills, and information. Their expertise gains them respect and compliance. Knowledge of the organization and its rules, regulations, and work flow helps one to acquire power over others who need the knowledge to meet their responsibilities.

Informal sources of power.   Informal sources of power are related to one's personal power rather than position power. Some people have situational power because they happen to be in the right place at the right time. Others have personal power because of their unique characteristics.

Education, experience, drive, and decisiveness are viewed positively and help establish credibility. The person with these qualities may be viewed as reliable, and therefore others are willing to cooperate. Attractiveness gains an individual access to people who will help promote the cause, because people enjoy being around others who have a happy temperament, generate a sense of well-being, and foster goodwill in others. Location also influences others, because individuals communicate more with people who are located near them in the organization, and communication increases their opportunities to influence. For instance, full voting membership on powerful committees places one in close proximity for persuading other members and provides the opportunity to confront, negotiate, and solve problems. In general, people are most comfortable with others who share similar values, beliefs, and customs. Social pressure from people who share social norms encourages others to conform to those norms. Coalitions strengthen one's power base. Consequently, friendships and associations with people can be a source of power.

Interpersonal relationships also provide access to the informal communication network. Doing favors for others so that they owe you favors creates an obligation-based power. One may gain power by default when there is no one else available or by autonomy when the decision is one's own to make. Control of resources, such as information, procedures, equipment, and personnel, also strengthens one's power base. Religion, politics, race, and national origin are bases for establishing power in some situations but interfere with power bases in others. For example, a nurse of a certain faith may be given priority for a job on the staff of an institute run by that faith, but religion may be held against the person seeking position at a hospital affiliated with another religion or denomination.

Power Relations

Power is interpersonal. It is a dependence relationship. Person x has power over person y to the extent that y depends on x for goal attainment. The power varies inversely to the availability of goals outside the particular interpersonal relationship. If nurses want to work for a hospital but do not care whether they work for one head nurse or another, they reduce the head nurses' power. Motivational investment in the goals being mediated is a variable. The nurse who wants to work in intensive coronary care is far more dependent on one head nurse than the nurse who is willing to work on several units. Cost of goal achievement is also a factor. Nurses may not be willing to work straight nights to work on the unit of their choice. A staff nurse may not be willing to hassle with a grievance procedure to get what is deserved. Sources of dependence are numerous: knowledge, skills, interpersonal relations, and organizational authority.

Predictable behaviors occur when there is a conflict of interest among people with power. Coalition is a technique to strengthen one's power. It involves uniting to gain a sense of strength. Whether coalition occurs or not, there will probably be bargaining in an attempt to negotiate the conflict. One may leave the situation if bargaining is ineffective or adjust to lessened power if alternative positions are not readily available.

It is useful to assess one's power in a relationship before engaging in conflict. Although there is no magic formula to assess one's power, there are considerations that help identify one's power in relation to that of others. Who is the most powerful? The person who appears the most powerful may not be. Communication patterns help assess who actually has the power. The person who structures the options has more power, whereas the person who does more accommodating probably has less power. The person with the least interest in maintaining the relationship has more power. Those who gain the most from ritualized patterns have the most power, because institutionalized norms reinforce the existing power structure, and people who try to maintain the status quo are probably protecting their own power. People who are aware of their sources of power can use that knowledge, but people are often unaware of their sources of power and consequently are unable to use those sources effectively.

Kinds of Power

In *Power and Innocence* Rollo May has identified five kinds of power. Exploitative power is the most destructive type. It subjects people to whatever use the power holder chooses. Slavery is an example. Manipulative power is influence over another person that may have been invited because of the person's desperation and anxiety. Operant conditioning is an example of manipulative power. Competitive power is energy used against another. One person wins and another loses, although neither the gain nor the loss is necessarily related to merit. An example is the competition of several people for one position. One person wins, and the others lose—even if they were well qualified for the job. Nutrient power, such as parents' caring for their children, teachers' caring for students, and politicians' caring for their constituents, is influence used for others. Integrative power is cooperative power with others. A person can possess the five types of power at different times.

Authority

Authority is legitimate power. It is determined by structure, which involves rules, roles, and relations. Rules legitimize authority and tend to suspend the subordinate's critical faculties. Subordinates tend to do unquestioningly what the superior with legitimate authority tells them to do. Role is position or office. Authority is inherent in the position, not in the person. Relations are related to credibility, which is obtained through knowledge and expertise.

Authority is traditionally structured as line or staff. Line authority refers to levels of authority and superior-subordinate relationships, and it therefore provides the framework for the organization. Staff authority has no command privileges. It has only the right to advise or assist managers in the performance of their duties. Staff members provide assistance when requested, must sell their ideas to the manager over whom they have no authority, and must sell their ideas up the line to managers who have the line authority to implement the ideas. More recently, functional authority, or authority of the specialist, has emerged. Functional authority is normally limited to the performance of defined duties for a limited period of time.

It is preferable for a manager's power to be equitable to the authority of the position. Knowledge, experience, drive, and decisiveness help achieve power. Being attractive, visible, and available are sources of informal power. More formal sources of power available to nurse managers are control of resources, reward and coercive power, association with other powerful people, and legitimate power derived from the managerial position. The nurse manager's knowledge of sources of power can help assess and use them.

Politics

Politics is the authoritative allocation of scarce resources. It requires legitimate power to distribute goods, services, and other resources that are less abundant than desired. A political system is a social system that gets people to do what they would not ordinarily want to do. There are several theories that help explain the dynamics of political systems. According to *game theory,* politics is a fascinating game with rules, referees, and players on opposing sides. *Elite theory* purports that political power is concentrated with people who hold top positions in large centralized institutions. These people tend to have a unified purpose because of similar social backgrounds and interests and consequently have stable power. *Pluralist theory* explains that political life is based on competition between interest groups. The influence of political groups is determined by their political organization, strategies, and leadership. These competitive relationships are unstable because interest groups and related alliances are short-lived and new coalitions and interest groups develop as old ones decline. The power of interest groups is limited by dependence on other groups and the need for compromises. *Exchange theory* states that political behavior is based on the exchange of resources. People decide what they want, what it will cost, and whether they have the resources to exchange for it.

Levels of political participation.   There are levels of political participation ranging from apathetic inactivists who engage in no political activity to complete activists who engage in numerous activities. As nurses become involved in politics, they can expand their influence beyond a single vote. Spectator political activities include gathering political information, displaying bumper stickers or wearing buttons, initiating political discussions, trying to persuade others, and voting. As one becomes increasingly involved, one can make financial contributions, attend political meetings, and contact political leaders. Activists become active members in political parties, attend caucus meetings, contribute time to political campaigns, solicit funds, and run for offices.

Nurse managers can encourage others to become more politically active by educating them in issues, posting and circulating information, and encouraging staff discussion of political topics. They can educate and encourage others to work with legislators by providing formal classes on the legislative process, a list of key contacts, and information about voting records. The nurse manager can encourage participation in professional organizations, consumer groups, boards, legislative committee meetings and hearings, and political functions. Staff members can be sent to testify at hearings and be assigned to attend political activities. The manager can generally support political activities, exemplify political involvement, encourage others to vote, and grant release time for political participation.

Communicating with legislators.   Nurse administrators have found that communicating with legislators, building coalitions, being knowledgeable about current issues, providing testimony, solving problems, educating and involving other nurses, and knowing the legislator before needing help are the most successful political strategies. Less effective political strategies include mass mailings, petitions, demonstrating, and relying on others to protect nurses' interests. Factors that have contributed to unsuccessful political outcomes include emotionalism, lack of preparation, lack of unity among nurses, failure to build an adequate power base, failure to attend political meetings, failure to contact policymakers until too late, lack of publicity, and lack of feedback from politicians, other nurses, and community members.*

Legislators spend so much time in sessions and at committee meetings that it can be difficult to reach them by telephone. A letter is a written record that requires a written reply and is more likely to reach the legislator. Letters should be kept brief, preferably one and not more than two pages. A personal letter is more effective than a form letter or a petition. The title and number of the bill one is addressing and a brief interpretation of it should be included. One's position should be stated succinctly. The name and address of the writer need to be legible, and when possible writers should identify themselves as nurses and voters in the legislator's district. One must use discretion in selecting a time to discuss an interest with a legislator. It is preferable not to talk to legislators who are engrossed in activities related to another bill; wait until they can give their full attention to one's concerns. Appointments are set up ahead of time. The nurse should prepare a short, well-written statement of what legislative action is preferred and why, specifying the direct impact it will have on the legislator's constituents. The points should be concise and accompanied with news clippings,

---

* Political strategies are reported in Archer SE, Goehner PA: Acquiring political clout: guidelines for nurse administrators, *JONA* 11:49-55, Nov-Dec 1981.

research reports, and other supportive documentation. It is preferable to deal with one issue at a time.

One should know the party of which the legislator is a member and address him or her as a representative or senator, as appropriate, to show respect. One should be specific and reasonable about what is wanted and should ask legislators to do only what is within their power. A dialogue can be continued by writing to express gratitude for the meeting and by sending new information as it becomes available.

Organizing political meetings.   Nurse managers can take the initiative to organize political meetings. It is best to start with a small group with political and organizing experience. The group should include all organizations and important people willing to be involved. One should compile lists of members of organizations, agency directories, officers, names from newspaper articles, and so on. Personal time and money will be needed to type, copy, and mail invitations as well as for refreshments, room rental, supplies such as name tags and agendas, and follow-up correspondence.

The meeting should be held at a neutral meeting site. A map should be included with the invitation. A self-addressed, stamped response postcard and request for correction of address and telephone number should also be enclosed. Brief handouts and name tags should be prepared in advance of the meeting. A minimum of food should be served. The atmosphere of the political meeting should be kept comfortable and professional.*

The legislative process.   Because the legislative process is complex and technical, nurses need to know the process to determine when to intervene. The state legislative process is similar to the national process that follows. First, legislation is introduced. These legislative proposals originate in a number of ways, but most originate in the executive branch. However, either individuals such as members of Congress or groups such as interest groups may introduce legislation.

Next, there is committee referral. A bill is considered read for the first time when it is referred to a committee. Only a member of Congress can introduce legislation. There is no limit to the number of bills a member may introduce. In the House of Representatives and the Senate, a bill is numbered according to its place in the order of introduction, referred to committee, labeled with the sponsor's name, and printed by the Government Printing Office. Bills are prefixed with HR when introduced in the House of Representatives and S when introduced in the Senate. After referral to a standing committee, most legislation is referred to a subcommittee. Most bills go no further. Each bill introduced must pass the House of Representatives and the Senate in identical form within 2 years to become a law.

After referral to a standing committee and a subcommittee, hearings are held by the subcommittee. Often only a few members of the subcommittee who have a special interest in the subject will participate in the hearings. The chairperson uses the agenda, funds, and staff to expedite, delay, or modify legislation. The subcommittee usually schedules public hearings and invites testimony from private and public witnesses.

---

*From Davis CK, Oakley D, Sochalski JA: Leadership for expanding nursing influence on health policy, *JONA* 12:15-21, Jan 1982.

Interested individuals submit written requests to testify. Once they are informed of when to testify, rescheduling is not allowed. If one cannot be present at the designated time, one may file a written statement for the record of the hearing. Witnesses who share common positions are urged to consolidate testimony and designate a single spokesperson. Groups with similar concerns that are unwilling to have a single spokesperson may form panels. Panelists are allowed a 6-minute presentation of the key points in their written documents and are urged to avoid repeating other presentations. All witnesses are required to file a written statement with the committee at least a day before the scheduled appearance or the preceding Friday if the testimony is to be on Monday or Tuesday. The statement should be typed on letter-sized paper and include a summary of the principal points. Witnesses should not read their written statements but should summarize the key points in no more than 6 minutes. Once the testimony has been given, each subcommittee member may ask questions.

If, after the hearing, the subcommittee members decide the legislation should go further, they consider the language line by line and section by section to determine the language of the final bill, which is then recommended to the full committee.

When presenting the bill to the floor of the House or Senate, the full committee justifies its actions in a written report that accompanies the bill. Bills that are unanimously voted out of committee have a good chance on the floor. However, dispute is likely to occur on the floor if there has been a divided committee.

After a bill has passed one house, it is sent to the other, where the same process takes place. If the second house approves the bill as it was passed by the first, it is sent to the president for his signature. However, if the bill was revised or amendments added, the bill must be returned to the originating chamber for approval of the changes. If that body refuses to approve the revised bill, both versions are sent to a conference committee. The bill is sent to the president for signature or veto after the differences are reconciled and there is a final vote of acceptance by the conference committee. In the case of a presidential veto, both houses can override the veto to make the bill law.*

Negotiation

Two major ways of negotiating have been identified: hard and soft. The hard negotiator wants to win and believes that the side that takes an extreme position and holds out longer benefits more. Unfortunately, hard negotiators often exhaust themselves and their resources and harm relationships. On the other hand, the soft negotiator prevents conflict and makes concessions quickly to reach an agreement. The soft negotiator ultimately feels exploited and bitter.

Principled negotiation is another option for negotiation that is neither hard nor soft. This method decides issues on their merits, looks for mutual gains, and insists on fair standards. It is hard on merits and soft on people. There are four basic points to principled negotiations: (1) separate the people from the problem, (2) focus on interests instead of positions, (3) generate a variety of options before deciding what to

---

*The legislative process is discussed in more detail in Kalisch BJ, Kalisch PA: *Politics of nursing,* Philadelphia, 1982, JB Lippincott.

**Box
18-2** **PRINCIPLED NEGOTIATIONS**

---

1. Separate the people from the problem

2. Focus on interests, not positions

3. Generate a variety of options before deciding what to do

4. Insist on objective data

---

do, and (4) insist that the result be based on an objective standard (see Box 18-2). Fisher and Ury discuss these strategies in detail in *Getting to Yes*.

Positional bargaining is typical; each side takes a position and argues for it. Negotiations then involve taking and giving up positions successively. The more one defends a position the more committed one becomes to it and the more difficult it becomes to revise the position. Egos become involved, and "saving face" is an issue. Besides producing unwise agreements, positional bargaining is inefficient. The more extreme the opening position and the smaller the concessions, the longer it takes to reach an agreement. Positional bargaining also damages ongoing relationships.

During the analysis phase, one tries to gather and organize data and to diagnose the situation. One notes the people problems, hostile emotions, unclear communications, interests, and options and standards already identified. During the planning phase, each of the four principles is again considered and additional options and criteria are generated. During discussions, differences in perceptions, feelings such as frustration and anger, and difficulties in communication can be identified and addressed. There can be mutual exploration of how to meet each party's concerns by using objective standards. Negotiations that focus on interests, mutually satisfying options, and fair standards are likely to reach sound agreements.

When separating the people from the problem, understanding others' thinking is critical because that thinking is the problem. Activities include discussing each other's perceptions, trying to put yourself in their shoes, avoiding blaming them for your problem, getting them involved and committed through participation, and making your proposal consistent with their values. It is also important to understand both your and their emotions; make the emotions explicit and acknowledge them as legitimate; let them ventilate; do not react to their emotional outbursts; and use symbolic gestures of friendship such as shaking hands, embracing, eating together, apologizing, and sending a note of congratulations or sympathy.

Communications are critical to negotiations. One should listen actively and acknowledge what is being said. Speak calmly to be understood. Speak about yourself instead of about them. Speak with a purpose. Build working relationships and face the problem, not the people.

Focus on interests instead of positions because the conflicts among needs, desires, concerns, and fears are the problem. Look for shared and compatible interests as well as conflicting ones. Realize that each side has multiple interests and that the most

Box 18-3   **THREE STEPS IN NEGOTIATING**

1. Recognize the tactic
2. Raise the issue explicitly
3. Question the tactic's legitimacy and desirability

powerful interests are the basic human needs for security, belonging, recognition, and control.

Next, invent options for mutual gain. Separate inventing options from judging them. During brainstorming generate as many ideas as possible without judging them. After brainstorming note the most promising ideas and invent improvements on them. Later, evaluate the ideas and the ramifications of implementing them. Then decide on the best options. Each side may want different things from the same item so look for ways to dovetail differing interests. Try to make the desired option so appealing that the decision is easy.

Finally, insist on objective criteria for reaching wise agreements amicably and efficiently. Look for fair standards and fair procedures such as parliamentary procedure.

Some players will not play fairly. Some assert their position, attack your ideas, and even attack you. First, do not attack the idea: look behind it to see what the person's interest is. Second, do not defend your idea; invite criticism and advice instead. Third, reframe the attack on you as an attack on the problem. When attacked, do not counterattack. Break the vicious cycle by refusing to attack. Avoid pitting your strength against theirs directly. Instead of resisting their force, channel their energy into exploring interests, generating options that are mutually acceptable, and finding independent standards.

Some negotiators use dirty tricks such as deliberate deception by misrepresenting the facts, using ambiguous authority, and seeking dubious intentions. They employ psychological warfare by using stressful situations, personal attacks, and threats. Positional pressure tactics such as refusal to negotiate, extreme demands, escalating demands, and calculated delay are also common devices. There are three steps in negotiating the rules when the other side uses dirty tricks (see Box 18-3): (1) recognize the tactic, (2) raise the issue explicitly, (3) question the tactic's legitimacy and desirability by using principled negotiations. Separate the people from the problem. Focus on interests instead of positions. Invent options for mutual gain and insist on objective criteria (Fisher and Ury).

Peter Block describes negotiating with allies and adversaries in *The Empowered Manager*. He presents a grid with agreement increasing up the vertical axis and trust increasing to the right of the horizontal axis (see Fig. 18-1). Adversaries are represented by low agreement and low trust in the lower left quadrant; opponents are represented by low agreement and high trust in the lower right quadrant. Allies are indicated by high agreement and high trust in the upper right quadrant, and

TRUST ⟶

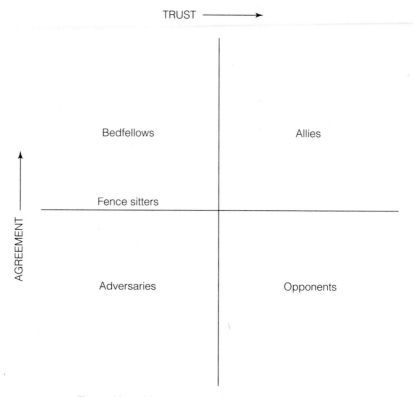

Figure 18-1 Negotiating with allies and adversaries.

bedfellows are indicated by high agreement and low trust in the upper left quadrant. Fence sitters are represented by low trust and medium agreement between adversaries and bedfellows on the left side of the grid.

Adversaries with whom we have low agreement and low trust use much of our time and psychic energy. They become adversaries only after our attempts to negotiate agreement and trust have failed. Steps in dealing with adversaries include the following: (1) State your vision of the project. (2) State in a neutral way your best understanding of the adversary's position. (3) Identify your own contribution to the problem, such as having lobbied against them, discounted their position, gone around them, or talked to a higher authority. (4) End the meeting with your plans and no demand.

Opponents are people whom we trust but who disagree with our goals and purposes. Opponents can bring out the best in us by challenging us and making us clarify our beliefs and strategies. The steps for dealing with opponents are as follows: (1) Reaffirm the quality of your relationship and mutual trust. (2) State your position. (3) State in a neutral way what you think your opponent's position is. (4) Do problem solving.

One has high agreement and high trust with allies. They should be treated as friends; one can discuss doubts and vulnerabilities with them. The basic strategy when dealing with allies is to bring them into the organization and treat them as members.

Steps include (1) affirming agreement, (2) reaffirming the quality of the trusting relationship, (3) acknowledging doubts and vulnerabilities related to the project, and (4) asking for advice and support.

One has high agreement and low trust with bedfellows. There is a tendency to become manipulative toward people we do not trust. One is careful about how much information to share. The issue is trust, not agreement. To work with bedfellows, (1) reaffirm the agreement; (2) acknowledge caution; (3) be clear about what one wants from the bedfellow, such as keeping one informed; (4) ask what the bedfellow wants and expects; and (5) try to agree about how to work together.

Fence sitters do not take a stand for or against us; they exhibit doubt, risk, and uncertainty. To deal with fence sitters, (1) state your position, (2) ask for the fence sitter's position, (3) apply gentle pressure to get a decision and express frustration with neutrality, and (4) ask what it would take to get the fence sitter's support (Block, 1987).

Using our power in organizations and politics through principled negotiations with people with whom we have more or less agreement and trust can advance nursing.

BIBLIOGRAPHY

Anderson W: The New York needle trial: the politics of public health in the age of AIDS, *Am J Publ Health* 81:1506-1517, November 1991.

Barry CT: Profiles of nurses professionally involved in public policy, *Nurs Econ* 8:174-176, 187, May-June 1990.

Burns M, Thornam CM: Broadening the scope of nursing practice: federal programs for children, *Pediatr Nurs* 19:546-552, November-December 1993.

Canada EP: Power, influence, and the development professional, *Econ Dev Rev* 11:42-45, September 1993.

Carlson-Catalano JM: Application of empowerment: theory for CNS practice, *Clinical Nurse Specialist* 7:321-325, November 1993.

Castledine G: Winter of discontent . . . the significance of politics in nursing, *Geriatric Nursing and Home Care* 8:8, March 1988.

Cunningham N: Identity, metaphors, and power, *AWHONN's Clinical Issues in Perinatal and Women's Health Nursing* 4:634-640, 1993.

Dean HE: Political and ethical implications of using quality of life as an outcome measure, *Semin Oncol Nurs* 6:303-308, November 1990.

Doering L: Power and knowledge in nursing: a feminist poststructuralist view, *Adv Nurs Sci* 14:24-33, June 1992.

Drory A, Romm T: The definition of organizational politics: a review, *Hum Relat* 42:1133-1154, November 1990.

Erlen JA, Frost B: Nurses' perceptions of powerlessness in influencing ethical decisions, *West J Nurs Res* 13:397-407, June 1991.

Farmer B: The use and abuse of power in nursing, *Nursing Standard* 7:33-36, February 24-March 2, 1993.

Feldman SP: Symbolism and politics in organizational change, *Hum Relat* 43:809-828, September 1990.

Feldman SP: Stories as cultural creativity: on the relation between symbolism and politics in organizational change, *Hum Relat* 43:809-828, September 1990.

Frederick SL: Nursing management according to Goren, *Nurs Manage* 20:47-50, September 1989.

Geese T: Political participation behaviors of nurse midwives, *J Nurse Midwifery* 36:184-191, May-June 1991.

Glen S: Power for nursing education, *J Adv Nurs* 15:1335-1340, November 1990.

Hanley BE: Political participation: how do nurses compare with other professional women? *Nurs Econ* 5:179-185, July-August 1987.

Hawks JH: Power: a concept analysis, *J Adv Nurs* 16:754-762, June 1991.

Hayes, E, Fritsch R: An untapped resource: the political potential of nurses, *Nurs Adm Q* 13:33-39, Fall 1988.

Hoelzel CB: Using structural power sources to increase influence, *JONA* 19(11):10-15, November 1989.

Jongbloed L, Crichton A: A new definition of disability: implications for rehabilitation practice and social policy, *Can J Occup Ther* 57:32-38, February 1990.

Kari N, Michels P: The Lazarus Project: the politics of empowerment . . . nursing home models of governance, *Am J Occup Ther* 45:719-725, August 1991.

Kelly S: Nursing in politics: future hope, *Pennsylvania Nurse* 46:16, June 1991.

Keys B, Case T: How to become an influential manager, *Academy of Management Executive* 4:38-51, November 1990.

Kippenbrock TA: Power at meetings: strategies to move people, *Dermatology Nursing* 4:382-385, October 1992.

Krouse HJ, Roberts SJ: Nurse-patient interactive styles: power, control, and satisfaction, *West J Nurs Res* 11:717-725, December 1989.

Lapierre L: Mourning, potency, and power in management, *Human Resource Management* 28:177-189, Summer 1989.

Larson E: Nursing research and societal needs: political, corporate, and international perspectives, *J Prof Nurs* 9:73-78, March-April 1993.

Manthey M: Trends: shifting patterns of authority, *Nurs Manage* 21:14-15, October 1990.

Mason DJ: Nursing and politics: a profession comes of age, *Orthop Nurs* 9:11-17, September-October 1990.

Mason DJ, Backer BA, Georges CA: Toward the feminist model for the political empowerment of nurses, *Image: Journal of Nursing Scholarship* 23:72-77, Summer 1991.

Maurin JT: Research utilization in the social-political arena, *Appl Nurs Res* 3:48-51, May 1990.

McMahon R: Power and collegial relations among nurses on wards adopting primary nursing and hierarchical ward management structures, *J Adv Nurs* 15:232-239, February 1990.

Miller I: Executive leadership, community action, and the habits of health care politics, *Health Care Manage Rev* 17:81-84, Winter 1992.

Palich LE, Hom PW: The impact of leader power and behavior on leadership, *Group and Organization Management* 17:279-296, September 1992.

Pfeffer J: Understanding power in organizations, *California Management Review* 34:29-50, Winter 1992.

Pfeffer J: Manage with power, *Success* 40:112, November 1993.

Pinchot ES: Balance of power, *Executive Excellence* 9:3-5, September 1992.

Pitts CE: For project managers: an inquiry into the delicate art and science of influencing others, *Project Management Journal* 21:21-23, March 24, 1990.

Porter S: A participant observation study of power relations between nurses and doctors in a general hospital, *J Adv Nurs* 16:728-735, June 1991.

Raatikainen R: Power or the lack of it in nursing care, *J Adv Nurs* 19:424-432, March 1994.

Ray MA: Transcultural caring: political and economic visions, *Journal of Transcultural Nursing* 1:17-21, Summer 1989.

Reimer, JM, Morrissey N, Mulcahy KA et al: Power orientation: a study of female nurse and non-nurse managers. *Nurs Manage* 25:55-58, May 1994.

Rienzo BA, Button JW: The politics of school-based clinics: a community-level analysis, *J Sch Health* 63:266-272, August 1993.

Robinson J: Politics and professional power, *Health Visitor* 63:236-238, July 1990.

Robottom I, Colquhoun D: The participatory research, environmental health education and the politics of method, *Health Educ Res* 7:457-469, December 1992.

Schultz MC: Leadership and the power circle, *Human Systems Management* 11:213-217, 1992.

Skelton R: Nursing and empowerment: concepts and strategies, *J Adv Nurs* 19:415-423, March 1994.

Smith JP: The politics of American health care, *J Adv Nurs* 15:487-497, April 1990.

Smith LS: The history of nursing and politics in the United States, *Adv Clin Care* 6:6-7, July-August 1991.

Sneed NV: Power: its use and potential for misuse by nurse consultants, *Clinical Nurse Specialist* 5:58-62, Spring 1991.

Temple JS, Saul RA, Calvin RL: First impressions! The power of language in the health care setting, *Journal of National Black Nurses' Association* 6:27-32, 1993.

Titchen A, Binnie A: Changing power relationships between nurses: a case study of early changes towards patient centered nursing, *J Clin Nurs* 2:219-229, July 1993.

Tjosvold D, Andrews IR, Struthers JT: Power and interdependence in work groups—views of managers and employees, *Group and Organization Studies* 16:285-299, September 1991.

Velthouse BA: Creativity and empowerment: a complementary relationship, *Review of Business* 12:13-18, Fall 1991.

Wilson B, Laschinger HKS: Staff nurse perception of job empowerment and organizational commitment: a test of Kanter's theory of structural power in organizations, *JONA* 24(suppl 45):39-47, April 1994.

Wing DM: A cross-cultural field study of nurses and political strategies, *West J Nurs Res* 12:373-385, June 1990.

Winter K: Educating nurses in political process: a growing need, *Journal of Continuing Education in Nursing* 22:143-146, July-August 1991.

CASE STUDY

Everyone on your unit wants a raise, but you have a limited amount of money to use. Describe how you will apply principled negotiations to the situation.

CRITICAL THINKING AND LEARNING ACTIVITIES

1. Using Worksheet 18-1, identify your sources of power and make a list of those sources.

2. Form a small group in class. Develop a scenario of a situation that requires negotiations. Choose sides and practice principled negotiations.

3. Using Worksheet 18-2, identify strategies for negotiating with parties in each quadrant.

✍ **Worksheet 18-1**

Sources of Power

List your sources of power.

1.

2.

3.

4.

5.

6.

7.

8.

✍ **Worksheet 18-2**

Negotiating Strategies

Using the following grid, identify strategies for negotiating with parties with differing amounts of agreement and trust.

	High agreement	Low agreement
Trust	1.	1.
	2.	2.
	3.	3.
	4.	4.
	5.	5.
Distrust	1.	1.
	2.	2.
	3.	3.
	4.	4.
	5.	5.

Chapter

19

Conflict

Chapter Objectives

◆ Identify at least five sources of conflict.

◆ Identify at least five kinds of conflict and describe them.

◆ Describe reactions to conflict.

◆ Identify five approaches to conflict resolution, describe each, and identify appropriate times to use each.

◆ Describe nominal group technique.

◆ Explain role negotiations.

Major Concepts and Definitions	
Conflict	clash, fight, battle, struggle
Role ambiguity	person does not know what is expected
Role overload	person is unable to accomplish what is expected within the allotted time frame
Nominal group technique	a group participation method for making decisions
Role negotiations	the process of preventing role conflicts, role ambiguities, and role overload

CONFLICT THEORY

Conflict, which is closely related to power and political issues, is inevitable and can be constructive or destructive. It may offer an individual personal gain, provide prestige to the winner, be an incentive for creativity, and serve as a powerful motivator. Indeed, there seems to be an optimal level of conflict or anxiety necessary for effective functioning. Conflict that is managed instead of avoided, ignored, or suppressed can be used effectively. If conflict goes beyond the invigorating stage, it becomes debilitating. Conflict is a warning to management that something is amiss, and it should stimulate a search for new solutions through problem solving, the clarification of objectives, the establishment of group norms, and the determination of group boundaries. However, eliminating conflict is not necessary. If managers learn the sources and types of conflicts and how to manage them, they can minimize stress on individuals and the organization and maximize effectiveness.

Sources of Conflict

Conflict can arise because the individuals involved do not have the same facts. They define the problem differently, have different pieces of information, place more or less importance on various aspects, or have divergent views of their own power and authority. Varying goals and objectives or contrasting procedural strategies for accomplishing mutually acceptable goals produce conflict. Variations in personal value systems or in perceptions of ethical responsibilities can lead to divergence in choices of both goals and methods, thus producing conflict.

When people work together in a complex organization, there are numerous sources of conflict. Conflict increases with both the number of organizational levels and the number of specialties. It is greater as the degree of association increases and when some parties are dependent on others. Competition for scarce resources, ambiguous jurisdictions, and the need for consensus all contribute to conflict. Communication barriers impede understanding, and separations in time and space foster factionalism rather than mutual cooperation. Although standardized policies, rules, and procedures regulate behavior, make relationships more predictable, and decrease the number of arbitrary decisions, they impose added controls over the individual. Men and women who value autonomy are likely to resist such control. Clearly, the sources of conflict are endless, and the number of conflicts increases as the number of unresolved differences accumulates.

Types of Conflict

Structurally based conflict is either vertical or horizontal. Differences between managers and staff associates (vertical conflict) are often related to inadequate communication, opposing interests, and lack of shared perceptions and attitudes. In vertical situations, managers often attempt to control staff associates' behavior, and the staff associates resist, often causing managers to apply their position power through impersonal bureaucratic rules. Line-staff conflict, usually horizontal, is commonly a struggle between domains related to activities, expertise, and authority and is often related to interdepartmental strife.

Interdepartmental differences are related to the degree of interdependence between departments. Interdependence demands collaboration, and the latter provides the occasion for conflict. The need for consensus, the work sequence, and common use of shared facilities or services are areas of interdependence aggravated by differing departmental goals. Both the personalities and the status of the individuals involved affect attitudes such as trust and cooperation and are just as important as the communication and interaction structures.

There are several types of role conflict (see Box 19-1). *Intrasender* conflict originates in the sender who gives conflicting instructions or expects conflicting or mutually exclusive behavioral responses. For example, the same supervisor may demand a higher quality of nursing care, refuse to allow the head nurse to fire incompetent help, and, in an effort to cut costs, refuse to increase an inadequate staff or to permit overtime.

Intersender conflict arises when an individual receives conflicting messages from two or more sources. For example, management may implement an incentive plan to stimulate production and peer pressures may discourage rate busting. In university settings, the dean may expect department chairpersons to function as administrators, and the faculty may expect them to act as their advocates. The matrix organization that imposes project management on a functional structure creates intersender role conflict. Any time one is responsible to more than one person, one can anticipate intersender role conflict.

Box 19-1   TYPES OF CONFLICT

Intrasender	Person-role	Intergroup
Intersender	Interperson	Role ambiguity
Interrole	Intragroup	Role overload

Interrole conflict can occur when an individual belongs to more than one group. Simultaneous, multiple roles within the same organization or the conflicting expectations that result from being a member of more than one organization are sources of such conflict. For example, a person may be expected to attend two different committee meetings at the same time. Job expectations can easily interfere with one's family life. The individual has to develop a system of trade-offs to determine how to behave at certain times.

Person-role conflict is the result of disparity between internal and external roles. An individual has perceived roles and expectations based on ones values and perceptions of oneself. When one's values, needs, or capabilities are incompatible with the role requirement, person-role conflict is created. Behavioral expectations that exceed one's current level of knowledge and skill are also stressful. If the nurse believes that people are important but must process patients through a large clinic in a relatively impersonal manner, the nurse is bound to suffer person-role conflict.

Interperson conflict is common between people whose positions require interaction with other persons who fill various roles in the same organization or other organizations. Interperson conflict is usually not personal but rather the result of each person's acting as a protagonist for that person's department. For example, the director of nursing competes with other departmental heads for resources. Occasionally, the conflict arising from the nature of the roles involved is complicated by personal animosity.

Intragroup conflict occurs when the group faces a new problem, when new values are imposed on the group from outside, or when one's extragroup role conflicts with one's intragroup role. In an academic setting, pressures to have baccalaureate nursing students prepared by faculty with master's degrees and graduate students prepared by faculty with doctoral degrees produces intragroup conflict. Faculty members are caught in a conflict over their teaching responsibilities, continuation of their own education, and fulfillment of expectations for community service and scholarly work. A group facing a new problem may require a change in role relationships that requires role negotiations. When intragroup conflict becomes intense, two new groups may form and give rise to intergroup conflict.

Intergroup conflict is common where two groups have different goals and can only achieve their goals at the other's expense. The conflict may be between groups on the same level or between groups on different levels within an organization. Competition between groups also produces conflict. Resolution may be reached by the dominance of one group over the other, by a compromise that rarely satisfies either group, or by an integration of goals attained when each group recognizes the role of the other group in the system. Intergroup conflict need not be dysfunctional. It can stimulate creativity, innovation, and progress. A conflict-free organization suggests stasis, a situation that offers little challenge for group members.

Role ambiguity, a condition in which individuals do not know what is expected of them, frequently occurs in organizations. Inadequate job descriptions, incomplete explanations of assigned tasks, rapid technological change, and the increasing complexity of organizations contribute to role ambiguity and produce uncertainty and frustration.

If individuals cannot meet the expectations placed on them, they will experience *role overload*. This does not involve a questioning of the legitimacy of the request or of what is expected. Rather, the person is simply unable to accomplish so much within a limited time period. As a result, quality is sacrificed for quantity, the ego is threatened, and frustration develops.

Reactions to Conflict

Numerous psychological mechanisms exist for coping with one's own behavioral reactions to conflict, but such stress contributes to somatic reactions, for example, cardiovascular diseases and gastric disorders. Box 19-2 lists some common reactions to conflict.

Sublimation is one of the most constructive psychological mechanisms whereby unacceptable feelings are repressed and channeled into socially acceptable activities. Energy from hostility and anger that would be destructive if expressed directly is diverted with positive results into other activities such as jogging, tennis, or community service. *Vigorous physical activity* often reduces interpersonal aggression.

People who are displeased with the results of their behavior may *increase* their *efforts*. Working longer and harder is likely to increase productivity. Flight into activity, a defense mechanism whereby a person keeps busy to avoid thinking about problems, provides some temporary relief but does not solve the problems.

Identification is the practice of enhancing one's self-esteem by imitating another's behavior. The values and beliefs of the other person are internalized, and both achievements and suffering are experienced vicariously. This illustrates the adage, "If you can't beat them, join them." An individual may compensate for a real or imagined inadequacy in one area by substituting a high degree of proficiency in another area. For example, one who lacks social skills may excel academically.

Goals may be *reinterpreted* to attain an unmet goal, or the goal may be lowered or another goal *substituted*. A person promoted to vice president with little hope of

Box 19-2   **REACTIONS TO CONFLICT**

Sublimation	Rationalization	Displacement
Vigorous physical exercise	Attention getting	Fixation
Increase efforts	Reaction formation	Withdrawal
Identification	Flight into fantasy	Repression
Reinterpret goals	Projection	Conversion
Substitute goals		

becoming president may decide that the vice presidency is a satisfactory position. A rejected job applicant may find another job the applicant enjoys more.

Rationalization provides acceptable explanations for undesirable beliefs or behaviors. Managers may find reasons to fire someone they do not like or pad the expense account because "everyone does it."

Attention getting may involve seeking highly visible jobs, engaging in loud or excessive talking, wearing bright or sexy clothing and unusual hair styles, or driving flashy cars. These displays are destructive only if they divert attention from problem solving.

When individuals repress unacceptable behaviors and values and substitute the opposite attitudes and behaviors, they are using a coping mechanism called *reaction formation*. For example, an employee who was denied a merit pay increase may defend the manager and vigorously support the related policies.

Another mechanism people use to cope with stress is *flight into fantasy*. Flight into fantasy allows one to think about something else. For example, the nurse's aide may daydream about being the charge nurse. Although daydreaming, watching television, and going to the movies are constructive forms of relaxation, engaging in excessive fantasy interferes with one's productivity.

People may protect themselves from their undesirable feelings and traits by attributing them to others. This defense mechanism is called *projection*. For example, a student who is unable to answer a test question may claim that the question is unclear. An unsuccessful person who wants to block another's success claims that the colleague is hostile and uncooperative. Projection is a destructive way to meet needs.

Displacement redirects emotions toward ideas, people, or objects other than the source of the emotions. For example, after the director corrects the head nurse, the nurse manager may displace aggression by snapping at the staff. Some individuals reacting to conflict may resort to negativism, picking apart every idea and action and putting everything in the worst light.

Fixation is the maintenance of a certain maladaptive behavior even though it is obvious that it is not effective in this situation. One who depends on this escape mechanism will make the same mistake repeatedly.

Withdrawal removes one from the area of frustration. For example, a staff nurse who is frustrated by hospital working conditions may go into teaching. This mechanism can be constructive if the person withdraws from a dangerous situation.

Repression pushes painful information and memories into the subconscious, but the material is not truly forgotten. An individual may revert to earlier, even childish behavior. When regressing, staff members may transfer their attitudes toward their parents to their manager and expect the manager to act like a parent. Some people may even have temper tantrums. Regression moves one away from the present and is rarely constructive.

An individual may unconsciously convert an emotional conflict into physical symptoms, for example, the common tension headache. Paralysis of an arm to avoid writing a report or losing one's voice to avoid discussing an unpleasant topic are extreme forms of the coping mechanism called *conversion*.

Latent—antecedent conditions predict conflict behavior
Perceived—cognitive awareness of stressful situation exists
Felt—feelings and attitudes are present and affect the conflict
Manifest—overt behavior results from three earlier stages

Everyone uses psychological mechanisms. They are our unconscious defenses against impaired self-esteem, anxiety and guilt, and other threatening or uncomfortable feelings. Defense mechanisms serve a purpose. They become harmful only when excessive.

Stages of Conflict

Conflict may be divided into four progressive stages (see Box 19-3): latent, perceived, felt, and manifest. *Latent conflict* is a phase of anticipation in which antecedent conditions, such as scarcity of resources, predict conflict behavior. When change is required, the manager anticipates differences of opinion about the desirability of the change, how it should be implemented, and how the consequences should be handled.

Perceived conflict, which may or may not be discussed, indicates a cognitive awareness of a stressful situation. One's personal perceptions can contribute to either an accurate or inaccurate assessment of the situation and affect the amount of threat and potential loss the individual anticipates. Conflicts can be perceived when antecedent conditions do not exist, as when individuals have a limited knowledge of the facts or do not know others' opinions and values. For instance, a manager may think there are limited resources or that someone else wants to use the same materials when, in fact, there is plenty for everyone or no one else is interested anyway. Personal perceptions also can help to avoid conflict. A suppression mechanism may be used to ignore conflict that involves low potential loss or is only minimally threatening. An attention-focus mechanism helps the individual select which conditions to change and which to ignore.

Affective states such as stress, tension, anxiety, anger, and hostility are present during the *felt conflict.* Feelings and attitudes may create or avoid conflict. Trust, for example, is a significant factor in the development of a manifest conflict. If the individuals involved possess trusting attitudes, they share information and control and recognize their mutual vulnerability. In the absence of trust, individuals may withhold information so it cannot be used against them or distort communications to their advantage. They may scheme to increase their control over others and strive to decrease others' control over them. Clearly, trusting attitudes may prevent potential conflict, and the lack of them may actually create conflict. Two self-serving individuals are more likely to have manifest conflict than a dominant and submissive pair.

The personalization or depersonalization of the situation affects the evolution of conflict. When the situation is personalized, the individual is threatened or judged negatively. With a depersonalized approach, the behavior rather than the individual is identified as creating the problem. "You are wrong" is personalized, whereas "your views are very different from mine" is depersonalized. Personalized comments increase anxiety; a depersonalized approach is conducive to problem solving.

Manifest conflict is overt behavior resulting from the antecedent, perceived, and felt conflict. It can be either constructive or destructive to problem solving. Unfortunately, aggression, competition, and other defenses are learned unconsciously, whereas problem solving requires a more deliberate, conscious effort.

CONFLICT RESOLUTION

Approaches to Conflict Resolution

Some common approaches to handling conflict are avoiding, accommodating, compromising, collaborating, and competing (see Box 19-4). *Avoiding* creates lose-lose situations through unassertive and uncooperative means. The conflict is simply not addressed. This approach may be appropriate when the other party is more powerful, the issue is unimportant, one has no chance of meeting the goals, or the cost of dealing with the conflict is higher than the benefit of the resolution. It may also be used when it is more appropriate for others to solve a problem, when more information is needed, or when one wishes to reduce tension and gain composure. Withdrawing from a conflict does not resolve it, and the individual who retreats frequently harbors a gnawing anger over a situation that drains energy needed for more constructive purposes.

Accommodating is cooperative but unassertive. It is self-sacrificing—the opposite of competing. One neglects one's own needs to meet the goals of the other party. It is appropriate when the opponent is right, the opponent is more powerful, or the issue is more important to someone else. It can be used when preserving harmony is important or when collecting social credits is necessary for later, more important issues. By complimenting one's opponent and accentuating points of agreement, one may smooth out an agreement on minor issues, but the real problems still have to be dealt with.

Compromising moderates both assertiveness and cooperation. It addresses a problem more effectively than avoidance but less than collaboration. Compromisers are willing to yield less than accommodaters but more than competitors as they seek expedient, mutually acceptable answers. Because both parties feel that they sacrifice something, they are only partially satisfied, and a lose-lose atmosphere results. Compromising is useful for reaching expedient answers for limited periods when the goals are only moderately important and the parties have equivalent power.

Collaborating is assertive and cooperative. It is a win-win strategy. It contributes to effective problem solving because both parties try to find mutually satisfying solutions. This method integrates insights from different perspectives with the commitment developed through participation and the resolution of hard feelings. Problems are identified, alternatives explored, and ramifications considered until difficulties are resolved. Unfortunately, it may take more time than the results are worth. Generally this is a most effective method of conflict resolution.

Box 19-4   **APPROACHES TO CONFLICT RESOLUTION**

Avoiding—unassertive and uncooperative
Accommodating—cooperative but unassertive
Compromising—assertive and cooperative
Collaborating—assertive and cooperative
Competing—assertive but uncooperative

Competing is a power-oriented mode that is assertive but uncooperative. In competition one is aggressive and pursues one's own goals at another's expense. This creates a win-lose situation. Nevertheless, it is appropriate when a quick or unpopular decision is needed, when the person is very knowledgeable about the situation and able to make a sound decision, or when one must protect oneself from other aggressive people. If this strategy is used too often, colleagues may become afraid to admit mistakes and may simply say what they think the aggressor wants to hear. A manager can always fall back on authority and give orders to a subordinate, but because the resolution is forced, it almost certainly will be unsatisfactory.

A foundation of mutual trust must underlie any attempt to understand alternative views and to actively seek solutions that will allow each party to achieve its goals. This trust creates an atmosphere conducive to successful conflict resolution.

Strategies for Conflict Resolution

There are three ways of dealing with conflict: the win-lose, lose-lose, or win-win strategy (see Box 19-5). *Win-lose* methods include the use of position power, mental or physical power, failure to respond, majority rule, and railroading a minority position over the majority. *Lose-lose* strategies include compromise, bribes for accomplishing disagreeable tasks, arbitration by a neutral third party, and resortion to the use of general rules instead of considering the merits of individual cases. In win-lose and lose-lose strategies, the parties often personalize the issues by focusing on each other instead of on the problem. Intent on their personal differences, they avoid the more important matter of how to mutually solve their problem. Solutions are emphasized instead of goals and values. Rather than identifying mutual needs, planning activities for resolution, and solving the problem, the parties involved look at the issue from their own point of view and strive for total victory.

By contrast, *win-win* strategies focus on goals. They emphasize consensus and integrative approaches to decision making. The consensus process demands a focus on the problem (instead of on each other), on the collection of facts, on the acceptance of the useful aspects of conflict, and on the avoidance of averaging and self-oriented behavior. The group decision is thus often better than the best individual decision.

Problem-solving strategies include identifying both the problem and each party's needs, exploring alternatives, choosing the most acceptable alternative, planning, defining roles, implementing, and evaluating the decision.

Box 19-5 STRATEGIES FOR CONFLICT RESOLUTION

Win-lose	Lose-lose	Win-win
position power	compromise	consensus
mental or physical power	bribes	problem-solving
failure to respond	arbitration	
majority rule	general rules	
railroading		

Interpersonal Conflict

Interpersonal conflict is inevitable, but the manager can lessen its impact by coaching staff associates in assertive communication and fair fighting. Engaging in a fair fight demands that individuals with a complaint first ask their opponent for a meeting. Once a time and place are agreed on, both parties should determine whether or not their manager should be present. Moreover, a fair fight demands that both parties know the purpose of the meeting so neither will be caught off guard—each can be prepared. The encounter should begin with a statement of the problem. The manager, if present, should act as a mediator, asking the complainer to explain the perceived problem to the opponent. Opponents then should relate their understanding of how the complainer perceives the problem. After each has spoken, each can clarify any differences over the statement of the problem. Next, opponents describe their perception of the problem; this description then should be followed by the complainers' repeating their understanding of how the opponent perceives the problem. Again, there is a pause for clarification.

A clear statement of the problem helps to shed light on the negative effects of each person's behavior. This feedback process, which requires each party to repeat what the other has just said, forces each to listen carefully. Were it not for such interaction, one might be so busy thinking of what one is going to say next that one fails to hear what is being said. Feedback does not imply parroting, because an understanding of meaning is more important than sheer memorization of words. Differences often begin to disappear when both parties really hear each other for the first time.

By exploring the alternatives to the problem and the ramifications of their options, the parties can identify and request changes in each other's behavior and respond to the other's requests. The discussion should close with an agreement on whether to change and the establishment of the accompanying conditions. A follow-up engagement should be set to discuss the success or failure of the agreement.*

---

* Nine steps in a fair fight are presented in Bach GR, Goldberg H: *Creative aggression: the art of assertive living*, New York, 1974, Avon Books.

Box 19-6   **NOMINAL GROUP TECHNIQUE**

List ideas on paper
Round-robin session
Serial discussion for clarification
Preliminary vote
Analysis of votes
Discussion of preliminary vote
Revote

Group Conflict

Team development can help prevent and resolve conflict. Planning, goal setting, and rating goals represent the first step in team development. The statement of the core mission of the team is developed by brainstorming and sharing individual mission statements.

The *nominal group technique** is very effective for developing team-performance goals and priorities (see Box 19-6). First, individual group members list on separate pieces of paper what they think team-performance goals should be. The group leader helps keep the group problem centered by presenting the question and prevents interruptions of thoughts by asking participants to work silently and independently. This step allows time for thinking, avoids status and conformity pressures, prevents focusing on a particular idea because of a vocal person, and helps avoid choosing among ideas prematurely.

Next, during a round-robin session, each person in turn states one team-performance goal, which is then written on a chalkboard or paper for all to see. It is probable that equalization of participation and sharing of all ideas fosters group creativity. By citing one goal, each member is encouraged to participate equally. By the second round, each member has participated and the precedent is set, and thus competition from aggressive or high-status members is minimized.

If all an individual's listed goals have been cited, that individual passes, and other members continue to offer listed goals in turn until all are exhausted. Ideas are not repeated. However, "hitchhiking" may occur. An idea listed by one member may stimulate another member to have an idea not previously listed. That idea can be added to the member's list and cited during the round-robin session.

It is common for many of an individual's ideas about a problem to remain unspoken because of fear of self-disclosure and embarrassment. When one person states several ideas at once, those ideas tend to be associated with that person.

---

* The nominal group technique is described in detail in Delbecq AL, Van de Ven AH, Gustafson DH: *Group techniques for program planning: a guide to nominal group and Delphi processes*, Glenview, Ill, 1975, Scott, Foresman.

However, with the round-robin method, it is difficult to remember who presented what ideas, and full disclosure is encouraged.

The written list can be the basis of recorded minutes and serve as a source of information from which the group continues to work. During this step, the group leader should see that ideas are recorded as rapidly as possible and in the words used by the contributor. The entire list should be made visible to all group members. Tearing completed sheets from a flip chart and taping them on the walls works well, and it is an early reward in that the group can see the array of ideas generated. The written ideas are more objective and less personal than oral comments because the personality and position of the contributors are separated from the written statement. The group leader should encourage the simple listing of ideas by explaining that a discussion period will follow. Discussion of the ideas, arguments about them, and side conversations while the list is being made should not be allowed.

The third step is a serial discussion for clarification. During this step, each listed idea is discussed in order. This provides an opportunity to clarify ideas, state differences of opinion, provide the logic behind ideas, and prevent undue focusing on any one idea. The group leader's responsibility is to clarify the purpose of this step and to pace the group. Arguments can be curtailed by stating that both points of view have been noted and then moving on to the next point. It is better not to ask the contributors to clarify their own items, because such a request can put them on the spot. Instead, the group members can be asked what the items mean to them. The contributor can clarify when appropriate. This method helps reduce identification of items with specific individuals.

The preliminary vote on item importance is the fourth step. In the nominal group process, individuals make independent judgments, express their judgments mathematically by ranking items, use the mean value of the independent judgments for the group's decision, talk over the results, and revote.

Alternative ways to determine a group decision are consensus, majority rule, and independent listing. When using consensus, group members may distort their judgments to maintain group cohesion, and consequently a regression toward the mean may occur. A showing of hands for majority rule is subject to social pressure, and minority positions do not count. Consequently, it may not truly reflect group preference. Independent listing, however, overcomes status, personality, and conformity pressures but does not indicate degree of importance. For example, an item listing might look like the one shown in Box 19-7. An analysis of the votes in Box 19-7 suggests that items 1, 4, 5, and 6 are considered the most important by frequency. Information about degree of importance can be obtained by having the items ranked. Ranking of the list might look like the one shown in Box 19-8. Using a scale of 5 as most important and 1 as least important, an analysis of the votes reveals that items 6, 4, 1, 5, and 8 are considered most important in descending order from 6 to 8. This method is more likely to reflect the true group preference.

The group leader asks each individual to select a specific number of most important items from the list. Individuals seem most able to accurately list five to nine items. Each member is asked to take that specific number of 3×5 index cards, identify that number of items from the list, place the item number in the upper left-hand corner, and write some identifying words in the middle of the card (Fig. 19-1). Then the participants are asked to spread out the cards, choose the item they consider most

Box 19-7   **ANALYSIS BY FREQUENCY**

Item	Votes
1	5
2	1
3	2
4	5
5	5
6	5
7	1
8	2

Box 19-8   **ANALYSIS BY RANKING**

Item	Votes	Totals
1	1-2-5-5-1	14
2	2	2
3	3-2	5
4	4-3-2-4-2	15
5	1-2-1-3-1	8
6	5-5-4-5-4	23
7	1	1
8	3-3	6

6 (item number from original list)

Setting goals for the unit
(identifying words)

2
(rank order number)

Figure 19-1   Index card illustrating rank order.

```
┌─────────────────────────────────────────────────────────────┐
│                    ROLE MESSAGE FORM                          │
│                                                               │
│       To:_____                                        │
│       From:_____                                       │
│                                                               │
│       In order for me to _____, I need you to do     │
│                                                               │
│          Less of:                                             │
│                                                               │
│                                                               │
│                                                               │
│          Same of:                                             │
│                                                               │
│                                                               │
│                                                               │
│          More of:                                             │
│                                                               │
│                                                               │
└─────────────────────────────────────────────────────────────┘
```

Figure 19-2 Role message form.

important, and put the high number in the lower right-hand corner of the card and underline it. If five items are being selected, 5 would be the high number. For nine items, 9 would be the high number. That card is turned over, the remaining cards are assessed, and a 1 is put in the lower right-hand corner and underlined for the least important card. That card is turned over and the next most important item is selected and rated as one less than the highest number: for instance, 8 for nine items or 4 for five items. Then the next to the lowest item is chosen and marked as 2, and so on, until the middle item is left and numbered. This process encourages careful decisions.

When the card ranking is complete, the group leader collects and shuffles the cards and records the votes on the written list of items.

The fifth step is a discussion of the preliminary vote. Inconsistent voting patterns can be examined, and items receiving many or few votes can be discussed. A discussion will probably allow for correction of misinformation, misunderstandings, and unequal information, thereby offering a more accurate indication of preferences than voting only.

The final step is the revote, which determines the outcome of the process, documents the group judgment, and closes the nominal group process.

Role negotiations—the process of preventing role conflicts, role ambiguities, and role overload—become important once priorities have been set. During this process group members clarify each individual's role on the team and help to resolve any disagreements over the team members' roles. Members initially send one written message to each team member indicating that for them to act, they need the other team members to do more, less, or to continue their previous performance (see Fig. 19-2). *To whom* and *from whom* are essential parts of the message. The number of role messages sent to any one individual should be limited to prevent an information overload. The message must clearly state how the sender wants the receiver to behave and how a change will help the sender. Each role message must indicate the need for

ROLE CONTRACT

1. Problem:

2. Person **x** agrees to:

3. Person **y** agrees to:

4. Others agree to:

We agree that a follow-up check will be done by _____.
                                                              (date)

                                                    Signatures

                                                    _____
                                                    x
                                                    _____
                                                    y
                                                    _____
                                                    others

Figure 19-3   Role contract.

more, less, or the same of some activity. More than one message in the "same" category indicates support for the other person.

Receivers respond by indicating what they can or cannot do, explaining why, and offering alternative solutions, for example, "I can't do x, but I can do y, which should help solve your problem," or "If I do x, I would like you to do y." Receivers analyze the role messages they receive in the "do more, do less, and do the same" categories and according to who sent the message and their response to that message. Do the receivers know what is expected of them? Do different people want them to do more *and* less of the same activity at the same time? Do the receivers have time to meet all the demands made of them? Role definition helps identify role ambiguity, role conflict, and role overload. After roles are negotiated, a contract (Fig. 19-3) is written that defines the problem, identifies what each involved person will do, and sets a date for a follow-up check.

Negotiating involves good communication skills. One can identify needs, ideas, and information by using open-ended probes to clarify. Closed probes can be used to pinpoint specifications and to confirm understanding. One should indicate one's intent ("I support your idea") when one offers ideas of information. It is preferable to present reasons before conclusions, because they seem to be heard better that way, and

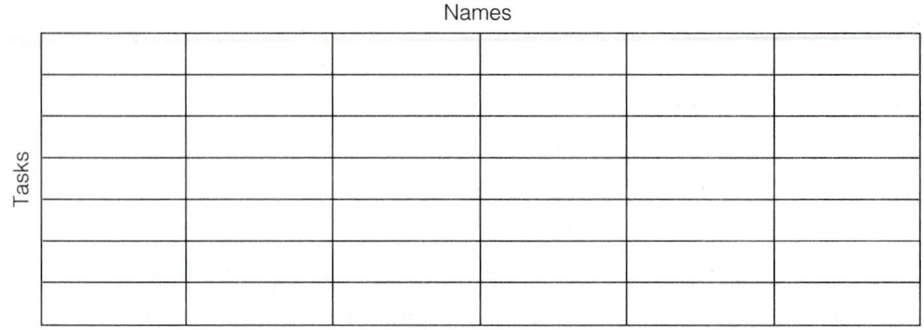

Names

Tasks

M, manages the process; C, consulted before the decision; D, makes the decision; I. informed of the decision.

Figure 19-4 Decision chart.

the speaker is more likely to be considered reasonable. To build on ideas, one should acknowledge the connection ("Bill's comment made me think of . . .") and then add value. To criticize constructively, merits should be stated before concerns. One should then ask for ways to retain merits and eliminate concerns. Confront counterproductive tactics by confirming the behavior and expressing its impact. ("That seemed like a personal attack. Is that what you intended? I feel angry when I am treated that way.") To break an impasse, one can indicate one's desire to continue and then initiate a change of pace: "Let's go get a cup of coffee and then try to solve this problem."

To come to an agreement, the purpose of the meeting and a review of the situation should be discussed. The needs and restrictions to develop, examine ideas from both points of view, and to determine the best alternative should be explored. The discussion can be closed by summarizing the agreement and confirming the next steps.*

Decision charting is the next major phase of team development and is concerned with who should be involved in decision making and with the nature of that involvement. To determine who should be involved in decision making, one should assess who has the information necessary to make a sound decision and who is responsible for implementing that decision. The latter needs to understand the decision and be committed to it.

People can be involved in decision making in a variety of ways. Some are directly involved because they have the necessary information and are responsible for implementing the decision. The involvement of some may be limited to input or consultation. Others need to be informed about the decision, and someone must be responsible for managing the overall decision-making process.

A decision chart helps one to visualize the decision-making process (Fig. 19-4). Decisions to be made are listed down the side of the page and the involved people across the top in a grid pattern: placing an *M* in a square indicates who manages the process; *D* indicates who is directly involved; *C* indicates who should be consulted;

* Negotiating skills can be practiced in *Negotiating self-taught,* Stamford, Conn, 1984, Learning International.

and *I* indicates who should be informed. Anyone who is expected to implement the decision obviously must be informed.*

Intergroup Conflict

Intergroup conflict is common and can be dysfunctional. As with interpersonal conflict, intergroup resistance may result from low trust, poor communications, and false assumptions. People resist what they perceive as threatening. Intergroup actions may threaten territorial rights and contribute to role overload and conflict. By preventing win-lose situations, emphasizing the organization's goals and effectiveness, rotating personnel among groups to facilitate understanding, and increasing interaction and communication between groups, one can help reduce intergroup conflict.

When a group recognizes its need to solve some intergroup conflict, it must first decide how to begin. A study of the organizational chart will determine who should be involved. Who should represent the group—a person or a committee? Someone who is already friendly with members of the other group? Someone with strong or moderate feelings about the position? What is the group's position and how much negotiation is acceptable? It helps to emphasize common goals and discuss constraints. The same process used in interpersonal conflict should be used in group conflict situations: setting and rating goals, negotiating roles, and making decisions.

Organizational Conflict

Organizations in conflict display the collective symptoms of their members. Personnel feel frustration at work. If they do not think their skills are being used, they experience a loss of self-esteem and a sense of powerlessness, both of which lead to withdrawal from the situation instead of an attempt to solve the problems. Group members also engage in backbiting and blame others for the problems. Subgroup formations are common. Members of the organization identify the same task and group maintenance problems but act contrary to the information, thereby increasing their frustrations. However, personnel do not have the same frustrations or exhibit the same dysfunctional behavior outside the organization.

Consultation may be sought to deal with organizational conflict. The consultant must analyze the organization's structure, the leadership and authority of the institution, the communication patterns, the amount of intergroup cooperation and competition, the group's norms and goals, the group's problem-solving and decision-making processes, and various individual roles and functions within the group. Organizational research can help provide the information necessary to solve the problem.

After data have been collected and analyzed, the consultant offers feedback. Members of the organization can publicly vote whether or not they agree with the

---

* Team development is described in detail in Rubin IM, Plovnick MS, Fry RE: *Improving the coordination of care: a program for health team development,* Cambridge, Mass, 1975, Ballinger; and *Managing human resources in health care organizations: an applied approach,* Reston, Va, 1978, Reston, by the same authors.

consultant's views. A public vote facilitates ownership of ideas. If there is disagreement, the consultant helps the group clarify the reasons for the differences and modifies the statement until it reflects the group's thinking.

The consultant then asks all members to write a few sentences about how they contribute to the situation so that they can recognize their own part in the problem. Individuals are likely to maintain the status quo for fear of serious consequences if they confront the issues. The consultant shares his or her theory with the group, helps develop an awareness of dysfunctional behavior, helps individuals cope with their feelings, encourages fantasy and reality testing, and coaches group members toward new behaviors.

Prevention of Conflict

Careful development of an organization's structure, strategic and comprehensive planning, management and organizational development, and careful selection and placement of personnel help prevent organizational conflict. The same strategies also prevent intergroup, group, and interpersonal conflict. Although conflict can be reduced, it cannot be totally avoided. Conflict can be constructive or destructive. By capitalizing on the positive aspects, the negative features can seem more bearable.

BIBLIOGRAPHY

Alter C: An exploratory study of conflict and coordination in interorganizational service delivery systems, *Academy of Management Journal* 33:478-502, September 1990.

Bedi H: Guidelines for referees, *Asian Business* 29:4, February 1993.

Brandt P: Negotiation and problem-solving strategies: collaboration between families and professionals, *Infants and Young Children* 5:78-84, April 1993.

Broom C: Conflict resolution strategies: when ethical dilemmas evolve into conflict, *DCCN: Dimensions of Critical Care Nursing* 10:354-363, November-December 1991.

Collyer ME: Resolving conflicts: leadership style sets the strategy, *Nurs Manage* 20:77-80, September 1989.

Fowler AR, Bushardt SC, Jones MA: Retaining nurses through conflict resolution, *Health Progress* 74:25-29, June 1993.

Hayes, PM: Team building: bringing RNs and NAs together, *Nurs Manage* 25:52-54, May 1994.

Holly CM, Lyons M: Increasing your decision making role in ethical situations, *DCCN: Dimensions of Critical Care Nursing* 12:264-270, September-October 1993.

Jackson LE: Understanding, eliciting and negotiating clients' multicultural health beliefs, *Nurse Pract* 18:30,32,37-38, April 1993.

Jones ML: Role conflict: cause of burnout or energizer? *Soc Work* 38:136-141, March 1993.

Lees S, Ellis N: The design of a stress-management programme for nursing personnel, *J Adv Nurs* 15:946-961, August 1990.

Maher CA: A systems approach to managing conflict in orthopaedic nursing, *Orthop Nurs* 10:35-36, May-June 1991.

Marriner A: Conflict theory, *Superv Nurse* 10:12-16, April 1979.

Marriner A: Conflict resolution, *Superv Nurse* 10:46-54, May 1979.

Marriner A: How do you spell relief of conflict? F-L-E-X-I-B-I-L-I-T-Y, *Nurs 87* 17:113-114, March 1987.

Marriner A: Managing conflict, *Nurs Manage* 13:29-31, June 1992.

Martin K, Wimberly D, O'Keefe K: Resolving conflict in a multicultural nursing department, *Nurs Manage* 25:49-51, January 1994.

Proffitt CJ, Byrne ME, Namei SK et al: The nurse clinician: role conflict in research, *Clinical Nurse Specialist* 7:309-311, November 1993.

Rahim M, Afzalur G, Edward J et al: Ethics of managing interpersonal conflict in organizations, *Journal of Business Ethics* 11:423-432, May 1992.

Schwartz AE: How to handle conflict between employees, *Superv Manage* 37:9, June 1992.

Sitkin SB, Bies RJ: Social accounts in conflict situations: using explanations to manage conflict, *Hum Relat* 46:349-370, March 1993.

Watson RE, Burkholder JS: Conflict resolution: coping skills, empowerment, and decision making strategies for today's nurses, *Dermatology Nursing* 2:29-30,37, February 1990.

CASE STUDY

Two staff nurses on the team want the same weekend off. You need someone to work. How are you going to go about resolving the conflict?

CRITICAL THINKING AND LEARNING ACTIVITIES

1. Think of a situation in which you have had to deal with conflict. What were the sources of conflict? Would avoiding, accommodating, compromising, collaborating, or competing be the best way to deal with the conflict? What would be symptoms if you used the chosen mode too much?

2. Form a small group in class and use nominal group process to solve a problem, decide on class content, decide on possible class activities, set goals, and so forth.

3. Do role negotiations for a small group project.

4. Using Worksheet 19-1, make a decision chart for a small group project.

✎ Worksheet 19-1

Decision Chart

Make a decision chart for a small group project, inserting the appropriate code in the blocks for each group member's tasks.

Names

Tasks

Codes:
    M   Manages the process
    C   Consulted
    D   Makes decision
    I   Informed of the decision

Chapter

20

Motivation

Chapter Objectives

◆ Put Maslow's five needs into Alderfer's three categories of growth, relatedness, and existence needs.

◆ Identify at least five hygiene and five motivation factors in Herzberg's theory.

◆ Describe Vroom's expectancy theory.

◆ Explain how Skinner's positive reinforcement theory works.

◆ Describe ways people deal with perceived inequities.

◆ List at least three beliefs each for McGregor's Theory X and Theory Y.

Major Concepts and Definitions	
Motivation	given impetus to incite or impel or to spur on
Intrinsic	essential, inherent, not dependent on external circumstances
Extrinsic	not inherent, not essential, external, extraneous
Job satisfaction	contentment with one's work

MOTIVATION

Why do people work? Why do some employees achieve high productivity while others are content with mediocrity or less? What can a manager do to stimulate intrinsic and extrinsic motivation? These questions are important to the manager. They elicit complex and uncertain answers. Unfortunately, there are no simple rules that a manager can follow to stimulate the staff.

Taylor's Monistic Theory

Monistic theory is derived from the principles of scientific management. Frederick Taylor, a pioneer in this field, believed that if energetic people with high productivity learned that they earned no more than a lazy worker who did as little as possible, they would lose interest in giving optimal performance. Taylor argued that an incentive was needed to prevent this loss. It should be possible to earn more by producing more, so that pay would depend on productivity. Incentives such as merit increases, bonus systems, profit sharing, savings sharing, and piece rates are examples of monistic methods. With implementation of payment by piece rate, the employer must be certain that wage costs do not increase more rapidly than production. This system can place considerable pressure on the worker and create tensions that lead to undesirable behavior. Payment by piece rate almost certainly guarantees that some workers will be paid more than others. A larger paycheck may increase one's self-esteem and even serve as a status symbol, but the amount of motivation provided by money is questionable.

Maslow's Hierarchy-of-Needs Theory

In contrast to Taylor's belief that money is a primary motivator, A.H. Maslow maintained that people are motivated by a desire to satisfy a hierarchy of needs. Maslow hypothesized that satisfaction of the basic physiological needs triggers the emergence of more abstract needs and that a satisfied need is no longer a motivator. The five basic needs he identified are physiological, safety, love, esteem, and self-actualization.

Physiological needs. The body needs water, food, oxygen, elimination, rest, exercise, sex, shelter, and protection from the elements. People have a strong drive for self-preservation, and whenever their basic physiological needs are threatened, the needs become prepotent. These needs are relatively independent and must be met repeatedly to remain fulfilled. In an affluent society, the physiological needs are probably not the most common motivators. The nurse manager should determine whether physiological needs are being met. Personnel should not be overworked. Meal breaks and rest breaks should be provided. Pay should be adequate for food, shelter, health care, and recreation.

Safety needs.   People need physical, emotional, and financial safety. They need a stable environment in which they are protected against the threats of danger and deprivation. People do not want to worry about inadequate income because of loss of job, accident, or old age. Arbitrary management actions, favoritism toward or discrimination against employees, and unpredictable administration of policy are dangerous to safety needs and should be avoided.

Love needs.   Love needs include a feeling of belonging, acceptance by one's peers, recognition as an accepted member of a group, being an integral part of the operation, giving and receiving friendship, and affectionate relations with others. A cohesive work group is likely to be more effective than an equal number of people working separately. Yet management, fearing hostility toward its objectives, may control situations to prevent esprit de corps. Thwarting of the social needs, however, may stimulate resistance and antagonism that further defeat management's objectives.

Esteem needs.   Achievement, competence, knowledge, independence, status, recognition, prestige, appreciation, reputation, and respect contribute to one's self-confidence and self-esteem. Management can help meet these needs by giving praise when it is deserved and through the use of constructive evaluations, pay raises, and titles. Unlike the lower physiological and safety needs, the esteem needs are not so easily satisfied.

Self-actualization.   It is doubtful that one ever achieves all that of which one is capable. Feelings of accomplishment, responsibility, importance, challenge, advancement, and new experiences and opportunities for growth contribute to self-fulfillment.

Alderfer's Modified Need Hierarchy

Clayton Alderfer proposes a modified need hierarchy theory that collapses Maslow's five hierarchical levels into three (see Box 20-1). His existence-relatedness-growth (ERG) theory suggests that in addition to a satisfaction-progression process, in which people are constantly frustrated in their attempts to satisfy one level of needs, they can redirect their energy toward a lower-level need. Alderfer's model is less rigid than Maslow's and suggests that more than one need may be operative.

McClelland's Basic Needs Theory

David McClelland has identified three basic needs that all people have in varying degrees: the need for achievement, power, and affiliation. The need for achievement

Box 20-1   MASLOW AND ALDERFER HIERARCHIES

MASLOW	ALDERFER
Self-actualization Esteem needs	Growth needs
Love needs	Relatedness needs
Safety needs Physiological needs	Existence needs

involves a desire to make a contribution, to excel, and to succeed. People with high achievement needs are eager for responsibility, take calculated risks, and desire feedback about their performance. People who have a high need for power want to be in control and desire influence over others. They are more interested in personal prestige and power than effective performance. For contrast, people with high affiliation needs desire working in human environments and seek out meaningful friendships. They want to be respected and avoid decisions or actions that oppose group norms. They are more interested in high morale than productivity. Managers should match personnel needs with assignments. If a project has well-defined objectives and specific tasks, a person with a high achievement need may be appropriate. If a project involves unpleasant tasks with personnel (such as retrench-ment), a person with high power needs may do the job best. A person with high affiliation needs would not want to make decisions that would alienate peers but would be good for fostering morale.

Herzberg's Motivation-Hygiene Theory, or Two-Factor Theory

Frederick Herzberg found that work motivators include achievement, growth, responsibility, advancement, recognition, and the job itself. According to Herzberg, if people are satisfied with their job, they are receiving positive feedback, develop-ing skills, and improving their performance. Herzberg maintains that employees can be motivated by giving them challenging work in which they can assume respon-sibility.

Dissatisfaction results when people perceive that they are being treated unfairly in pay, benefits, status, job security, supervision, and interpersonal relationships. Herzberg classifies all of the above as hygiene factors and argues that they are not motivators because they do not cause any improvement in attitudes or per-formance. They can only prevent dissatisfaction and poor morale. Hygiene fac-tors do not make a job more interesting. If people are highly motivated and find their job interesting and challenging, they can tolerate dissatisfaction with hygiene factors.

Argyris's Psychological Energy Theory

Chris Argyris believes that people will exert more energy to meet their own needs than those of the organization. The greater the disparity between the individual's and the organization's goals, the more likely it is that the employee will feel dissatisfaction, tension, conflict, apathy, or subversion. Argyris suggests that management match personnel and jobs by taking advantage of people's talents and interests, make jobs interesting and challenging, help personnel satisfy their needs for self-actualization, improve interpersonal relationships, and use a management style consistent with Theory Y (discussed later).

Vroom's Expectancy Theory

Victor Vroom popularized the expectancy theory during the 1960s. It is based on Kurt Lewin's field theory and has been expanded by Lyman Porter and others. Expectancy theory states that motivation is dependent on how much people want something and their estimate of the probability of getting it.

$$\boxed{\text{Motivation}} = \boxed{\text{Valence}} \times \boxed{\text{Expectancy}}$$

Valence is the strength of one's preference for something. It may be negative or positive. If one does not want something, there is a negative valence. If the person is indifferent, the valence is 0. A positive valence indicates a desire for something.

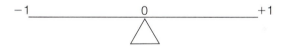

Expectancy is the probability of getting something through specific actions. If a person believes that an action will result in an outcome, expectancy has a value of 1. If no probability is perceived, the expectancy is 0. Expectancy varies from one situation to another.

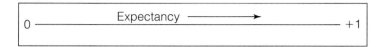

If someone has a high valence and a high expectancy, the motivation will be high. If there is a low valence and a low expectancy, the motivation will be low. If one is high and the other low, moderate motivation will result.

$$\boxed{\text{M}} = \boxed{\text{EP}} \times \boxed{\text{PO}} \times \boxed{\text{V}}$$

M = Motivation
EP = Belief that effort will lead to desired performance
PO = Anticipation that performance will lead to a particular outcome
V = Value of reward

The expectancy theory has been further developed to include the value of the outcome factor. To be highly motivated, a person needs to find an outcome attractive, believe that certain actions will lead to the desired outcome, and assess that the result is worth the effort. Consequently, to motivate personnel, managers should clarify connections between work and outcome and should reward desirable behavior.

Skinner's Positive Reinforcement Theory

Operant conditioning or behavior modification are other names for Skinner's positive reinforcement theory. Behavior may be strengthened or weakened depending on what follows it. Positive reinforcement strengthens behavior. Withholding positive reinforcers weakens behavior, whereas intermittent reinforcement increases resistance to extinction. Punishment will help reduce behavior, but it cannot teach new behaviors, and it may condition avoidance.

Accentuating the positive with plenty of praise and positive feedback may increase the frequency of desired behavior. If, however, a subordinate admits to less than desirable behavior, the manager may respond, "I appreciate your honesty," while reminding the worker of the goal. When desired results are not obtained, managers should analyze the situation. First they should assess the working environment for interference. Does the employee have adequate time to complete the task? Does the system allow nurses to maximize their efficiency, or must they spend most of their time running to central supply to gather materials that should have been readily available? If managers do not locate the cause of the problem in the environment, they must ask themselves if the employee has been properly utilized. Do they have the knowledge and skills necessary to do the job? If not, can they be taught? If they cannot be taught, can they be replaced and assigned other duties?

Equity Theory

During the 1960s, Jo Stacy Adams and others studied perceptions of equity and inequity. They found that employees assess fairness by considering their input and the psychological, social, and financial rewards in comparison with those of others. Perceived inequity causes tension. The amount of the tension was found to be proportional to the magnitude of the perceived inequity. Tension motivates people to reduce its cause. Consequently, the strength of the motivation to reduce the perceived inequity is proportional to the cognitive dissonance. To reduce the inequity, people may alter input or outcome, cognitively distort input or output, change the basis for comparison, or leave. If people feel overworked and underpaid, they are likely to decrease their productivity. Less often, employees feel overrewarded and strive to improve their performance. People resist changing their bases of comparison or distorting their perceptions. People do not usually leave an organization unless there is extreme inequity. If the comparison is equal, people feel that they are treated fairly. If not, they are motivated to take corrective action. Managers should be attentive to the perceived equity of the reward system.

Intrinsic Motivation

Edward L. Deci has studied intrinsic motivation. He found that some activities are ends in themselves, not just means to ends. There is no apparent reward except the activity itself. Intrinsically motivated behavior seems to be stimulated by people's needs for feeling competent and self-determining. When there is no stimulation, people will seek it. When they are overstimulated, they back away, regroup, and reaffirm competence. People engage in a process of seeking and conquering to feel competent and self-determined. When peoples' feelings of competence and self-determination are enhanced, their intrinsic motivation will increase. If their perception of competence and self-determination are diminished, their intrinsic motivation will decrease. Extrinsic rewards have a controlling aspect that may decrease intrinsic rewards. Insufficient extrinsic rewards tend to increase intrinsic motivation because people try to reduce cognitive dissonance. Consequently, managers should foster stimulation through means such as continuing education and special projects.

McGregor's Theory X and Theory Y

Douglas McGregor has classified traditional management theories as Theory X. They are based on the assumption that people will avoid work if possible because they dislike it; consequently, most people must be directed, controlled, coerced, and threatened. Theory X assumes that people want direction, have little ambition, avoid responsibility, but want security. A manager with a Theory X philosophy would probably use fear and threats to motivate personnel, supervise closely, delegate little responsibility, and not consider personnel participation in planning.

McGregor maintains that if people behave as described in Theory X it is because of what the system has done to them—not because of their inherent nature. He believes that as long as managerial strategies are based on Theory X, managers will fail to discover, let alone use, the potentials of their personnel.

McGregor classifies the newer developments in management as Theory Y. In this theory McGregor makes the assumption that people like and enjoy work, are self-directed, and seek responsibility. It maintains that most people have imagination, ingenuity, creativity, and other intellectual capacities that are only partially utilized. A manager with a Theory Y philosophy will use positive incentives such as praise and recognition, give general supervision, provide opportunities for individual growth, delegate responsibilities, and encourage participation in problem solving. Job enlargement and decentralization are additional motivational techniques that may stimulate personnel's performance to the extent that it exceeds the requirements stated in the job description.

Likert's Participative Management Theory

Rensis Likert believes that effective managers are highly sensitive to their staff associates, use communication to keep the group working as a unit, and foster supportive relationships among all group members. Participative management is a human relations theory that may use management by objectives and job-enrichment approaches.

Theory Z

The Japanese form of participative management is known as Theory Z. The major firms of Japan are organized into *Zaibatsu,* small groups of 20 to 30 firms representing each important industrial sector. Each firm hosts satellite companies that provide a service or manufacture a subassembly for the host firm. Employees are hired to work for the host firm until retirement. After slow evaluation and promotion in nonspecialized careers, employees are retired at age 55. They then work on a part-time basis for a satellite company. Women work temporarily and serve as a buffer to the job security of the male work force. Their schedules are flexible so they can care for their families, and they are laid off in slack periods.

Concern for the worker is apparent. Japanese companies form inclusive personal and professional relationships and provide social support. Because personnel anticipate lifetime relationships, they are cautious about interpersonal conflicts. Cooperation is stressed. Collective decision making is practiced. Through the ritual of *ringi,* ideas pass from manager to manager for approval. This helps establish trust and cooperation. Objectives and the procedures to achieve them are implicitly described. Quality circles are formed when two to ten employees meet to identify problems, explore options, and make decisions. Quality circles have increased worker productivity, enhanced job satisfaction, and reduced turnover in addition to solving identified problems. Decisions are made by consensus. Because it takes so much time to reach a consensus, only policy and behavior changes are dealt with. Responsibility is also collective. An emphasis is placed on developing all aspects of the employees, and they are rewarded with regular pay bonuses based on the company's performance.

The Japanese Theory Z managers focus on the four soft S's of management: staff, skills, style, and superordinate goals. Staff is the workers. Skills are the capabilities of the organization or key personnel. Style refers to the cultural style of the organization or how managers achieve goals. The superordinate goals are the guideposts as determined by the personnel.

Less attention is given to the hard S's: system, structure, and strategy. The system is the mechanism whereby information circulates through the organization. Structure is the organization, and strategy is the plan of action.

Historical Development of Motivation Theory

Traditional management theory is based on McGregor's Theory X. Traditional theory addresses itself to Maslow's primary physiological and safety needs and employs the monistic theory for reinforcement. The latter, according to Herzberg, helps meet some of the hygiene needs but does not provide motivation.

Newer developments in management are based on McGregor's Theory Y. Maslow's secondary needs of love, esteem, and self-actualization are more prepotent than the primary needs for most personnel. Because a satisfied need is no longer a motivator, hygiene factors such as money and working conditions do not serve as motivators. People are more interested in autonomy, responsibility, achievement, recognition, variety in work, and efforts for self-actualization. Argyris has suggested that personnel may become more self-actualized if their personal goals are consistent with the goals of the organization. Talents and interests should be considered when assigning jobs. And then, according to Skinner, positive reinforcement will further increase desired behaviors.

Participation is a major factor in newer management techniques. Personnel are encouraged to contribute to decisions, goals, and plans. Decentralization is supported to the point of management by objectives, allowing personnel to define their own objectives and to determine how they plan to achieve them. The supervisor approves the goals, makes sure they are consistent with the organization's goals, and evaluates personnel using their own objectives as the standard. Modern managers delegate duties and assist others to work more effectively. They help each person develop their own talents and try to maintain a close relationship between the interests and skills of the individual and the requirements of the job. Job enrichment and job rotation may be used to help develop personnel fully. When personnel are actively striving toward esteem and self-actualization and when their goals are consistent with those of the organization, there is likely to be a noticeable effect on the accomplishment of the organization's goals and productivity.

Job Satisfaction*

Job dissatisfaction contributes to higher turnover rates and decreased productivity. Considerable time and money are required to recruit and select a replacement for someone who leaves a position. It takes time to socialize the new employee to the organization's norms. This orientation period is expensive because of educational expenses and decreased productivity. Other employees must carry more than their share of the load until the new individual can work to capacity, and group redevelopment is necessary after each change in membership. For all these reasons job satisfaction is a concern for nursing administrators.

Job dissatisfaction has been shown to be correlated with absenteeism and turnover. Herzberg maintains that satisfiers and dissatisfiers are mutually exclusive; he classifies the sense of achievement, recognition for achievement, the work itself, responsibility, advancement potential, and possibility of growth as motivators or satisfiers and matters such as working conditions, policies, supervision, interpersonal relations, salary, status, and job security as hygiene factors or dissatisfiers. He concludes that hygiene factors cannot motivate employees but can only prevent dissatisfaction. Herzberg's work remains controversial.

Maslow's theory shows insight into Herzberg's findings. It suggests that hygiene factors can be motivators and that only when hygiene factors are satisfied do satisfiers such as responsibility become motivators. Several research studies have indicated that people at lower educational, socioeconomic, and occupational levels and minority members tend to place more emphasis on hygiene or extrinsic job factors, whereas people at higher educational, socioeconomic, and occupational levels and whites are more concerned with motivators or intrinsic factors. In accordance with Maslow's theory, physiological and safety needs are apparently prepotent for lower socioeconomic groups, whereas these needs have probably been satisfied for people at higher

---

* From Marriner A: *Contemporary nursing management,* St Louis, 1982, CV Mosby.

educational and occupational levels, such as nurses, for whom esteem and self-actualization needs have become prepotent.

Researchers disagree about the effects of supervision on job satisfaction. Employees' attitudes toward supervision are influenced by their perception of the supervisor's role, their self-perception, and their level of development. These individual differences necessitate that supervision be an adaptive leadership process.

The desire for influence in decision making is also affected by individual differences. Even though people presumably desire some control over their environment, this desire is not equally strong for all people. Vroom found that authoritarians are relatively unaffected by participating in decision making but that participation in decision making generally has a favorable effect on job satisfaction. Role ambiguity, the result of a failure to inform an individual of what is needed to do the job, is relatively common. Even if the role is clear, an employee in that role may resign if role conflict is present and persists. Role conflicts may result from a number of factors and are affected by individual differences. Likewise, job satisfaction is multidimensional and subject to individual differences.

Women seem to show more variation than men in their job attitudes. Women emphasize working conditions, hours and ease of work, supervision, and social aspects of the job, whereas men emphasize wages, opportunity for advancement, company management and policies, and task interest. College-educated women rank the importance of motivators such as achievement, recognition, and responsibility significantly higher than female clerical workers without college degrees. People tend to have more job satisfaction before the age of 20 years and after the age of 35 years than during the period between. Younger people tend to be more interested in income, whereas older people are interested in security.

Nurses surveyed about their sources of satisfaction identify a sense of achievement, recognition, challenging work, responsibility, advancement potential, autonomy, authority, pleasant work environment, agreeable working hours, and adequate staffing all as satisfiers. Nurses stress the importance of respected hospital administrators, supportive nursing administrators, trustful managers, fair evaluations, and adequate feedback. Poor planning, poor communication, inadequate explanations of decisions affecting jobs, unclear rules and regulations, unreasonable pressure, excessive work, workload negatively affecting work quality, understaffing, uncooperative physicians, nonnursing duties, and unqualified managers are all sources of dissatisfaction. Reduced productivity, increased absenteeism, and rapid turnover are expensive consequences of job dissatisfaction but can be reduced if the nursing administrator fosters job satisfaction through organization and management.

BIBLIOGRAPHY

Burkes M: Identifying and relating nurses' attitudes toward computer use, *Comput Nurs* 9:190-201, September-October 1991.

Chacko SB, Huba ME: Academic achievement among undergraduate nursing students: the development and test of a causal model, *J Nurs Educ* 30:267-273, June 1991.

Coombs M: Motivational strategies for intensive care nurses, *Intensive Care Nurs* 7:114-119, June 1991.

Dake SB, Taylor JA: Motivating adult learners with effective feedback, *Journal of Extra Corporeal Technology* 24:64-68, 1992.

Dixon EA: Characteristics of registered nurses' self-directed learning projects for professional development, *J Prof Nurs* 9:89-94, March-April 1993.

Fleury JD: Empowering potential: a theory of wellness motivation, *Nurs Res* 40(5):286-291, September-October 1991.

Garfink CM, Kirby KK, Bachman SS: The University Hospital nurse extender program: what have we learned? Part 4, *JONA* 21:26-31, April 1991.

Havens DS, Mills ME: Professional recognition and compensation for staff RNs: 1990 and 1995, *Nurs Econ* 10:15-20, January-February 1992.

Hellman EA: Analysis of a home health agency's productivity system, *Public Health Nurs* 8:251-257, December 1991.

Henderson MC: Measuring motivation: the power management inventory, *J Nurs Manage* 1:67-80, Spring 1993.

Herzberg F: One more time: how do you motivate employees? *Harv Bus Rev* 46:53-62, January-February 1968.

Hudy JJ: The motivation trap, *HR Magazine* 37:63-67, December 1992.

Hurst KL, Croker PA, Bell SK: How about a lollipop? A peer recognition program, *Nurs Manage* 25:68-72, September 1994.

Lufkin SR, Herrick LM, Newman DA et al: Job satisfaction in the head nurse role, *Nurs Manage* 32:27-29, March 1992.

Hughes KK, Marcantonio RJ: Recruitment, retention, and compensation of agency and hospital nurses, *JONA* 21:46-52, October 1991.

Marriner A: Motivation of personnel, *Superv Nurse* 7:60-63, October 1976.

Mueller CW, McCloskey MC: Nurses' job satisfaction: a proposed measure, *Nurs Res* 39:113-117, March-April 1990.

Simpson P: Motivational theories: reflections on their application by nursing managers, *Canadian Journal of Nursing* 1:16-19, March-April 1988.

Smith R: Motivation is the key to effective performance, *Management Accounting* 71:50, March 1993.

Stachnik T, Brown B, Hinds W et al: Goal setting, social support, and financial incentives in stress management programs: a pilot study of their impact on adherence, *Am J Health Promotion* 5:24-29, September-October 1990.

Valadez AM, Lund CA: Mentorship: Maslow and me, *Journal of Continuing Education in Nursing* 24:259-3, November-December 1993.

Webb D, Tour C, Hurt R et al: Recognizing excellence: giving your AWE, *J Nurs Adm* 22:54-56, September 1992.

Wineman NM, Durand E: Incentives and rewards for subjects in nursing research, *West J Nurs Res* 14:526-531, August 1992.

CASE STUDY

You have identified that Ann has a high need for achievement, Betty for power, and Carl for affiliation. What assignments will you give them to meet those needs to motivate them?

CRITICAL THINKING AND LEARNING ACTIVITIES

1. List five needs that you have now and place them in Maslow's classification.

2. Place those same needs in Alderfer's classification.

3. Make two columns on a sheet of paper. In one column list what was happening when you had job satisfaction. In the second column list what was happening when you had job dissatisfaction. Do these lists support Herzberg's theory or not?

4. Using Worksheet 20-1, identify the valence and expectancy of something you want. How do they affect your motivation?

5. Think about something you need to do. Do you receive any reinforcement for doing it? How does the response you get affect your motivation?

6. Have you ever felt you were being treated inequitably? If so, how did you respond? Was your behavior consistent with equity theory?

7. Review the list of beliefs in McGregor's Theory X and Theory Y. How do you classify your philosophy?

Worksheet 20-1

Valence, Expectancy, and Motivation

List three things that you want, and then identify the valence, expectancy, and motivation of each.

Want	Valence	Expectancy	Motivation

Chapter

21

Communication

Chapter Objectives

◆ List the six steps in the communication process.

◆ List at least six barriers to communication.

◆ Describe ways to improve communication.

◆ Describe how to deal with hostile-aggressive people.

◆ Plan strategies for dealing with a sniper.

◆ Describe how to handle complainers.

Major Concepts and Definitions	
Communication	giving and receiving information via talk, gestures, writing, and so forth
Ideation	decision to share an idea
Encoding	putting meaning into symbols
Transmission	sending the message
Receiving	seeing and hearing transmitted message
Decoding	defining words and interpreting gestures
Feedback	an evaluative response
Grapevine	informal communication system

COMMUNICATION PROCESS

All of the manager's functions involve communication. The communication process involves six steps.

$$\text{Ideation} \rightarrow \text{Encoding} \rightarrow \text{Transmission} \rightarrow \text{Receiving} \rightarrow \text{Decoding} \rightarrow \text{Response} \,\rceil$$
$$\text{Response} \leftarrow \text{Decoding} \leftarrow \text{Receiving} \leftarrow \text{Transmission} \leftarrow \text{Encoding} \leftarrow\!\!\rule{1cm}{0.4pt}$$

The first step, ideation, begins when the sender decides to share the content of a message with someone, senses a need to communicate, develops an idea, or selects information to share. The purpose of communication may be to inform, persuade, command, inquire, or entertain. Whatever the reason, the sender needs to have a goal and think clearly, or the message may be garbled and meaningless.

Encoding, the second step, involves putting meaning into symbolic forms: speaking, writing, or nonverbal behavior. One's personal, cultural, and professional biases affect the goals and encoding process. Use of clearly understood symbols and communication of all the information that the receiver needs to know are important.

The third step, transmission of the message, must overcome interference, such as garbled speech, unintelligible use of words, long complex sentences, distortion from recording devices, noise, and illegible handwriting.

Receiving is next. The receiver's senses of seeing and hearing are activated as the transmitted message is received. People tend to have selective attention (hear the messages of interest to them but not others) and selective perception (hear the parts of the message that conform with what they want to hear) that cause incomplete and distorted interpretation of the communication. Sometimes people tune out the message because they anticipate the content and think they know what is going to be said or are so busy formulating their response that they do not hear the message. The receiver may be preoccupied with other activities and consequently not be ready to listen. Poor listening is one of the biggest barriers in the communication process.

Decoding of the message by the receiver is the critical fifth step. The receiver defines words and interprets gestures during the transmission of speech. Written messages allow more time for decoding, as receivers assess the explicit meaning and implications of the message based on what the symbols mean to them. The symbols are subject to interpretation based on one's personal, cultural, and professional biases and may not have the same meaning to the receiver as to the sender. The communication process is dependent on the receiver's understanding of the information.

Response, or feedback, is the final step. It is important for the manager or sender to know that the message has been received and accurately interpreted.

COMMUNICATION SYSTEMS

Study of small-group process has revealed various communication networks (Fig. 21-1). The chain system is fast and accurate for simple problems. The middle person in the chain emerges as the leader, and the leadership position is stable. Unfortunately, morale is low and so is the flexibility for problem solving.

The leader emerges at the location of highest centrality, which is the fork of the Y and the hub of the wheel. Both provide fast, accurate problem solving. The coordinator, who is centrally located, is generally satisfied, but the peripheral members are less satisfied than members in less efficient systems. The wheel is an efficient, effective communication structure for simple problems.

The circular structure is slow and inaccurate. The structure does not influence the emergence of a leader. Because no one can communicate with everyone, there is no coordinator. However, morale is high, and there is considerable flexibility for problem solving.

When free to do so, groups tend to evolve to the all-channel network as problems become complex and shift back to a wheel structure as problems become simple.

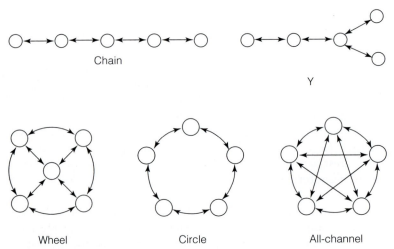

Chain

Y

Wheel   Circle   All-channel

Figure 21-1 Communication systems: chain, Y, wheel, circle, all-channel.

Greater amounts of information must be processed as task uncertainty and complexity increase. Consequently, an adaptive structure such as the all-channel system is best for completing complicated and unpredictable tasks. Essentially, the right network is the structure that facilitates the communication necessary to accomplish the task.

DOWNWARD COMMUNICATION

The traditional line of communication is from the manager down through the levels of management (Fig. 21-2). This downward communication is primarily directive and helps coordinate the activities of different levels of the hierarchy by telling staff associates what to do and by providing the information needed by staff associates to relate their efforts to the organization's goals. It includes oral and written indoctrination, education, and other information to influence the attitudes and behaviors of staff associates. Common forms of downward communications are employee handbooks, operating manuals, job description sheets, performance appraisal interviews, employee counseling, a loudspeaker system, letters, memos, messages circulated with paychecks, posters, bulletin boards, information racks, company newspapers, annual reports, the chain of command, the grapevine, and unions. Downward communication contributes to greater staff associate dissatisfaction than upward communication, regardless of the quality of the message.

UPWARD COMMUNICATION

Newer management techniques encourage delegation of authority and more personal involvement in decision making, thus creating a need for accurate upward communication (Fig. 21-3). Upward communication provides a means for motivating and

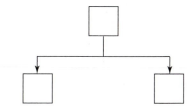

Figure 21-2   Downward communication.

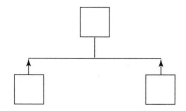

Figure 21-3   Upward communication.

satisfying personnel by allowing employee input. The manager summarizes information and passes it upward to the next level for use in decision making. That level then summarizes its action and transmits information to the next level. Because each level tends to bias the report by embellishing it with information that puts that level in the best light, there is a natural filtering process as information moves upward. By the time it reaches top management, it is highly refined.

In spite of this bias, staff associates are often in a position to assess the situation more accurately than are their managers. An employee may have a better solution to a problem than the first-line manager, who may know more about a situation than a middle manager, and so on. Consequently, accurate upward communication is important for effective problem solving. Staff associates must feel free to communicate both solicited and unsolicited information upwardly and must have opportunity to do so, or management will lack needed information, and both managers and staff associates will become frustrated. Common means for upward communication include face-to-face discussions; open-door policies; staff meetings; task forces; written reports; performance appraisals; grievance procedures; exit interviews; attitude surveys; suggestion boxes; counseling; the chain of command; ombudsmen; informers; the grapevine; unions; and participative, consultative, and democratic management in general.

LATERAL COMMUNICATION

Lateral, or horizontal, communication is between departments or personnel on the same level of the hierarchy and is most frequently used to coordinate activities (Fig. 21-4). The need for lateral communication increases as interdependence increases. For instance, it becomes more important when one worker starts a job and someone else finishes it. It is also used by staff to transmit technical information to line authorities, and it may contain subjective and emotional aspects. Committees, conferences, and meetings are often used to facilitate horizontal communication.

DIAGONAL COMMUNICATION

Diagonal communication occurs between individuals or departments that are not on the same level of the hierarchy (Fig. 21-5). Informal in nature and frequently used between staff groups and line functions and in project-type organizations, it is another facet of multidirectional communication, which is common when communications often flow in all directions at the same time.

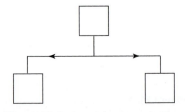

Figure 21-4   Lateral communication.

THE GRAPEVINE

Informal methods of communication coexist with formal channels and are referred to as the grapevine. Informal communication is often rapid and subject to considerable distortion. The grapevine transmits information much faster than the formal channels because it uses cluster chain pathways involving three or four individuals at a time instead of going from one person to another as in manager-staff associate relationships. Communication passes at an increasing rate as individuals from clusters inform other small groups of people who work near each other or have contact with each other. Information spreads most quickly through the grapevine when it is recent, affects personnel's work (for example, pay increases or changes in policies), and involves people they know. People who work near each other or come in contact with each other are likely to be on the same grapevine.

Information becomes distorted for a number of reasons. Grapevine information is often fragmentary and incomplete. Consequently, there is a tendency to supply the missing pieces. Some people seize this opportunity to express feelings of self-importance, thus compensating for feelings of insecurity but also distorting the message. Because the grapevine is informal, with no formal lines of accountability, individuals do not have to answer to their manager for misinforming others.

Managers can learn much by listening to the grapevine and can remedy distortions by using the informal channels to pass on correct information.

BARRIERS TO COMMUNICATION

Faulty reasoning and poorly expressed messages are major barriers to communication. Lack of clarity and precision resulting from inadequate vocabulary, poorly chosen words, platitudes, jargon, awkward sentence structures, poor organization of ideas, and lack of coherence are common. Talking too fast or too slow, slurring words, and not emphasizing important points lead to the faulty transmission of ideas. Memos that are poorly organized, ramble, and lack summaries also complicate the communication process. Words mean different things to different people. Communication is complicated when the sender uses words with which the receiver is not familiar, does not communicate on the receiver's level, or makes the message long and complicated.

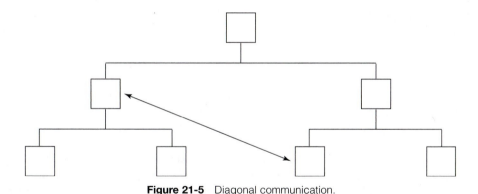

Figure 21-5   Diagonal communication.

If senders lack information or omit facts they do know, they will pass on a distorted or filtered message. Filtering, whether intentional or unintentional, involves a biased choice of what is communicated. For instance, distortion is more likely when subordinates desire promotion, for they may pass on information about their merits and suppress less successful aspects of their work. Fear of the consequences of full disclosure contributes to such omissions. At other times individuals may not communicate some information because they do not believe it is important enough to do so. The receiver becomes confused when nonverbal cues, such as facial expressions and posture, conflict with the verbal communication or when the sender does not admit to the intent of, or to the emotions underlying, the message.

People use selective perception to hear what they want to hear in terms of their biases. Values, attitudes, and assumptions affect one's perception of the message. Making a value judgment about the worth of a message based on one's opinion of the sender or the expected meaning of the message allows the receiver to hear what she wants to hear. An attitude is a feeling toward someone or something that is based on experience or the lack thereof, and it is a common barrier to communication because of its screening effect. Uncommunicated assumptions are common and can make a considerable difference between the message sent and the one received. For instance, when program evaluation is mandated, personnel may fear that the results will be used to terminate workers, whereas management's actual intention is to use the results for recruiting purposes. Trust or distrust of the sender also influences how the message is received.

The sender is judged along with the message because the receiver has difficulty separating what one hears from how one feels about the sender. In fact, nonexistent motives can be attributed to the sender. Messages from higher echelons are often considered authoritative, even when they are not intended to be. The higher in the hierarchy a message originates, the greater are its chances of being accepted because of the status of the sender. If the sender has status with the listener, the message is usually considered credible. If the sender does not, the message may be discounted.

Staff associates tend to pay attention to communications from managers, thus facilitating downward communication. Unfortunately, managers may give verbal and nonverbal cues about how busy and unapproachable they are. They probably value communications from higher-level managers more than those from staff associates and may not reward associates for communications. In fact, staff associates are sometimes punished for communicating. Staff associates will be reluctant to report problems or potential problems when they believe these will be viewed as a weakness in their performance appraisal. Similarly, middle managers may not report problems that would reflect unfavorably on their managerial skills.

Status symbols magnify role and status barriers by increasing the psychological distance and the perceived organizational distance. Time pressures also become barriers that prevent communication. Managers do not have time to see all of their staff associates as much as desired, and staff associates may not take the time to report to the manager. Time pressures are also used as an excuse for not listening. Premature evaluation of what is going to be said, preoccupation with oneself, lack of readiness to hear, lack of receptivity to new ideas, and resistance to change interfere with listening. Physical distance, organizational complexity, temperature, noise, physical facilities (such as offices, meeting rooms, and an informal coffee shop), and technical facilities (such as telephones, loudspeakers, and duplicating equipment) also affect communications.

IMPROVING COMMUNICATION

Ideas should be clear before one speaks. What is the purpose of the message? Is it to seek information, inform, persuade, or initiate action? To formulate a message, one must gather the information needed and seek consultation from others as appropriate. Considering the goals and attitudes of the receivers helps the sender convey something of help or value to the receivers. One must also determine the mode of communication—by written or oral messages or through gestures. Face-to-face contact involves nonverbal behavior that further clarifies intent and allows for feedback to validate understanding of the message. Feedback through mutual exchange decreases the chance for misunderstanding. A climate that allows people to say what they think facilitates feedback.

One must also consider the setting in which one communicates and time one's messages for maximal impact. Should the communication be made in public or private? What is the social climate and what effect will that have on the tone of the communication? What are the customs and practices of the audience, and how does one's message conform to its expectations? It is helpful for the message to refer to something the person has experienced and for it to be timed for immediate use by the receiver. For example, a building evacuation plan will be better received during fire prevention week, when personnel are expecting a fire drill, than at most other times.

Communications should be well organized and expressed in simple words, a clear style, and the shortest sentences possible. Redundancy—the repetition of the message verbatim or its presentation in several different ways—ensures that the message is understood. The amount of redundancy depends on the content of the message and the experience and background of the receiver. Repetition is especially important when the information is important and the directions are complicated. However, redundancy can become a barrier to communication if the message is simple and personnel are familiar with it. Employees are likely to stop listening because they know what is going to be said.

Because actions speak louder than words, the message is more forceful if the sender acts congruously. Communications should be followed up to make sure they were understood, and one should seek to understand as well as to be understood.

Listening, an active process that requires conscious attention, is critical to good communication. Trust is a prerequisite, because nurses will not share feelings with people they do not trust. The speaker must be convinced that disclosures will be kept confidential, that feelings will be respected and not judged, and that the information will be used appropriately and not used against the speaker.

Once trust is established, empathetic listening is needed. We think faster than we talk. Consequently, when listening to another talk, we have time left over for thinking, time that is frequently misused. There is less time for irrelevant thoughts when one concentrates on what is being said. One can think ahead of the speaker, try to guess the points that will be made next, consider what the conclusion will be, listen between the lines, try to understand the speaker's point of reference, review, and summarize the points made.

Active listening involves refraining from talking while trying to understand the speaker's attitude and feelings. One should listen to the whole story, talking as little as possible and avoiding leading questions, arguing, or giving advice. Silent pauses encourage the speaker to continue. Attentiveness is indicated by comments such as "yes," "uh huh," "go on," restatement (repeating what was said), paraphrasing (saying what was said in different words), clarifying (asking the speaker what was meant), reflecting (responding to the feelings communicated), and summarizing (reviewing the major points made). By saying little, receivers can concentrate on listening instead of on what they are going to say in return.

Written communications usually have the advantage of being more carefully formulated than oral communications. They also may save time and money and can be retained as legal records and reference sources. Written communications are sent downward, upward, or horizontally. Policies, procedures, handbooks, annual reports, bulletin boards, and house newspapers are usually directed downward. Attitude and morale surveys, suggestion systems, and written grievances are directed upward. Letters, memos, and reports may be upward, downward, or horizontal communication. Between department heads they are horizontal.

Before writing, one must first consider the purpose of the communication. For a planned and organized message, the writer develops thoughts logically, gives evidence to back up statements, and carefully selects words. Writers must ask themselves whether the communication answers who, what, when, where, and why questions and should appraise the tone of the document. Because writing is not easy, one should expect to edit original drafts.

Dictation is a valuable communication skill. Dictating probably requires more effort at first, but it can soon become easier than writing in longhand. In dictation one must again consider the purpose of the communication and plan and organize one's remarks. One starts dictation by indicating who is dictating what (letter or memo), the subject, type of paper needed (letterhead stationery, memo pad), and the number of copies needed. One should state the format (headings, double space, tabular outline, new paragraph), punctuation (capitalization, hyphen, period, commas, question marks, italics), and spell out unusual or unfamiliar words. Conversational instructions are given as one dictates. For example, "Mary, list the following statements and precede each with a dash." One should not smoke, eat, or chew gum while dictating. Background noises should be reduced as much as possible. Closing the office door during dictation can eliminate interference. Dictation should be given at a normal talking speed, with the words pronounced clearly and correctly. The sender can conclude dictation by saying "end of memo." If one cannot complete the dictation, instructions for the incomplete correspondence should be dictated. The dictator may want to keep a list of what is dictated and mark the items off as they are processed.

Communications are critical for the functioning of an organization. Nurses need to be familiar with the communication process, communication systems, and directions communications can take. There are numerous barriers to communication. Managers need to know them and ways to overcome them.

COMMUNICATING WITH DIFFICULT PEOPLE

One requires special communication skills in order to deal with some personalities, including hostile-aggressive, complaining, negative, unresponsive, and overly nice. Some hostile-aggressive types seem to attack in an abrupt, abusive, intimidating manner that pushes others to acquiesce against their better judgment. These people tend to know what others should do, need to prove themselves right, and lack trust and caring. One must stand up to a hostile-aggressive person or feel overrun and frustrated. It is important to do this without fighting, or the conflict will escalate. It can be advantageous to give the hostile-aggressive person time to run down for a while and then interrupt to stand up for oneself. There may be no opportunity to speak between sentences, thus making it necessary to interrupt before the other person has finished speaking. It is also likely that one may interrupt. Then one must state firmly, "You interrupted me," and start again, preferably with a smile. One needs to get the other person's attention to do problem solving. Calling the person by name may help get the person's attention. Deliberately dropping a book is a more dramatic way to get attention. By standing up, one may also get attention. In addition, the other person may be less aggressive when sitting down. Then one needs to state ideas forcefully in a friendly manner that does not belittle the other person. It is important to avoid fighting with the hostile-aggressive person because such a battle will likely be lost. Even if the battle is won, the hostile-aggressive person's righteous anger will likely increase, and the war may be lost. When one stands up to a bully, one may become a friend. When dealing with hostile-aggressive people, it is important to stand up for oneself without fighting.

Exploders are another type of hostile-aggressive personality. Adult tantrums are the grown-up version of childhood tantrums that are a defense mechanism to cope with fear, helplessness, and frustration. Adult tantrums are sudden, almost automatic, responses to feeling threatened. The exploder typically feels angry first and then blaming or suspicious. People act on their perceptions, but people are likely to perceive the same situation differently. Consequently, the other person may be unaware that the exploder has been threatened and be surprised by the outburst. The exploder should be given time to finish the tantrum and regain self-control. If the exploder does not finish, a neutral statement such as "Stop" may interrupt the tantrum. Then show that the person is taken seriously by a comment such as, "I can see this is important to you. I want to discuss this with you, but not like this." Possibly change the pace by getting a cup of coffee and seeking a private place for a problem-solving session.

Sniping is an aggressive response to an unresolved problem. It causes distress rather than positive actions. Unfortunately, the unsolved problems become worse, and the resulting stress causes more difficult behavior such as innuendoes, not-too-subtle remarks, and nonplayful teasing.

First of all, it is important to expose the attack by such comments as, "That sounded like a put-down; did you mean it that way?" Usually snipers will deny any attack. Sniping is not possible without a camouflage that works. Standing up to the attack without escalating it will help one proceed with problem solving. It gives the sniper an alternative to a direct contest. It is appropriate to get other points of view that confirm or deny the sniper's criticism, then try to solve any problems that have surfaced. Sniping can be prevented by establishing regular problem-solving meetings.

Complainers may dump on you directly or may complain about other "awful" people. Complaining helps people appear blameless and innocent, at least to themselves. One should listen attentively to the complaints, paraphrase as acknowledgement of what you heard, and confirm one's perception of how the complainer feels. One should not agree with or apologize for the allegations and avoid the accusation-defense-reaccusation pattern. It is preferable to simply state and acknowledge the facts without comment, then proceed with problem solving.

Negatively thinking people believe that any task that is out of their hands will fail and that others do not care and are self-serving. One should beware of being dragged down by their despair. One can make optimistic but realistic comments about past successes in similar situations but should not try to argue negativists out of their pessimism. It is better not to offer solution-alternatives until the problem has been thoroughly discussed or to ask people to act before they feel ready. During the problem-solving session, the negative events that could occur if the option were implemented should be explored. Be ready to take independent action if the group refuses to do so, and announce these plans without equivocation.

Unresponsive people cannot or will not speak when input is needed from them. It is difficult to know what their silence means. The most important strategy is to get the silent person to speak by asking open-ended questions, waiting calmly for a response, and not talking to fill the silence. If an open-ended question gets no response, one should comment on what is happening, for example, "I'm not getting any feedback from you," and end the observation with another open-ended question such as "What are you thinking?" Attention should be given when the person does speak. If the person never speaks, one should terminate the meeting by stating what will be done because no discussion occurred.

Superagreeable people are equally difficult people because they lead one to believe that they are in agreement but let one down when it comes to taking action. They have strong needs to be liked and accepted and help others feel approved in order to get approval themselves. They run into trouble when their need for approval conflicts with negative aspects of reality. They commit themselves to actions that they do not complete. Once again, problem solving is important. One must try to learn what prevents people from taking action and let them know that they are valued by telling them so and by asking questions about their interests, hobbies, and family to get to know them better. One should ask them what is not as good as they would like it to be and what could interfere with good relationships. Listening to their humor for hidden messages in teasing remarks and being prepared to do problem solving is also important.*

BIBLIOGRAPHY

Anthonypillai F: Cross-cultural communication in an intensive therapy unit, *Intensive Critical Care Nurs* 9:263-267, December 1993.
Armstrong MA, Kelly AE: Enhancing staff nurses' interpersonal skills: theory to practice, *Clinical Nurse Specialist* 7:313-317, November 1993.

---

* For a more extensive discussion, see Branson RM: *Coping with difficult people*, Garden City, NY, 1981, Anchor Press.

Brown SJ: Communication strategies used by an expert nurse, *Clinical Nursing Research* 3:43-56, February 1994.

Brunner NA: That was a good meeting! *Orthop Nurs* 12:35-39, July-August 1993.

Carlson-Catalono JM: Said another way: what is the language of nursing? *Nurs Forum* 28:22-26, October-December 1993.

Davis LL, Cos RP: Looking through the constructivist lens: the art of creating nursing work groups, *J Prof Nurs* 10:38-46, January-February 1994.

Dienemann J, Shaffer C: Nurse manager characteristics and skills: curriculum implications, *Nurs Connections* 6:15-23, Summer 1993.

Ehrenfeld M: A learning experience in communication: psychosocial expansion, *J Clin Nurs* 1:77-82, March 1992.

Ferraro-McDuffie A, Chan JSL, Jerome AM: Communicating the financial worth of the CNS through the use of fiscal reports, *Clinical Nurse Specialist* 7:91-97, March 1993.

Fowler AR, Bushardt SC, Jones MA: Retaining nurses through conflict resolution, *Health Progress* 74:25-29, June 1993.

Grinde T: Implementing a nursing administration local area network, *Nurs Manage* 25:36-37, July 1992.

Kolber R: Team building: a strategy to enhance cohesiveness, *Recruitment and Retention Report* 7:1-6, January 1994.

Laing M: Gossip: does it play a role in the socialization of nurses? *Image J Nurs Sch* 25:37-43, Spring 1993.

McClellan MA, Henson RH, Schmele J: Introducing new technology: confusion or order? *Nurs Manage* 25:38-39, July 1994.

McMahon B: The functions of space, *J Adv Nurs* 19:362-366, February 1994.

Mertens R, Jans B, Kurz X: A computerized nationwide network for nosocomial infection surveillance in Belgium, *Infect Control Hosp Epidemiol* 15:171-179, March 1994.

Piscopo B: Organizational climate, communication, and role strain in clinical nursing faculty, *J Prof Nurs* 10:113-119, March-April 1994.

Roberts GW: Nurse/patient communication within a bilingual health care setting, *Br J Nurs* 3:60-64, 66-67, January 27-February 9, 1994.

Simpson RL: Technology: nursing the system: ensuring patient data, privacy, confidentiality and security, *Nurs Manage* 25:18-20, July 1994.

Sviden G, Saljo R: Perceiving patients and their nonverbal reactions, *Am J Occup Ther* 47:491-497, June 1993.

Sweeney T, Sheahan N, Rice I et al: Communication disorders in a hospital elderly population, *Clinical Rehabilitation* 7:113-117, 1993.

Teasdale K: Information and anxiety: a critical reappraisal, *J Adv Nurs* 18:1125-1132, July 1993.

VanCott ML: Communicative competence during nursing admission interviews of elderly patients in acute care settings, *Qualitative Health Research* 3:184-208, May 1993.

Wilkinson S: Good communications in cancer nursing, *Nursing Standard* 7:35-39, November 1992.

Williams D, Brown DL: Automation at the point of care, *Nurs Manage* 25:32-35, July 1994.

CASE STUDY

The institution where you work is rightsizing and carefully evaluating productivity. The workers know that something is going on but are not informed. Consequently, they are imagining scenarios and rumors are rampant. One day a normally quiet, shy person explodes in your presence. She screams about the unfairness of cutting wages and laying off people. What might be the causes of her behavior? How should you deal with her behavior as it is occurring? What will you do regarding rumors?

CRITICAL THINKING AND LEARNING ACTIVITIES

1. Draw five squares connected differently on each of two pages. One person stands with her back to the class and describes how the squares are connected. Classmates are to draw squares as described without feedback. A second person stands facing the class and describes how five squares are connected. Classmates are to draw the squares as described. Questions and answers are allowed. Compare the accuracy of both methods. Was there a difference? If so, which method produced the more accurate outcomes?

2. In class, write scenarios for working with hostile-aggressive people. Assume roles and role-play how to handle hostile-aggressive people. Use Worksheet 21-1 to help you plan your responses.

3. In class, write scenarios for working with negative complaining people. What might be the causes of their behavior? How should you handle it as it is occurring? Assume roles with classmates and role-play how to handle difficult people, again using Worksheet 21-1.

✎ **Worksheet 21-1**

Working with Difficult People

Plan strategies for dealing with difficult people.

	Strategies
Hostile-aggressive	
Complaining	
Negative	
Unresponsive	
Overly nice	

Chapter

22

Assertiveness

Chapter Objectives

◆ List barriers to assertiveness.

◆ Describe complementary transactions.

◆ Describe crossed transactions.

◆ Describe three games people play.

◆ Identify the four life positions.

◆ Identify at least three assertive techniques and discuss how to use them.

Major Concepts and Definitions	
Assertiveness	the quality of being confident in stating one's opinions or needs
Transactional analysis	a technique for analyzing discussions
Life positions	an individual's assumption about self in relation to others
Passive	inactive, acted on
Aggressive	active, bold, pushy
Broken record	a technique involving repeating what one wants
Fogging	agreeing with the truth
Negative assertion	accepting negative aspects about oneself
Negative inquiry	asking for more information about oneself

ASSERTIVENESS

Barriers to Assertiveness

Communication styles are either passive, aggressive, or assertive. Assertiveness is the best style for nurse managers and the one they should foster in their personnel. However, there are barriers that nurses must overcome to become assertive. The most pervasive barrier is female sex role socialization. Whereas men are characterized as aggressive, competitive, independent, objective, analytical, task oriented, confident, self-disciplined, and emotionally controlled, women are expected to be passive, dependent, subjective, intuitive, empathetic, sensitive, interpersonally oriented, weak, inconsistent, and emotionally unstable.

The nursing socialization process and the nature of nursing are additional barriers. Both nursing schools and health agencies have organizational hierarchies with authority and power concentrated at the top. This arrangement usually promotes compliance and conformity. Nurses are taught to value sacrifice, humility, and service to others. They have been taught not to state their thoughts or feelings. Although they give intimate physical nurturing, they are not to become emotionally involved with clients. Nurses have been socialized into a subservient role. They are expected to follow physicians' orders and to be professional but not to anticipate equal financial reimbursement for their education and responsibilities. They are expected to be a part of the health team but not to make decisions or policies. They tend to keep so busy that they ignore their own rights.

In addition to these male-female role competition problems, nurses face female-female relationship problems. Men are more competitive with women than with other men, and women are more competitive with women than with men. Consequently, attempts to develop support systems for nurses are not usually successful. Instead, the queen bee and the trashing syndrome emerge.

The queen bee identifies with men, enjoys being told that she is different from most women, and feels superior to other women. The queen bee usually has to work very hard to become a success in a male-dominated society. She is likely to need to be cooperative and nonthreatening to achieve and maintain her successful position. She probably feels little animosity toward the system and the men who allowed her to become successful. Consequently, she is likely to identify with her male colleagues instead of with other women. However, protective of her own position and aware of the high price she paid for it, she makes it no easier for other women to succeed.

Trashing is a form of character assassination that divides women against one another. It is self-destructive and leads to impotent rage. Rather than exposing disagreements to resolve differences, trashing is done to destroy. It can be done to one's face or behind one's back, in public or in private. It questions one's motives, stresses one's worthlessness, and breaches one's integrity. The victim may be ignored, or anything she says or does may be interpreted in the most negative manner. Others' unrealistic expectations about her ensure failure. The trasher may give misinformation to others about what the victim does and thinks or tell her lies about what others think of her. Whatever method is used, it is manipulative, dishonest, and destructive. Women in general and nurses specifically need to become aware of what they are doing to each other, commit themselves to supportive instead of destructive behavior, learn to analyze interpersonal communication, and learn assertive behavior.

Transactional Analysis

Transactional analysis is a technique that can be used by nurses for analyzing and understanding behavior. It was developed by Eric Berne and popularized by Thomas Harris, Muriel James, and Dorothy Jongeward. Transactional analysis is an outgrowth of the Freudian concepts of id, ego, and superego: elements of the psyche that stimulate, monitor, and control behavior. Berne calls these ego states parent, child, and adult.

Ego states. The parent ego state controls and is the source of values, opinions, rules, regulations, and social conscience. The two major types of parent ego states are nurturing parent and critical parent. The nurturing parent guides, teaches, advises, and supplies "how to" information. The critical parent prohibits and supplies "should" and "should not" information. The parent ego state is a result of cultural traditions, social programming, and responsibilities. Parental judgments are drawn heavily from natural parents, older siblings, teachers, and other parent figures.

The child ego state is dominated by emotions and is the feeling state. It is the id ego state where strong feelings are triggered by immediate experiences. People are in the child state when they are experiencing childlike natural impulses, such as joy, delight, and gaiety or anger, hostility, and rage. The child ego state may be happy or destructive. The natural child is spontaneous, trusting, joyful, living, creative, and adventurous. The adapted child is suppressed and may express anger, rebellion, fear, or conformity.

The adult is the ego state that monitors one's behavior. It is the unemotional, thinking, problem-solving state. The adult ego state collects information, sets goals, compares alternatives, makes decisions and plans, and tests reality. The adult ego state is an unemotional state in which rational decision making takes place.

Every individual exhibits behavior from the three ego states at different times. A healthy individual maintains a balance among them. Unfortunately, some people are dominated by one or two of the ego states and are likely to create problems for managers. Parent-dominated individuals may not participate in problem solving because they think they already have the answer and know what is right and wrong. Child-dominated individuals do not engage in rational problem solving either. Screaming and being emotional have helped them get what they wanted before. It is likely to be difficult to reason with someone dominated by the child ego state. Working with adult-dominated individuals may be boring because they work so hard. A balance among the three ego states produces the healthiest worker.

Transactions. When people interact, they participate as parent, child, or adult (Figure 22-1). A transaction or an observation unit is an exchange between people that consists of at least one stimulus and one response. Transactional analysis is done to identify the participant's ego state and consists of complementary or crossed types. The basic principle of the complementary type is that the response to the stimulus is predictable and expected.

Adult-to-adult transactions are the manner in which much business is conducted (Figure 22-2). For instance, a supervisor says, "Would you please give Mr. Jones his PRN medication before you give Mrs. Smith her 8 AM medications?" A staff nurse replies, "Yes, I understand that Mr. Jones is complaining of surgical pain."

Parent-to-parent interaction is often a short-term sharing of opinions (Figure 22-3). One staff nurse says to another, "Those new graduate nurses certainly don't know how to function." The other nurse replies, "That's for sure."

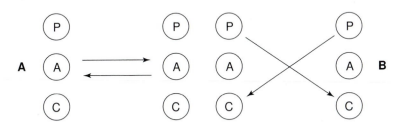

Figure 22-1 Transactions. A, Complementary; B, crossed.

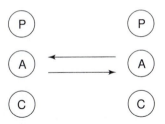

Figure 22-2 Adult-to-adult complementary.

Child-to-child interactions usually involve an emotional exchange (Figure 22-4). As long as both parties are in a child ego state, they are unable to think rationally and solve problems. The first staff nurse says, "I just gave Mrs. Smith her 8 AM medications, and when I went to chart them, you had signed for giving them. Why don't you sign right after you give medications so they won't be repeated!" The second nurse answers, "Why don't you give me a chance to sign before you go and give them again!"

In parent-to-child interactions, one person takes a psychologically superior position over the other (Figure 22-5). Manager says, "I want to see you in my office." Staff nurse answers, "Yes, ma'am."

Crossed transactions result in closing communications at least temporarily (Figure 22-6). The response may be inappropriate or unexpected and may confuse or threaten the sender of the stimulus. Supervisor says, "Miss Jones, could I see you about this in my office right away?" Miss Jones replies, "No! Can't you see I'm busy? You'll have to wait."

Transactions usually proceed in a programmed series with rituals and procedures being the simplest kinds. Rituals are a series of simple complementary transactions

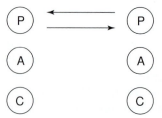

Figure 22-3   Parent-to-parent complementary.

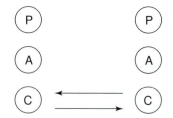

Figure 22-4   Child-to-child complementary.

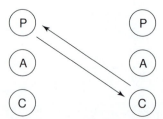

Figure 22-5   Parent-to-child complementary.

that provide mutual stroking with no real commitment. Most rituals have been used so often that the form has become more important than the content, but they provide structure for greeting people and expressing religious beliefs. Greeting rituals, such as "Hi," "How are you?" "I am fine," are not intended to supply information. The person who goes from office to office participating in rituals may get promoted because he or she is "a good guy." Rituals work for the person who can still get the job done. People who work hard to develop themselves may become apathetic when they realize socializing is more effective for obtaining promotions than hard work. Rituals may have started as a series of complementary adult transactions intended to manipulate reality, but they have lost their procedural validity over time.

Pastimes are pleasant ways to pass time with others to learn if you have enough in common to warrant further interaction. Common small talk includes topics such as cooking, fashions, costs, sports, recreation, and mutual acquaintances. There is no goal or emotional closeness involved. People who spend too much time participating in pastimes may sense that their lives are happy but empty, while the person who spends too little time making small talk may not have much fun and may feel harassed. Pastimes become a problem for the organization when they are an alternative to work.

Game-playing.   In *Games People Play,* Eric Berne writes: "A game is an ongoing series of complementary ulterior transactions progressing to a well-defined, predictable outcome."* Games have a high stroke or recognition potential, but the payoff is usually negative. Games have hidden agendas that prevent both people and organizations from becoming winners. While playing games, people dwell on their own sorrows and inadequacies, make mistakes, catch others making mistakes, pass the buck, and fail to meet their obligations. People receive negative strokes and get hurt while real problems go unsolved. Productivity is limited because people use their energies to play games instead of to get the job done. Attention is given to past events rather than to the present. While realities of the current situation go unperceived, problems go unsolved.

People need strokes, and negative strokes are better than no strokes. Consequently, in work environments that do not provide positive strokes, people have a need to play games. People who are bored with their jobs are also likely to play games.

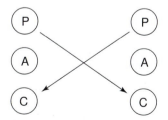

Figure 22-6 Crossed transaction.

---

* Berne E: *Games people play,* New York, 1964, Grove Press.

Games discourage openness, honesty, and intimacy. They take many forms. Games that blame others include "If it weren't for you" and "See what you made me do." Games that attack others include "Blemish," "Now I've got you, you SOB," "Bear Trapper," "Corner," "Rapo," "Uproar," and "Let's You and Him Fight." Self-pity is reinforced by games such as "Poor me," "Kick me," "Stupid," "Wooden leg," "Harried," and "Lunch bag."

"If it weren't for you" is a blaming game in which people who feel inadequate blame others for their inability to achieve. People who blame their inability to be innovative on rigid policies may fear their own creative abilities. "If it weren't for . . ." is a clue that the game is being played. When managers hear an employee say this, they should suspect that the complainer would not function better under different circumstances but would likely become frustrated and request a transfer or quit. Changes may be made on a trial basis to test suspicions.

"See what you made me do" and "You got me into this" are closely related blaming games. The player avoids responsibility by being vindictive. It is common for workers to blame managers for problems, and for democratic managers to blame workers for mistakes or poor decisions. The manager decides whether or not to use the input from the workers and needs to accept that responsibility.

Many games attack others. The "Blemish" player looks for inconsequential, unimportant flaws. Instead of looking at purposes, the player concentrates on minutiae and zeroes in on trivial mistakes. Any positive stroke is discounted with a blemish. "Blemish" players also play "I was only trying to help you." The victims become resentful and may become the persecutor by playing "Now I've got you, you SOB." In this game the persecutor waits for the victim to make a mistake or sets the victim up for failure. The manager may be indulging in this game by setting standards too high to achieve, assigning people to work they are not qualified for, creating impossible working conditions, or giving incomplete or unclear instructions. The worker may use grievance procedures or lawsuits against managers playing this game.

The "Bear trapper" often baits someone with false promises and then lets the trap fall. Organizations play this game in hiring practices when glamorous job descriptions are presented. This tends to result in high turnover. Workers learn the shortcomings of the job and become disillusioned. Presenting both the advantages and disadvantages of jobs is a more realistic approach.

The "Corner" player's victim is in a lose-lose situation. No matter what the victim does, it is wrong. A woman manager is damned if she is aggressive because that is not considered feminine and damned if she is not because aggressiveness is a desired managerial quality. A manager can corner someone into not completing work on time by not accepting the work that is done.

"Corner" can lead to "Uproar." Uproar often starts with a critical remark and results in an attack-defense dialogue that is often loud.

"Rapo" is a sexual game. A woman may wear revealing clothing and move in provocative ways. When a man responds, she rejects him. This game is problematic when men and women work together. Organizations need to concentrate on equality and use of human resources regardless of sex.

In "Let's you and him fight," one person gets a second and third person into a fight. When one person tells a second person the "bad" things a third person said about the second, the first person is fostering a fight.

There are several versions of self-pity games. "Kick me" players provoke put-downs and make comments such as, "I could kick myself for that." "Stupid" players collect put-downs about their intelligence. Managers need to give immediate feedback and take corrective actions to prevent the "Stupid" game. The "Wooden leg" player uses a physical or social handicap to avoid work. A deprived background may be used as an excuse to underachieve. The manager needs to set and maintain standards to minimize this game.

Managers play "Poor me" games also. "Harried" executives work hard to maintain the sense of being OK. They are likely to work nights and weekends to appear competent and confident. "I'm not OK" feelings are hidden by appearing super OK.

The "Harried" executive may also participate in the "Lunch bag game." Managers carry leftovers in a used paper bag and eat at their desk instead of going out to lunch with peers. This technique can be used to make other people feel guilty.

Games always involve putting someone down. To decrease games in organizations, one must stop putting oneself and others down. One should not play the complementary role, but should give and receive positive strokes and invest time in activities and intimacy. Managers should integrate the goals of the workers and the organization and decrease boredom through job enrichment and personnel development. With good organization and management, positive strokes can become an intrinsic part of the job. Managers should foster an "I'm OK, you're OK" atmosphere.

Activities such as working and learning are goal directed and have a high stroke potential. They are a highly rewarding way to spend time. Workers must be careful not to take on so many activities that they neglect rituals and pastimes, and managers should not overload themselves with activities and leave the workers with idle time.

Intimacy is an open sharing of experience with others, usually by people with close relationships but sometimes by strangers. It is the most rewarding way to spend time. It is also the most risky. Although intimacy is without ulterior motives or exploitation, one needs high self-esteem to risk the openness of intimacy. It requires and fosters the "I'm OK, you're OK" atmosphere.

Life Positions

Life positions are more permanent than ego states. As individuals mature, they make assumptions about themselves and others. They consider themselves as OK or not OK and see others as OK or not OK. Four positions result: "I'm OK, you're OK," "I'm OK, you're not OK," "I'm not OK, you're OK," and "I'm not OK, you're not OK." OK feelings are associated with a sense of power, personal worth, well-being, capability, and lovableness. Not-OK feelings result from a sense of inability, weakness, helplessness, worthlessness, anxiety, and a feeling of being insignificant and unlovable. Most people develop a basic life position early in childhood that tends to be reinforced by the person's selective perceptions and reactions to experiences.

In the I'm OK, you're OK position, individuals feel interdependent with others and the environment. They are happy, active people with a positive outlook on life who like reinforcement for being OK but are not dependent on it. They use the happy child and nurturing parent ego states. Because they feel OK about themselves, they have little difficulty feeling others are OK.

People in the I'm OK, you're not OK position do not believe they can rely on anyone but themselves. They think people are worthless and are likely to be enemies and consequently tend to blame others. The critical parent ego state is dominant. A manager in this position possesses a Theory X philosophy, implements a Likert type I system, and supervises people closely because they cannot be trusted.

People in the I'm not OK, you're OK position are burdened with self-defeating attitudes and a lack of confidence. They take a psychologically inferior stand to others and assume that they are less competent and less influential than others.

Individuals in the I'm not OK, you're not OK position are maladjusted. They think they are worthless and so are others. Lacking confidence in themselves and trust in others, they are suspicious and anxious, disconnected from others, alienated from the environment, miserable, and tend to give up.

During infancy individuals have a mixture of OK and not-OK feelings, with the not-OK feelings predominating. The infant feels OK when physical needs are met and positive strokes are received. Most of an infant's experiences provide negative strokes and not-OK feelings. Because adults can satisfy the infant's needs, they are viewed as OK. Consequently, for most people the I'm not OK, you're OK position is established early and continues into adulthood. Socialization of women and nurses particularly reinforces the position that they are not OK. Therefore they need a lot of positive reinforcement to move to an I'm OK, you're OK position. Assertiveness can help one achieve and maintain that position. Once it is learned, there will be less passive-aggressive behavior.

Assertive Techniques

Communication styles are commonly passive, aggressive, or assertive. Passive persons are often self-denying, inhibited, and allows others to choose for them. Consequently, their goals are not achieved and they feel hurt, anxious, and frustrated. Aggressive persons are self-enhancing at others' expense. They are expressive, choose for others, deprecate others, and achieve their goals by using others. Aggressive behavior generates hatred and sometimes revenge. Assertive persons are self-enhancing. They are expressive, choose for themselves, and can achieve their goals. Consequently, they are likely to feel good about themselves.

Passive persons tend to be at a loss for words, do not say what they really mean, use many apologetic words, and hope people will understand what they want without telling them. They tend to have a weak, hesitant voice, downcast eyes, and fidgety hands, and they nod frequently.

The aggressive person is loud, uses loaded subjective words, makes accusations, and sends "you" messages that blame others. A flippant, sarcastic style with an air of superiority and rudeness is common. The person is likely to stand with hands on hips, feet apart, narrowed eyes, pointing a finger and talking in a superior, demanding, authoritarian manner.

Assertive persons say what they want in direct statements that say what they mean. They use objective words, send "I" messages, and make honest statements about their feelings. They are attentive listeners who give the impression of caring. They use eye contact and spontaneous verbal expressions with appropriate gestures and facial expressions while speaking in a well-modulated voice.

The style used governs how situations will be handled. Suppose, for instance, that a manager has noticed that a staff nurse has been arriving at work late for the past 3 days. The passive manager may not mention the problem at all. The aggressive manager might say, "How about getting here on time or looking for a new job? What do you think we pay you for anyway?" The assertive manager would be likely to speak to the staff nurse in private and might say, "I've noticed you have been late the past 3 days. Why haven't you been getting to work on time?" The last approach gives an impression of caring and facilitates problem solving.

Assertiveness is the most desirable style for a nurse manager. To achieve assertiveness, one must substitute verbal persistence for silent passivity or verbal abuse. *Broken record* is a technique managers can use to reach a compromise by indicating what they want and by keeping other people from talking them into what the others want to do. With the broken-record technique managers keep repeating what they want.

Manager: I expect you to get to work on time.
Staff nurse: But I'm a night person. I stay up late, and it's difficult to get up so early to come to work. I'm so tired that I shut off my alarm and go back to sleep. Then when I do get up, I stumble around in the dark to find my clothes so I won't wake my husband.
Manager: You are scheduled to work the day shift this rotation, and I expect you to be at work on time. If you are a night person, would you like to be assigned to the night shift permanently?
Staff nurse: No. I wouldn't be able to see my husband then. He works 9 AM to 9 PM and gets home about 9:30 PM. I would have to come to work at 10:30 and I could only see him for about an hour. I would get home just in time for him to go to work.
Manager: You are scheduled to work the day shift this rotation, and I expect you to be to work on time. However, we could assign you to the evening shift permanently. Would you want that?
Staff nurse: Working the evening shift would allow me to see my husband after work and to sleep in. Yes, I would prefer the evening shift.
Manager: I will see how quickly we can get your schedule changed to permanent evenings. I do expect you to be here by 7 AM until we get your schedule changed.

Fogging, negative assertion, and negative inquiry are techniques for dealing with criticism whether it is self-directed or from another source, real or imagined. They help minimize the negative emotional response of anxiety to criticism that manipulates us into defending what we want to do instead of doing it. Consequently, one feels less at conflict with oneself and more comfortable with both the negative and positive aspects of one's personality.

Fogging is agreeing with the truth, agreeing in principle, or agreeing with the odds rather than denying the criticism, getting defensive, or counterattacking with criticism. It helps desensitize one to criticism and leads to a reduction in the frequency of criticism from others. It sets up psychological distance, is a passive skill, and does not encourage the other person to be assertive. It also encourages a person to listen to what the critic says, to respond only to what the critic says rather than to what is implied, and to consider probabilities. For example:

Staff nurse: You scheduled me to double back from evenings to days twice in a 2-week time schedule.

Manager: I see that I scheduled you to double back the first Wednesday and the second Friday (agreeing with the truth).

Staff nurse: When I double back, I have less than 7 hours for sleep. I get tired, have trouble functioning, and fear making mistakes.

Manager: I understand that you get tired when you double back and fear making mistakes. It seems logical that one would make more mistakes when tired than when alert (agreeing with the odds).

Staff nurse: We need a policy to prevent having just one shift off between shifts.

Manager: I agree. We do need staffing policies that would provide for adequate rest periods between shifts (agreeing in principle).

With *negative assertion* people assertively accept negative aspects about themselves. This reduces the need to seek forgiveness for one's mistakes or the need to counterattack with criticism.

Staff nurse: Your new uniform really reveals how fat you are.

Manager: I'm overweight because I eat too much. I eat just about everything in sight except the kitchen sink. I've even seen the cat get worried (negative assertion).

Staff nurse: Well, that new uniform sure makes you look like a blimp.

Manager: These new styles don't compliment my figure (negative assertion).

Negative assertion is not appropriate for physical or legal conflicts or for relating to people on a close interpersonal basis. The persistence of the critic will determine if one needs to use other assertive techniques.

Negative inquiry fosters assertiveness in the critic. In an unemotional manner, the criticized person asks for more information that may be negative. This provides a basis for problem solving and consequently reduces repetitive criticism.

Staff nurse: You don't look good today.

Manager: Is it me or what I'm wearing?

Staff nurse: It's your face. You look so tired.

Manager: I don't feel tired. What about my face makes me look tired?

Staff nurse: Your eyes look so tired. They're so dark. There are bags under them.

Manager: What can I do to make them look less tired?

Staff nurse: If the problem isn't fatigue, I guess you could use a creme cosmetic over the bags and use light instead of dark-colored eye shadow.

Assertive behavior is more than demanding one's rights from others and keeping others from manipulating. In a social sense, assertiveness is the ability to communicate with others about who you are, how you live, what you do, and what you want and the ability to make them feel comfortable talking about themselves. Free information—information offered without being asked for—gives you something to talk about and reduces awkward silences. Self-disclosure reveals how you think, feel, and react to others' free information. This social conversation allows one to discover mutually rewarding relationships or to identify people with whom one has few common interests.

Nurse leaders should behave assertively to achieve positive self-images and maintain an I'm OK position. Assertiveness techniques facilitate professional productivity and social satisfaction.

BIBLIOGRAPHY

Brooking J: Doctors and nurses: a personal view, *Nurs Standard* 6:24-28, December 11-17, 1991.
Davidhizar R: The art of setting limits, *Adv Clin Care* 4:26-27, November-December 1989.
Gerry EM: An investigation into the assertive behavior of trained nurses in general hospital settings, *J Adv Nurs* 14:1002-1008, December 1989.
Johnson L: Nurses in OR are more assertive than radiographers, *Aust J Adv Nurs* 10:20-26, March-May 1993.
Kilkus SP: Assertiveness among professional nurses, *J Adv Nurs* 18:1324-1330, August 1993.
Mahat G, Phiri M: Promoting assertive behaviors in traditional societies . . . Malawi and Nepal, *Int Nurs Rev* 38:153-155, September-October 1991.
Marriner A: Assertiveness behavior for nursing leaders, *Nurs Leadership* 2:12-20, Fall 1976.
Munro KE: Assertion for nurses, *Recent Adv Nurs* 25:110-132, 1989.
Slater J: Effecting personal effectiveness: assertiveness training for nurses, *J Adv Nurs* 15:337-356, March 1990.

CASE STUDY

A staff nurse works with you who is frequently late to work. How will you assertively problem solve the situation with the nurse?

CRITICAL THINKING AND LEARNING ACTIVITIES

1. Keep a diary of some of your interactions with others. Do transactional analysis on them and analyze whether you were passive, aggressive, or assertive. If you were passive or aggressive, decide how you could have behaved assertively.

2. Write a script for the use of broken record and role-play it with a classmate.

3. Someone is criticizing the nursing staff and the institution in general. Write a script for using negative inquiry and role-play it with a classmate.

Bibliography
Part Four

Ackoff RL, Finnel EU, Gharajedaghi J: *A guide to controlling your corporation's future,* New York, 1984, Wiley.
Adams J, editor: *Transforming leadership: from vision to results,* Alexandria, Va, 1986, Miles River Press.

Adams JD, editor: *Transforming work: a collection of organizational transformation readings,* Alexandria, Va, 1984, Miles River Press.

Alberti RE, Emmons ML: *Stand up, speak out, talk back!* New York, 1990, Pocket Books.

Alberti RE, Emmons ML: *Your perfect right: a guide to assertive living,* ed 6, San Luis Obispo, Calif, 1990, Impact Publishers.

Ash MK: *Mary Kay,* New York, 1984, Harper & Row.

Ashley J: *Hospitals, paternalism, and the role of the nurse,* New York, 1976, Teachers College Press.

Bach GR, Goldberg H: *Creative aggression: the art of assertive living,* New York, 1993, NAL/Dutton.

Badaracco JL, Ellsworth RR: *Leadership and the quest for integrity,* Boston, 1989, Harvard Business School Press.

Baer J: *How to be an assertive (not aggressive) woman in life, in love, and on the job, the classic guide to becoming a self-assured person,* New York, 1991, New American Library.

Bagwell M, Clements S: *A political handbook for health professionals,* Boston, 1985, Little, Brown.

Bass B: *Leadership and performance beyond expectations,* New York, 1985, Free Press.

Bennis W, Nanus B: *Leaders: the strategies for taking charge,* New York, 1985, Harper & Row.

Bensimon EM, Neumann A: *Redesigning collegiate leadership: teams and teamwork in higher education,* Baltimore, 1993, The Johns Hopkins University Press.

Berne E: *Games people play,* New York, 1985, Ballantine Books.

Berne E: *What do you say after you say hello? New York, 1984, Bantam Books.*

Beyers M, Phillips C: *Nursing management for patient care,* ed 2, Boston, 1979, Scott, Foresman.

Bittel LR, Newstrom JW: *What every supervisor should know,* ed 5, New York, 1992, McGraw-Hill.

Blake RR, Mouton JS: *Executive achievement: making it at the top,* New York, 1989, McGraw-Hill.

Blake RR, Shepard HA, Mouton JS: *Managing intergroup conflict in industry,* Houston, 1964, Gulf Publishing.

Blake RR, Mouton JS: *The managerial grid: leadership styles for achieving production through people,* ed 3, Houston, 1994, Gulf Publishing.

Blau PM: *Exchange and power in social life,* New Brunswick, NJ, 1986, Transaction Books.

Block P: *The empowered manager: positive political skills at work,* San Francisco, 1991, Jossey-Bass.

Bradford DL, Cohen AR: *Managing for excellence: the guide to developing high performance in contemporary organizations,* New York, 1987, Wiley.

Bradford LP: *Group development,* ed 2, La Jolla, Calif, 1988, Dell.

Bramson RM: *Coping with difficult people,* Garden City, NY, 1988, Dell.

Britton PR, Stallings JW: *Leadership is empowering people,* Lanham, Md, 1986, University Press of America.

Brooks Ann Marie T: *Team building,* Baltimore, 1989, Williams & Wilkins.

Buchholz RA: *Essentials of public policy for management,* Englewood Cliffs, NJ, 1985, Prentice-Hall.

Burns JM: *Leadership,* New York, 1982, Harper Collins.

Byham, WC: *Zapp! The lightning of empowerment: how to improve productivity, quality, and employee satisfaction,* New York, 1988, Harmony Books.

Charns MP, Schaefer MJ: *Health care organizations: a model for management,* Englewood Cliffs, NJ, 1983, Prentice-Hall.

Chenevert M: *Special techniques in assertiveness training for women in the health professions,* ed 3, St Louis, 1988, Mosby.

Christain WP, Hannah GT: *Effective management in human services,* Englewood Cliffs, NJ, 1983, Prentice-Hall.

Clark CC, Shea CA: *Management in nursing: a vital link in the health care system,* New York, 1979, McGraw-Hill.

Claus KE, Bailey JT: *Power and influence in health care: a new approach to leadership,* St Louis, 1977, Mosby.

Cohen H: *You can negotiate anything,* New York, 1983, Citadel Press.

Conner D: *The art of winning,* vol 1, New York, 1990, St Martin's Press.

Covey SR: *Principle-centered leadership,* New York, 1991, Summit Books.

Covey SR: *The seven habits of highly effective people: powerful lessons in personal change,* New York, 1989, Simon & Schuster.

Cowart M, Allen RF: *Changing conceptions of health care,* Grove Road, 1981, Charles B Black.

Dale E: *Management: theory and practice,* ed 4, New York, 1978, McGraw-Hill.

Davis K, Newstrom J: *Human behavior at work,* ed 7, New York, 1985, McGraw-Hill.

Deci EL, Ryan RM: *Intrinsic motivation,* New York, 1985, Plenum Press.

Denton DK: *Horizontal management: beyond total customer satisfaction,* New York, 1991, Lexington Books.

Delbecq AL, Van de Ven AH, Gustafson DH: *Group techniques for program planning: a guide to normal group and Delphi processes,* Glenview, Ill, 1986, Green Briar Press.

Deloughery G, Gebbie KM: *Political dynamics: impact on nurses and nursing,* St Louis, 1975, Mosby.

De Pree M: *Leadership jazz,* New York, 1992, Doubleday.

Dilenschneider RL: *A briefing for leaders: communication as the ultimate exercise of power,* New York, 1992, Harper Business.

De Vito JA: *Communication: concepts and processes,* ed 3, Englewood Cliffs, NJ, 1981, Prentice Hall.

Di Vincenti M: *Administering nursing service,* ed 2, Boston, 1977, Little, Brown.

Dyer W: *Your erroneous zones,* New York, 1993, HarperCollins.

Eddy WB et al, editors: *Behavioral science and the manager's role,* ed 2, La Jolla, Calif, 1980, University Associates.

England GW, Negandhi AR, Wilpert B: *The functioning of complex organizations,* Cambridge, Mass, 1981, Oelgeschlager, Gunn, & Hain.

Epstein C: *The nurse leader: philosophy and practice,* Norwalk, Conn, 1982, Appleton & Lange.

Fensterheim H: *Don't say yes when you want to say no,* New York, 1975, Dell.

Ferguson M: *The Aquarian conspiracy: personal and social transformation in the 1980s,* Boston, 1981, Houghton Mifflin.

Fiedler FE: *A theory of leadership effectiveness,* New York, 1967, McGraw-Hill.

Fiedler FE, Chemers MM, Martin M: *Improving leadership effectiveness: the leader match concept,* ed 2, New York, 1984, Wiley.

Fisher K: *Leading self-directed work teams: a guide to developing new team leadership skills,* New York, 1993, McGraw-Hill.

Fisher R, Ury W: *Getting to yes: negotiating agreement without giving in,* rev ed, Boston, 1991, Penguin Books.

Flarnholtz EG, Randle Y: *The inner game of management: how to make the transition to a managerial role,* New York, 1987, American Management Association.

French WL: *The personal management process,* Boston, 1986, Houghton Mifflin.

Friday N: *My mother my self,* ed 6, New York, 1987, Dell.

Frieze IH et al: *Woman and sex roles: a social psychological perspective,* New York, 1978, Norton.

Fuszard B: *Self-actualization for nurses,* Rockville, Md, 1984, Aspen.

George CS Jr: *The history of management thought,* ed 2, Englewood Cliffs, NJ, 1972, Prentice Hall.

Glover SM: *Performance evaluations,* Baltimore, 1989, Williams & Wilkins.

Greenleaf RK: *Servant leadership: a journey into the nature of legitimate power and greatness,* New York, 1977, Paulist Press.

Gretz KF, Drozdeck SR: *Empowering innovative people: how managers challenge, channel and control the truly creative and talented,* Chicago, 1992, Probus.

Grove AS: *High output management,* New York, 1985, Random House.

Hagbug J: *Real power: the stages of personal power in organizations,* Minneapolis, 1984, Winston Press.

Hall RH: *Organizations: structure, process, and outcomes,* ed 4, Englewood Cliffs, NJ, 1987, Prentice Hall.

Hampton DR: *Contemporary management,* New York, 1980, McGraw-Hill.

Hand L: *Nursing supervision,* Norwalk, Conn, 1980, Appleton & Lange.

Haney WV: *Communication and interpersonal relations,* ed 6, Homewood, Ill, 1991, Irwin.

Harragan BL: *Games mother never taught you: corporate gamesmanship for women,* rev ed, New York, 1989, Warner Books.

Harris T: *I'm OK—you're OK,* New York, 1967, Harper & Row.

Heider J: *The Tao of leadership,* New York, 1992, Humanics Limited.

Hein EC: *Communication in nursing practice,* Boston, 1986, Little, Brown,

Henderson C: *Winners: The successful strategies entrepreneurs use to build new businesses,* New York, 1985, Henry Holt.

Hennig M: *The managerial woman,* Garden City, NY, 1988, Pocket Books.

Hersey P: *The situational leader,* New York, 1985, Warner Books.

Hersey P, Blanchard K: *Management of organizational behavior: utilizing human resources,* ed 5, Englewood Cliffs, NJ, 1988, Prentice Hall.

Hersey P, Duldt BW: *Situational leadership in nursing,* Norwalk, Conn, 1989, Appleton & Lange.

Herzberg F, Mausner B, Snyderman BB: *The motivation to work,* New York, 1993, Transaction.

Hickman CR, Silva MA: *Creating excellence,* New York, 1986, New American Library.

Hicks HG, Gullett CR: *The management of organizations,* ed 4, New York, 1981, McGraw-Hill.

Hodgetts RM: *Management: theory, process, and practice,* ed 5, Orlando, Fla, 1989, Dryden Press.

Hunt JG, Baliga BR, Dachler HP et al: *Emerging leadership vistas,* Lexington, Mass, 1988, Heath.

James M, Jongeward D: *Born to win,* Reading, Mass, 1991, New American Library.

Jamison K: *The nibble theory and the kernel of power,* New York, 1984, Paulist Press.

Jandt FE: *Conflict resolution through communication,* New York, 1973, Harper & Row.

Jongeward D: *Everybody wins: transactional analysis applied to organizations,* Reading, Mass, 1973, Addison-Wesley.

Jongeward D: *Women as winners: transactional analysis for personal growth,* Reading, Mass, 1976, Addison-Wesley.

Josefowitz N: *Paths to power: a woman's guide from first job to top executive,* Reading, Mass, 1990, Addison-Wesley.

Joos IM et al: Man, health, and nursing: basic concepts and theories, Norwalk, Conn., 1985, Appleton & Lange.

Kanter RM: *Teaching elephants to dance: the managers guide to empowering change.* Westminister, MD, 1991, Random House.

Karrass CL: *Give and take: the complete guide to negotiating strategies and tactics,* New York, 1993, Harper Business.

Karrass G: *Negotiate to close,* New York, 1987, Simon & Schuster.

Kelly J: *Organizational behaviour,* ed 3, Homewood, Ill, 1980, Richard D. Irwin.

Korda M: *Power! How to get it, how to use it,* New York, 1987, Ballantine Books.

Kotter JP: *The general managers,* New York, 1986, Free Press.

Kotter JP: *The leadership factor,* New York, 1988, Free Press.

Kouzes JM, Posner BZ: *The leadership challenge: how to get extraordinary things done in organizations,* San Francisco, 1990, Jossey-Bass.

Kriegel RJ, Patler L: *If it ain't broke . . . break it! And other unconventional wisdom for a changing business world,* New York, 1991, Warner Books.

Kurtz R, Prestera H: *The body reveals: how to read your own body,* New York, 1984, Harper & Row.

Lange A, Jakubowski P: *Responsible assertive behavior,* Champaign, Ill, 1976, Research Press.

Lawler CE: *High-involvement management: participative strategies for improving organizational performance,* San Francisco, 1988, Jossey-Bass.

Lecker S: *The success factor: an incisive study of the components of success and how to develop them,* New York, 1986, Sidney Lecker.

Levey S, Loomba NP: *Health care administration: a managerial perspective,* ed 2, Philadelphia, 1984, Lippincott.

Likert R, Likert JG: *New ways of managing conflict,* New York, 1976, McGraw-Hill.

Lundy JL: *Lead, follow, or get out of the way,* San Diego, Calif, 1993, Pfeiffer.

Maddux RB: *Successful negotiation,* rev ed, Los Altos, Calif, 1987, Crisp.

Manz C: *The art of self-leadership: strategies for personal effectiveness in your life and work,* Englewood Cliffs, NJ, Prentice Hall.

Manz CC, Simms HP: *Superleadership,* New York, 1990, Berkeley.

Margulies N, Wallace J: *Organizational change: techniques and applications,* Glenview, Ill, 1973, Scott, Foresman.

Marriner A: *Contemporary nursing management,* St Louis, 1982, Mosby.

Mason DJ, Talbott SW: *Political action handbook for nurses,* Menlo Park, Calif, 1985, Addison-Wesley.

May R: *Power and innocence: a search for the sources of violence,* New York, 1972, Norton.

McBride AB: *Living with contradiction: a married feminist,* New York, 1976, Harper & Row.

McCelland DC: *Power: the inner experience,* New York, 1979, Irvington.

McConnell CR: *The effective health care supervisor,* ed 3, Rockville, Md, 1993, Aspen Systems.

McGregor D: *The human side of enterprise,* New York, 1985, McGraw-Hill.

Meininger J: *Success through transactional analysis,* New York, 1974, New American Library.

Micheli LMJ, Cepedes FV, Byker D et al: *Managerial communication,* Glenview, Ill, 1984, Scott, Foresman.

Miller JB: *Toward a new psychology of women,* ed 2, Boston, 1986, Beacon Press.

Mintzberg H: *The nature of managerial work,* New York, 1990, HarperCollins.

Molloy JT: *The woman's dress for success book,* New York, 1987, Warner Books.

Morrison AM, White RP, Van Velsor E: *Breaking the glass ceiling: can women reach the top of America's largest corporations?* rev ed, Reading, Mass, 1992, Addison-Wesley.

Musashi M: *The book of five rings,* New York, 1994, Shambhata.

Myers IB: *Gifts differing,* Palo Alto, Calif, 1993, Consulting Psychologists Press.

Newman WH, Warren EK, Kirby E: *The process of management,* ed 5, Englewood Cliffs, NJ, 1981, Prentice Hall.

Osborne D, Gaebler T: *Reinventing government: how the entrepreneurial spirit is transforming the public sector from schoolhouse to statehouse, city hall to the pentagon,* Reading, Mass, 1992, Addison-Wesley.

Osborn RN, Hunt JG, Jaugh LR: *Organization theory: an integrated approach,* New York, 1984, RE Krieger.

Osborn SM, Harris GG: *Assertive training for women,* Springfield, Ill, 1978, Charles C Thomas.

Ouchi WG: *Theory Z,* New York, 1993, Avon Books.

Pascale RT, Athos AG: *The art of Japanese management,* New York, 1982, Warner Books.

Peters T: *Thriving on chaos,* New York, 1989, HarperCollins.

Peters T, Austin N: *A passion for excellence,* New York, 1989, Warner Books.

Peters T, Waterman RH: *In search of excellence,* New York, 1988, Warner Books.

Pfeffer J: *Organizations and organization theory,* Boston, 1986, Harper Business.

Pinkerton S, Schroeder P: *Commitment to excellence,* Rockville, Md, 1988, Aspen.

Porter LW, Lawler EE: *Managerial attitudes and performance,* Homewood, Ill, 1968, Dorsey Press.

Porter-O'Grady T: *Creative nursing administration: participative management into the 21st century,* Rockville, Md, 1986, Aspen.

Randolph WA: *Understanding and managing organizational behavior,* Homewood, Ill, 1985, Richard D Irwin.

Ringer RJ: *Winning through intimidation,* New York, 1991, Fawcett Books.

Robbins, SP: *Organizational behavior: concepts, controversies, and applications,* ed 6, Englewood Cliffs, NJ, 1992, Prentice Hall.

Robbins SP: *Organizational theory: the structure and design of organizations,* ed 3, Englewood Cliffs, NJ, 1983, Prentice Hall.

Roberts W: *Leadership secrets of Attila the Hun,* New York, 1990, Warner Books.

Rogers C: *On personal power,* New York, 1977, Delacorte Press.

Rowan R: *The intuitive manager,* New York, 1991, Berkeley Books.

Schaef AW: *Women's reality: an emerging female system,* New York, 1992, Harper.

Schein EH: *Process consultation: its role in organization development,* ed 2, Reading, Mass, 1988, Addison-Wesley.

Senge PM: *The fifth discipline: the art and practice of the learning organization,* New York, 1990, Doubleday.

Shaw ME, Constanzo PR: *Theories of social psychology,* New York, 1982, McGraw-Hill.

Sheehy G: *Passages,* New York, 1984, Bantam.

Sheridan RS, Bronstein JE, Walker DD: *The new nurse manager: a guide to management development,* Rockville, Md, 1984, Aspen.

Shivastva S: *The executive mind,* San Francisco, 1983, Jossey-Bass.

Silber MB, Marlborough JL, McLachlan EM: *Dynamic nurse management,* San Diego, Calif, 1988, Cabashon.

Smith MJ: *When I say no, I feel guilty,* New York, 1985, Bantam Books.

Srivastra S and associates, editors: *The executive mind,* San Francisco, 1983, Jossey-Bass.

Steers RM, Porter LW: *Motivation and work behavior,* ed 5, New York, 1991, McGraw-Hill.

Stevens BJ: *First-line patient care management,* ed 2, Germantown, Md, 1983, Aspen Systems.

Stevens BJ, Derfoot: *The nurse as executive,* ed 4, Rockville, Md, 1994, Aspen.

Strasen L: *Key business skills for nurse managers,* Philadelphia, 1987, Lippincott.

Swingle P, editor: *The structure of conflict,* New York, 1970, Academic Press.

Taubman B: *How to become an assertive woman,* New York, 1976, Pocket Books.

Terry GR, Rue RT: *Principles of management,* ed 4, Homewood, Ill, 1982, Richard D Irwin.

VanFleet JK: *Twenty-one days to unlimited power with people,* Englewood Cliffs, NJ, 1992, Prentice Hall.

Vogt JF, Murrell KL: *Empowerment in organizations: how to spark exceptional performance,* San Diego, 1990, Pfeiffer.

Voich D, Wren DA: *Principles of management: resources and systems,* New York, 1968, Ronald Press.

Watson DL, Tharp RG: *Self-directed behavior,* ed 6, Monterey, Calif, 1993, Brooks/Cole.

Wellins RS, Byham WC, Wilson JM: *Empowered teams: creating self-directed work groups that improve quality, productivity, and participation,* San Francisco, 1991, Jossey-Bass.

Wieczorek RR, editor: *Power, politics, and policy in nursing,* New York, 1984, Springer.

Williamson JN: *The leader manager,* New York, 1986, Wiley.

Wren DA: *The evolution of management thought,* ed 4, New York, 1993, Wiley.

Yukl GA: *Leadership in organizations,* ed 2, Englewood Cliffs, NJ, 1989, Prentice Hall.

Yura H, Ozimek D, Walsh MB: *Nursing leadership: theory and process,* ed 2, Norwalk, Conn, 1981, Appleton & Lange.

Zurlage C, editor: *The nurse as personnel manager,* Chicago, 1982, S-N Publications.

PART

Five

Control

Nature and Purpose of Controlling

Controlling is the last step in the management process. It involves setting standards, measuring performance against those standards, reporting the results, and taking corrective actions. Controls should be designed for specific situations and should report potential or actual deviations promptly enough for corrective action to be effective. Controls must be determinable, verifiable, and flexible, because alternative flexible plans help achieve flexible controls. Controls must also be understandable and economical and must lead to corrective action. Adequate control systems disclose deviations, identify who is responsible, and recommend corrections. They are justified by correcting deviations.

Chapter

23

Evaluation of Personnel

Chapter Objectives

◆ List at least five purposes of personnel evaluation.

◆ List at least six common errors in performance evaluation.

◆ Describe five methods of personnel evaluation.

◆ Explain various ways to arrange a room for performance evaluations.

Major Concepts and Definitions	
Evaluation	valuation, appraisal, determination of worth
Peer review	group evaluation of a group member
Appraisal interview	verbal evaluation
Appraisal report	written evaluation

PURPOSES

Performance appraisal is a periodic formal evaluation of how well personnel have performed their duties during a specific period. Purposes of the evaluation are (1) to determine job competence, (2) to enhance staff development and motivate personnel toward higher achievement, (3) to discover the employee's aspirations and to recognize accomplishments, (4) to improve communications between managers and staff associates and to reach an understanding about the objectives of the job and agency, (5) to improve performance by examining and encouraging better relationships among nurses, (6) to aid the manager's coaching and counseling, (7) to determine training and developmental needs of nurses, (8) to make inventories of talent within the organization and reassess assignments, (9) to select qualified nurses for advancement and salary increases, and (10) to identify unsatisfactory employees.

COMMON ERRORS IN EVALUATION

Criteria involving judgments are used for performance evaluation. Because human judgment is subject to the influences of prejudice, bias, and other subjective and extraneous factors, the attempt to get objective, accurate evaluations is extremely difficult. A number of errors may affect performance ratings. The manager should be aware of the most common ones and try to minimize them.

The halo error is the result of allowing one trait to influence the evaluation of other traits or of rating all traits on the basis of a general impression. A logical error is rating a nurse high on one characteristic because the nurse possesses another characteristic that is logically related. Sometimes employees are given a good rating in the recent past because they did good work in the distant past, or outstanding performance on a recent job may offset a mediocre performance during the rest of the evaluation period. A manager is likely to rate personnel who are compatible with the manager higher than they deserve and may not see certain types of defects that are like the managers. The person who does not complain is likely to have higher ratings than the person who does.

The horns error is the opposite of the halo effect. The evaluator is hypercritical. Managers who are perfectionists may rate personnel lower than they should. Managers may compare how they used to do the job with how it is done now and are more likely to rate people doing jobs with which they are familiar lower than those with whose jobs they are not familiar. Good workers on weak teams are likely to get lower ratings than if they were working on a better team. Persons who are not well known may be judged by the company they keep. A recent mistake may offset a year's good work. If the worker is contrary, managers may vent their irritation by lowering the rating. The nonconformist or person with a personality trait that is not appreciated is likely to be rated lower than that person's work merits.

The contrast error is produced by the tendency of managers to rate the nurse opposite from the way they perceive themselves. A small range of scores may be a result of the central tendency error. When the rating on a preceding characteristic influences the rating on the following trait, a proximity error exists. Because raters tend to have their own built-in set of standards or frame of reference on which to make evaluations, it becomes a major problem comparing different raters' scores. Some managers may be easy and lenient, whereas others may be severe in their judgments.

The manager can take precautions to minimize judgment errors. For instance, a forced-distribution technique may be used to overcome the leniency and central tendency errors. A critical incident checklist can reduce the halo effect and logical rating errors. Ranking systems, paired comparisons, and force-choice techniques may be used.

METHODS OF EVALUATION

Anecdotal Notes

Anecdotal records are objective descriptions of behavior recorded on plain paper or a form. The notations should include who was observed, by whom, when, and where. The notation comprises a description of the setting or background and the incident, and interpretation and recommendations may be included. Value-laden words such as *good* and *bad* should be avoided.

Characteristic behavior cannot be determined without several incidents depicting similar behavior. The director or patient care coordinator may use time sampling to accumulate observations. The time that is set aside specifically for observations may be divided by the number of staff to be observed. The manager then concentrates on the scheduled staff member for a short period. It is advisable to make several brief observations over a time span to allow for temporary variables and to identify patterns of behavior.

An advantage of anecdotal recordings is that the description is not coerced into a rigid structure. However, this latitude becomes a problem when the interpreter tries to develop relationships among notations that may have little or no relationship to each other. Although anecdotal records provide a systematic means for recording observations, they do not guarantee that observations will be made systematically or that specific, relevant behaviors will be observed. It also takes considerable time to record the observations.

Checklists

With a checklist the manager can categorically assess the presence or absence of desired characteristics or behavior. Checklists are most useful for tangible variables, such as inventory of supplies, but they can be used for evaluation of nursing skills as well. It is advisable to list only the behaviors essential to successful performance, and it is advantageous to determine the behavior to be observed in advance. The same criteria can then be used in each situation. Unfortunately, this does not guarantee that the observed behavior is a persistent one or that a representative situation is being observed. Nor is the checklist practical for evaluating interpersonal relations.

Rating Scales

The rating scale does more than just note the absence or presence of desirable behavior. It locates the behavior at a point on a continuum and notes quantitative and qualitative abilities. The numerical rating scale usually includes numbers against which a list of behaviors is evaluated:

Observation of working hours   1 2 3 4 5

Ability to get along with others   1 2 3 4 5

This is not a very reliable tool because of the inconsistent value attributed to the number. That fault can be partially overcome by adding a few quantitative terms, as shown in Figure 23-1.

The tool can be made even more reliable by developing a standard scale by using comparative examples to establish a set of standards. The difficulty is finding

---

```
                        RATING SCALE

        Rate the staff member on the items below.
        Responses have the following values:

                    1 = Never

                    2 = Sometimes

                    3 = About half the time

                    4 = Usually

                    5 = Always

        A. Observation of working hours      1 2 3 4 5

        B. Ability to get along with others   1 2 3 4 5
```

Figure 23-1 Example of numerical rating scale.

appropriate comparative standards. A nurse-to-nurse comparison scale might be developed:

Nurse	Observation of working hours				
	Lowest (1)	Below average (2)	Average (3)	Above average (4)	Highest (5)
Betty Green	X				
Sara Smith		X			
Pam Peterson			X		
Sue Jones				X	
Anita Anderson					X

As long as the managers can agree on the qualifications of a few nurses known to all of them, a comparison scale that gives a common reference for rating the rest of the staff nurses can be developed.

The graphic rating scale is different from the numerical rating scale in that words rather than numbers are used. For example:

Unsatisfactory   Below average   Average   Above average   Outstanding

Observation of working hours

Graphic rating scales usually list extremely broad and general personal characteristics that are to be rated from poor to excellent or from low to high. Raters are given little if any guidance about what work behavior qualifies a person for a particular rating and must consequently use their own judgment about how to classify the behaviors.

The following descriptive graphic rating scale is similar to the graphic rating scale except that it presents a more elaborate description of the behavior being rated:

Usually late   Sometimes late   Usually on time

Observation of working hours

BARS is an acronym for behaviorally anchored rating scales, sometimes known as BES, behavioral expectation scales. They are similar to graphic rating scales in that a person is rated on a series of dimensions or qualities. However, BARS differs from graphic rating scales in the ways that the criteria are identified and the alternative responses along the rating scale are anchored or described. BARS evaluates behavior relevant to specific demands of the job and provides examples of specific job behaviors corresponding to good, average, and poor performances. This reduces the amount of personal judgment needed by the rater.

The major disadvantage of BARS is the time and expense required to involve large numbers of employees in determining the dimensions of effective performance and behavioral examples of various levels of performance of each variable. Separate BARS are needed for each job. It is primarily applicable to physically observable behaviors rather than to conceptual skills. However, it should reduce rating errors and provide more reliable, valid, meaningful, and complete data. Employees give more acceptance and commitment to this appraisal system because of their involvement in designing it. They have full knowledge of the requirements of the job, and they evidence less defensiveness and conflict because people are evaluated on the basis of specific behaviors rather than personalities. This system thereby identifies performance deficiencies and needs for development.

BOS is an acronym for behavioral observation scales. This system capitalizes on some of the strengths of BARS while avoiding some of the disadvantages. BOS also uses critical incidents of worker behavior. The evaluator lists a number of critical incidents for each performance dimension and rates the extent to which the behavior has been observed on a five-point scale ranging from almost never to almost always. It too is relatively reliable, well accepted and understood, and provides useful feedback, but it is relatively time-consuming and expensive to develop.

BEHAVIORAL OBSERVATION SCALE

Circle the number that most closely approximates your assessment of the staff member on the following qualities:

Punctual	Almost never	1 2 3 4 5	Almost always
Gets along well with co-workers	Almost never	1 2 3 4 5	Almost always

---

Instead of a descriptive choice, a frequency-rating scale provides a quantitative choice. The manager may rank the employee's behavior on any given criterion as among the bottom 10% of staff, next 20%, middle 40%, next 20%, or top 10% of staff.

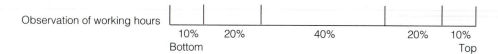

Observation of working hours

| 10% | 20% | 40% | 20% | 10% |
| Bottom | | | | Top |

Box 23-1   **EXAMPLE OF RANKING USING PAIRED COMPARISON**

Nurses	Possible Pairs	
Anita Anderson	AA with SJ	SJ with PP
Sue Jones	AA with PP	SJ with SS
Pam Peterson	AA with SS	PP with SS
Sara Smith		

To maintain perspective, the manager may list staff names down the side of a paper and the behavior to be rated across the top. Rating one behavior at a time, the manager checks for variation in evaluations because one expects variation in performance. Forced distribution should be used cautiously. It is based on a normal bell-shaped curve with a few people ranked high, a few ranked low, and the majority ranked in the middle. However, this assumes that the group is representative of the total population, and this is not true for a group of nurses.

Ranking

Ranking forces managers to rank staff in descending order from highest to lowest even if they do not feel there is a difference. Ranking implicitly requires the manager to compare each nurse with others, but that comparison is not systematically built into the method. Paired comparison forces the supervisor to compare each nurse with each other nurse. As shown in Box 23-1, if managers are ranking four nurses, they must deal with six possible pairs, or $N(N-1)/2 = 4(3)/2 = 12/2 = 6$.

Then each pair is presented to the manager, who must determine which of the two the manager feels is better. Choices should be marked. For example:

(AA) vs. SJ   (SJ) vs. PP

(AA) vs. PP   (SJ) vs. SS

(AA) vs. SS   (PP) vs. SS

Tally marks can be placed in a matrix to help visualize the ranking:

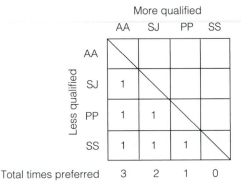

The major disadvantages of paired comparisons are that they do not lend themselves to large numbers of staff and demand considerable time of the manager.

Management by Objectives

Management by objectives (MBO) is a tool for effective planning and appraisal. It emphasizes the achievement of objectives instead of personality characteristics. It focuses attention on individual achievement, motivates individuals to accomplishment, and measures performance in terms of results. MBO is a managerial method whereby the manager and staff nurse identify major areas in which the nurse will work, set standards for performance, and measure results against those standards. It determines the results that the nurse is to achieve in a given time frame.

To develop management by objectives, nurses should first review the mission and group objectives. They can determine the mission and objectives by analyzing what they do or what they think they should do. They describe their job and clarify its purpose. This helps identify major job responsibilities.

Next they list their major job responsibilities. Results expected, rather than activities, should be listed. This can be accomplished by asking oneself why the activity is being done or why it is important. For example:

What is the task? To help team members organize their work for the day.

Why? To improve use of their time.

Why? To be as productive as possible.

Why? To give good, cost-effective nursing care by completing the work identified on nursing care plans efficiently.

Major job responsibilities of a nurse manager are related to productivity, quality of care, morale, turnover, staff development, self-development, and affirmative action.

Once the major job responsibilities are identified, expected levels of accomplishment are determined. Criteria for expected levels of accomplishment should be results oriented, established before the fact, time bound, realistic and attainable, measurable and verifiable, written, and agreed on by both the manager and the staff associate. Common errors to avoid when developing objectives are writing too many objectives or too complex objectives; having too high or too low standards; using too long or too short a time period; and having imbalanced emphasis, objectives that are not measurable, or objectives for which the cost of measurement is too high.

After staff associates have reviewed the mission and group objectives and determined their major job responsibilities and the expected levels of accomplishment, they should meet with the manager to establish priorities and to develop plans for the accomplishment of the objectives. The manager will determine whether the objectives are compatible with the overall goals of the organization. The manager and staff associate should hold periodic reviews to check the progress and make adjustments. An annual review should be held to compare the actual results with the expected levels of accomplishment and to set the objectives for the next period.

The underlying philosophy is a belief that people perform best and develop most in an environment of participative management, high performance standards that build on individual strengths, prompt feedback that accentuates the positive, and appropriate rewards. Staff is encouraged to "do their thing" while maintaining individual accountability. The manager is a listener and clarifier who readjusts responsibilities on the basis of individual differences.

Higher frequencies of appraisal are associated with a more favorable attitude toward MBO, higher goal success, improvement of manager-staff associate relationships, clarity of goals, an opinion that the manager was helpful and supportive, the attitude that staff associates had influence in matters affecting them, and esteem and satisfaction for the manager. More praise and less criticism of the objectives by the manager are associated with higher goal success. It is advisable to use an incentive system that rewards effective planning as well as goal achievement when using MBO.

Advantages of MBO for the staff nurse are that the standard of evaluation is based on the characteristics of a specific person and job; nurses have input and some control over their future; nurses know the standard by which they will be judged; nurses have knowledge of the manager's goals, priorities, and deadlines; staff nurses have a greater understanding of where they stand with the manager in relation to relative progress; there is a better basis for evaluation than personality traits; MBO emphasizes the future, which can be changed, instead of the past; and it stimulates higher individual performance and morale.

Advantages for the manager include a reservoir of personnel data and performance information for updating personnel files, an indication of personnel development needs within the agency, a basis for promotion and compensation, a relationship with the staff that makes the manager a coach rather than a judge, and better managerial planning and use of the employee.

MBO directs work activities toward organizational goals, facilitates planning, provides standards for control, provides objective appraisal criteria, reduces role conflict and ambiguity, and uses and motivates human resources.

MBO is limited because it is not an easy system to implement and requires hard work for maintenance; the process must be taught and reinforced for managers to become and remain proficient in applying the principles of the system; the MBO system assumes that staff nurses and managers will define suitable standards that will serve the agency; it presumes that managers understand their limitations; managers are responsible for assessing actual results rather than activities that seem to indicate results; some managers are unable to manage by objectives; some staff nurses may not want to be involved in setting goals; managers and staffs may give lip service to MBO while managers really set the goals; staff nurses may set their goals according to what they know their managers expect; MBO stresses results but does not supply the methods for achieving them; nurses can become frustrated if they believe that increasingly higher goals will be expected of them; overlapping objectives are difficult to evaluate; MBO lends itself to quantitative assessment but may neglect qualitative factors; and MBO does not provide comparative data for promotions and salary increases.

Peer Review

Peer review is a process whereby a group of practicing registered nurses evaluate the quality of another registered nurse's professional performance. It provides a feedback mechanism for sharing ideas, comparing the consistency of the nurse's performance with standards, recognizing outstanding performance, and identifying areas that need further development. This process can increase personal and professional growth and job satisfaction because of the recognition from peers.

Once it has been decided that an institution will use peer review, appraisal tools must be developed. A review of the evaluation tools currently used and the literature on evaluation tools is in order. Various standards may also be reviewed. The tool developed may address technical competence and human relationship, communication, organizational, leadership, and other skills. The process must also be determined, and then staff must be oriented to the system.

The staff should be oriented to the components of the peer review before it is implemented and thereafter during orientation. It is appropriate to give them copies of the peer review process and forms used for peer review. Opportunities to learn how to fill out the forms, how the peer review committee uses the materials, and what questions are to be expected during the peer review interview should be provided.

The peer evaluation process typically includes a review of an employee's self-evaluation form (including short- and long-term goals), reference letters, committee work, special projects, additional education, and contributions to nursing; a performance evaluation by the nurse's immediate manager; a review of past performance; care plans and charting done by the nurse; assessment; observation of the nurse; interviews with patients; a summary of the findings; a presentation of the findings; and recommendations to the nurse. It is appropriate to allow the candidate some agency time to prepare a review folder. A leader is assigned to the nurse to help clarify policy and procedures and to check the documents for completeness.

Who will evaluate whom must be determined. A committee may be appointed, elected, or randomly selected, but it should represent a number of job titles and a wide variety of specialty areas. The members should be familiar with committee responsibilities. The committee's recommendations should be made by consensus, with dissenting opinions recorded.

Once the candidate has been evaluated, there should be a peer review interview for feedback. All feedback must be well documented in the review materials. Hearsay reports are not permitted. The review committee chairperson or designee is responsible for arranging the interview and helping the candidate feel welcome and comfortable. The interview may provide recognition of outstanding performance, identification of areas that need further development, recommendations regarding learning needs, and possibly a recommendation for classification.

Peer review can be threatening and time-consuming. There is a risk of rating candidates too high or too low. However, nurses will be held accountable and responsible for their nursing performance when they are measured against realistic and attainable standards.

Appraisal Interview

There are several kinds of appraisal interviews. They include tell and sell, tell and listen, problem solving, and goal setting. When using the tell-and-sell technique, the manager does most of the talking while the staff associate listens. The manager reports the results of the evaluation to the employee and tries to persuade the staff associate to improve. This assumes that managers are qualified to evaluate staff associates and that staff associates will want to correct their weaknesses. In this role of judge, the interviewer risks losing the loyalty of the employee and inhibiting independent judgment. Face-saving problems are created. Employees usually suppress defensive behavior and attempt to cover their hostility to protect themselves. The tell-and-sell method uses positive and negative extrinsic motivation and is most likely to be successful when the employee respects the interviewer. It tends to perpetuate existing values and practices. The tell-and-sell method works best with young or new employees or individuals who are new to an assignment. These employees may want advice and assurance from an authority figure. Under these conditions, managers are most likely to be respected because of their position, knowledge, and experience. Unfortunately, the tell-and-sell method fosters either dependent and docile or rebellious behavior. After a tell-and-sell style evaluation, the employee often feels like looking for another job.

When using the tell-and-listen method, the manager speaks for about half the time and lets the staff associate speak for the remainder. The interviewer outlines the strong and weak points of the staff associate's job performance and then listens to the interviewee's response. Although still in the role of judge, the interviewer listens to disagreement and allows defensive behavior without attempting to refute any responses. This tends to remove defensive behavior. The employee expresses defensiveness and feels accepted while the interviewer listens, reflects, and summarizes. Thus resistance to change is reduced, and the staff associate develops a more favorable attitude toward the manager. Although this method fosters upward communication and allows the interviewer to learn and change views, the need for change may not be developed in the employee. Tell and listen works best when there is a good relationship between the interviewer and interviewee. Interviewers can learn about staff associates' needs and aspirations, but the latter may not know where they stand. There are no plans for personnel development.

With the problem-solving method, the interviewer assumes the role of helper to stimulate growth and development in the interviewee. It assumes that change can occur without correcting faults and that discussing problems can lead to improvements because the discussion develops new ideas and mutual interests. The staff associate does most of the talking while the interviewer listens, reflects ideas and feelings, asks exploratory questions, and summarizes. Intrinsic motivation is stimulated through increased freedom, increased responsibility, and problem-solving behavior; thus, change is facilitated. Both the manager and staff associate learn from each other. Staff associates may view their job in relation to others more accurately, and managers gain insights into staff associates' working conditions. Unfortunately, the employee may lack ideas, and change may be other than what the interviewer had planned. Although this method is excellent for problem solving and personnel development, it does not warn staff associates or let them know where they stand, evaluate them for lateral transfers or promotional purposes, provide a rating or furnish an evaluation record, or supply top administration with an inventory of talent.

Goal setting is future oriented. It focuses attention on the employee's achievement and consequently stimulates accomplishment. The philosophy behind MBO is teamwork. Top administration sets the organization's objectives, and employees set individual objectives. This method integrates institutional and personal achievement goals. It clarifies objectives and, because it focuses on results and not methods, encourages the person closest to a job to decide how to do it. MBO involves participative management. An autocratic leader is likely to dictate goals to a staff associate. Although that is not consistent with a participative management philosophy, it is better for staff associates to know what is expected of them than not to know.

Which appraisal interview style is used largely depends on the purpose of the evaluation, the manager's philosophy of management, and the institutional guidelines. The manager can create an atmosphere during the interview that is consistent with the appraisal interview style. To create an authoritative image for the tell-and-sell method, managers should have the interview in their office and sit behind a desk, preferably looking down on the staff associate.

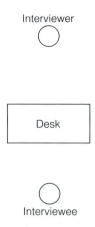

To create an atmosphere of equality for the tell-and-listen, problem-solving, or goal-setting style, the interviewer and employee may sit at a corner table looking at each other.

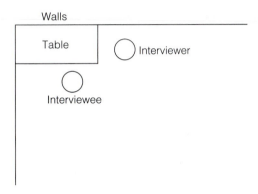

Sitting at a table helps create a working situation for problem solving and goal setting. Sitting either side by side or at the corner of the table helps create a sense of equality and a working relationship.

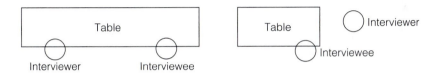

Nonverbal communication is important and should be consistent with verbal communication. Active listening can be expressed through eye contact, a responsive posture, and facial expressions and lets the interviewee know that the interviewer is trying to understand the employee's attitudes and feelings. Pauses give the employee time to think and respond. The interviewer may restate what the employee said. Although this helps the interviewee know the interviewer is listening, it does not guarantee that the meaning of the message was understood. Paraphrasing states the message in fewer and simpler words. If the interviewee says, "I don't understand! One minute she tells me to do it this way and the next minute she tells me to do it that way," the interviewer may paraphrase, "She confuses you." One should ask for clarification if the intent is not clear or say, for example, "Do you mean . . .?" Reflection of feelings, such as "You sound proud of that," helps show understanding. Summarizing what has been said at the end of the interview is particularly important.

The manager's assessment of the staff nurse's performance should be continuous rather than annual. This maximizes feedback for learning. The manager and staff nurse should have an appointment to do the appraisal interview when both are unhurried and should meet where they have privacy. Adequate time should be allowed and interruptions prevented. The purpose of the interview should be clear; both should enter it ready to compare notes, knowing that the counseling notes will not become part of the personnel file. Emphasis should be on the growth of the nurse and on accomplishments related to specific targets. Actual, observed behavior rather than broad personality traits should be discussed during the exchange of ideas between the manager and the staff nurse. The staff nurse should be encouraged to take the initiative in setting goals for improving performance, with the manager supporting, guiding, and validating the nurse's plans.

If managers find it necessary to make unfavorable comments, they should insert them between favorable comments. It is important that the manager not create an atmosphere in which they appear to be sitting in judgment. When the manager enumerates improvement needs, the staff nurse's self-esteem is threatened, and the nurse may become defensive. The greater the threat to the self-image, the poorer the attitude toward evaluations will be, and less improvement in job performance results. If the staff nurse becomes defensive or aggressive, the manager should accept comments without a fight. Keeping quiet and not exposing alibis can help the staff nurse save face.

Before the interview is terminated, ways in which the manager can help the staff nurse accomplish goals should be explored. Staff nurses will probably approach their work with more enthusiasm and confidence if they feel they have the respect and support of the manager.

Appraisal Reports

The appraisal report is to be written jointly by the manager and staff nurse. It should be reliable, valid, and accurate, showing progress made by the nurse and giving illustrations to substantiate value judgments. If both have kept notes that they have periodically assessed, and if the staff nurse believes the manager's intent is to help rather than to blame, the nurse will feel more free to be honest in an evaluation of strengths and weaknesses. If staff nurses have not been functioning satisfactorily, they will already be aware of it. If their performance has not improved adequately since previous interviews, they should be informed that the weakness will be included in the report. Any improvements are to be noted, and staff nurses should know exactly where they stand. It may be necessary to tell them they have to make certain improvements within a definite time period or they will be fired.

Permanent, cumulative evaluation records can be used to assess how the nurse can best be used in the agency. They can be used as a basis for pay increases and promotions or terminations. These records are frequently used as a source of information for letters of reference to be sent to other agencies.

BIBLIOGRAPHY

Buechlein-Telutki MS, Bilak Y, Merrick M, et al: Nurse manager performance appraisal: a collaborative approach, *Nurs Manage* 24:48-50, October 1993.

Gardner DL: Assessing career commitment: the role of staff development, *J Nurs Staff Dev* 7:263-267, November-December 1991.

Keyes MAK: Recognition and reward: a unit-based program, *Nurs Manage* 25:52-54, February 1994.

Marriner A: Evaluation of personnel, *Superv Nurse* 7:36-39, May 1976.

Vogel G, Ruppel DL, Kaufmann CS: Learning needs assessment as a vehicle for integrating staff development into a professional practice model, *Journal of Continuing Education in Nursing* 22:192-197, September-October 1991.

CASE STUDY

You do appraisal interviews with appraisal report follow-ups once a year with the personnel who work with you. You want to create an atmosphere of equality for planning and problem solving. What will you do to create that atmosphere?

CRITICAL THINKING AND LEARNING ACTIVITIES

1. Evaluate an evaluation tool and share your assessment with a classmate. Use Worksheets 23-1 and 23-2 to help you in this process.

2. Practice an appraisal interview with a classmate. Evaluate classroom participation by the appraisal interview style of your choice. Discuss how it felt to appraise and be appraised in that manner.

3. Fill out Worksheet 23-3 to help you distinguish among the various methods of personnel evaluation. Then write a script for an authoritative and an equal working relationship appraisal interview. Arrange furniture accordingly and role-play the scripts with a classmate.

✍ Worksheet 23-1

Purposes of Personnel Evaluation

List at least five purposes of personnel evaluation.
1.

2.

3.

4.

5.

✍ **Worksheet 23-2**

Errors in Performance Evaluation

List at least six common errors in performance evaluation.

1.

2.

3.

4.

5.

6.

✍ **Worksheet 23-3**

Methods of Personnel Evaluation

Describe five methods of personnel evaluation.

1.

2.

3.

4.

5.

Chapter

24

Discipline
of Personnel

Chapter Objectives

◆ List at least five principles of disciplinary action.

◆ Identify at least three components of a disciplinary action program.

◆ Explain behavior modification.

Major Concepts and Definitions	
Discipline	to train, control, punish
Penalties	punishment; negative consequences
Behavior modification	changes in behavior
Reinforcement	actions that strengthen a behavior or increase its probability
Shaping	reinforcing successive attempts at achieving the desired behavior
Extinction	annihilation, destruction, end

DISCIPLINE OF PERSONNEL

Need for Discipline

Lack of knowledge about policies and procedures is a major cause of the need for disciplinary action. Management should provide orientation from the first day of employment. Nurses cannot be expected to follow rules that are unknown to them, vague, or loosely enforced. Consequently, each new employee should be given an employee's handbook. The handbook itemizes the rules and procedures of the agency and specifies the type of discipline that will be imposed for infractions. New employees should be encouraged to read the handbook and ask questions about it.

During orientation, the manager should explain in detail the most frequently violated rules and discuss their significance and rationale. It is recommended that the manager conduct regularly scheduled meetings with staff to discuss changes or to review policies. Rules and regulations also may be posted in a consistent and conspicuous manner.

Most employees are not disciplinary problems, but a minority does exist that requires more than positive stimuli. These few cases are potentially explosive. About half of the grievance cases appealed to an arbitrator by labor unions involve disciplinary action. In about half of those cases, management either reversed or modified its decision when the individual's appeal was upheld. Consequently, it is of utmost importance that disciplinary action be undertaken in a judicious manner. The disciplinary action program and grievance procedure must be uniform for all personnel of a specific grade or classification. A standard disciplinary action program with procedures outlined and forms provided should be available to managers.

Principles of Disciplinary Action

Have a positive attitude.   The manager's attitude is very important in preventing or correcting undesirable behavior. If staff nurses are treated as suspect, they are more likely to provide the trouble that the manager anticipates. People tend to do what is expected of them; therefore, it is the manager's duty to maintain a positive attitude by expecting the best from the staff.

Investigate carefully.   The ramifications of disciplinary action are so serious that managers must proceed with caution. They should collect the facts, check allegations, talk to witnesses, and ask accused employees for their side of the story. Managers should accept the staff nurse's account until and unless the allegations are proven. The manager may wish to consult other managers or the director. If the situation is serious enough to require action before a full investigation can be conducted, it is better to suspend the staff nurse subject to reinstatement after investigation than to take more drastic action.

Be prompt.   Managers should not be so expeditious that they neglect to be thorough in ascertaining the facts. If a staff nurse is disciplined unfairly or unnecessarily, the effects on the entire staff may be severe. However, if the discipline is delayed, the relationship between the punishment and the offense may become less clear. Because of the distastefulness of disciplinary action, the manager may tend to postpone the punishment as long as possible. The longer the delay, the more the staff forget their actions, the more likely they are to feel that the discipline is not deserved, and the fewer are the positive educational effects for the future.

Protect privacy.   Disciplinary action affects the ego of the staff nurse. Thus it is better to discuss the situation in private. By helping the nurse save face, there is less possibility of future resentment and a greater chance for future cooperation. However, a public reprimand may be necessary for the nurse who does not take private criticism seriously.

Focus on the act.   When disciplining a staff nurse, the manager should emphasize that it was the act that was unacceptable, not the employee. If the employee is not acceptable, the person should be fired.

Enforce rules consistently.   Offending employees should be treated equally or consistently for similar transgressions. Equal treatment is based on rules with specific penalties for various acts and the number of offenses. Consistency reduces the possibility of favoritism, promotes predictability, and fosters acceptance of penalties.

Be flexible.   Consistent implementation is complicated by the fact that individuals and circumstances are never the same. A penalty should be determined only after the entire record of the employee is reviewed. The manager should consider length of service, past accomplishments or problems, level of skill, and expendability to the organization. The intent of the staff nurse, the extenuating circumstances, and whether this situation constitutes a test case and will set precedent for the future should also be taken into consideration. If managers enforce identical penalties for seemingly similar offenses, they may be excessively severe with one person and lenient with the other.

Advise the employee. The employees must be informed that their conduct is not acceptable. Personnel files containing anecdotal notes can be a useful management tool, but they are of little value in upholding disciplinary action if the staff nurse is not informed of the contents promptly.

Take corrective, constructive action. The manager should be sure that the staff nurse understands that the behavior was contrary to the organization's requirements and should explain why such regulations are necessary. The staff nurse should be counseled as to what behavior is required and how to prevent future disciplinary action.

Follow up. The manager should quietly investigate to determine whether the staff nurse's behavior has changed. If the staff nurse continues to invite disciplinary action, the manager should reevaluate the situation to try to determine the reason for the nurse's attitude. The manager must try to come to terms with the offender and the reasons for the transgression.

Penalties

Oral reprimand. For minor violations that have occurred for the first time, managers may opt to give an oral warning in private. They might tactfully correct the deviation by telling the staff nurse the proper way to deal with the situation or by rebuking the nurse. An oral reprimand is of limited value beyond alerting the nurse in a relatively friendly way to a need for correction. Because nothing is in writing and the reprimand is given in private, it is difficult to prove that a warning was given. Over time the manager may become unsure and inexact about what was said to whom and under what conditions. When an oral warning is given, the manager is advised to make an anecdotal note of the time, place, occasion, and the gist of the reprimand. Oral comments may be easily forgotten, but too formal handling of initial minor offenses can be counterproductive.

Written reprimand. If the offense is more serious or repeated, the reprimand may be written. It is suggested that the manager and staff associate develop a written plan for improvement that defines what the staff associate will do to make the performance acceptable and what the manager will do to change the environmental situation if appropriate. A time limit should be set. Additional penalties may be defined in case the employee's behavior does not adequately improve during the allowed time period. The written notice should include the name of the worker, the name of the manager, the nature of the problem, the plan for correction, and the consequences of future repetition. It is recommended that the worker sign the report to indicate that the employee has read it, received a copy of it, or both. A copy should be given to the employee and one retained for the personnel file. If personnel believe that signing such a document would be considered an admission of guilt and hence refuse to sign, the manager may ask another managerial person to sign as witness to the fact that the document was discussed with the worker and that a copy was given to the worker. It is appropriate for higher management and the personnel department to review this report. At the end of the designated time, the manager and worker should have another conference to determine if the terms of the agreement have been met. It is hoped that the nurse can be complimented for having made progress and that no further action is deemed necessary. However, if no change or inadequate change has occurred, the continuing nature of the problem should be identified and documented. Additional penalties will probably be necessary.

Other penalties. Fines may be charged for offenses such as tardiness. Loss of privileges might include transfer to a less desirable shift and loss of preference of assignment.

Layoff, demotion, and discharge are the most serious penalties and need approval beyond the manager. Layoff may be appropriate in situations where it is best to remove the nurse while an investigation is conducted. The staff nurse may be reinstated with no loss of pay if cleared through the investigation or may be suspended if found guilty of a serious offense. Demotion is a questionable solution. It creates hard feelings, which may be contagious, and more than likely places offenders in a position for which they are overqualified. Termination becomes necessary as a last resort.

Components of a Disciplinary Action Program

Codes of conduct. Employees must be informed of the nature and meaning of codes of conduct. Agency handbooks, policy manuals, and orientation programs may be used. The staff nurse must understand that the rules are reasonable and directly related to efficient, effective operation of the agency.

Authorized penalties. During disciplinary action, the personnel record should indicate that a fair investigation was made of charges before the assessment of guilt and determination of penalties. The agency's disciplinary action program should indicate that the current action is being administered without bias and is directly related to the offense.

Records of offenses and corrective measures. Records are of utmost importance when disciplinary action is appealed. The personnel record should clearly indicate the offense, management's efforts to correct the problem, and resulting penalties.

Right of appeal. Formal provision for the right of employee appeal is a part of each disciplinary action program. Appeal beyond the manager ensures equitable treatment and encourages more employee acceptance of the disciplinary process. At the same time, fair managers need not fear a review of their actions by others.

MODIFICATION OF EMPLOYEE BEHAVIOR

Can an employee's behavior be changed by changing the manager's behavior? Is behavior that recurs in the presence of the manager being reinforced by the manager? Is it possible that doing nothing is doing something? In all three instances the answer is yes. Behavior leads to consequences, and the consequences that follow the behavior affect the probability of recurrence of that behavior. Because behavior is a function of the consequence, it is important for nurse managers to identify the contingency relationship.

Consequences may be favorable, punitive, absent, or insufficient. Positive consequences increase the probability of recurrence of the behavior that preceded them. Absence of consequences decreases the probability, and insufficient consequences have little effect. Punishing consequences have varied and unpredictable effects. Punishment is not the opposite of a favorable consequence. No consequence is.

Reinforcement

Positive reinforcement increases the probability of a recurrence of desired behavior. It is more effective the sooner it follows the desired behavior, and it should be clearly connected to the behavior that the manager wishes to increase. Positive reinforcement may be as subtle as a smile or a nod of the head when someone speaks. Whatever is being said when the manager smiles or nods is reinforced and will recur with increasing frequency. Recognition is a powerful reinforcer. "Mr. Jones must feel so much better now since you have completed his morning care" and "You collected a lot of valuable information during your interview with Mrs. Smith" are examples. "I'm glad to see you here today" reinforces attendance, whereas "I see you were absent again yesterday" gives attention to the absence.

The nurse manager can even stimulate new behavior by verbal acknowledgment of the desired response. Words are used to describe the behavior the nurse manager wants to encourage. A comment such as "I really appreciate nurses' attending in-services" is likely to increase attendance at in-services. A number of stimuli—such as feedback, attention, praise, avoidance of punishment, merit pay increases, special assignments, assistance with tuition, or tickets to a ball game or play—can be used to reinforce behavior. However, nurse managers must consider that any stimulus can be reinforcing or aversive depending on the person and the situation, so they should carefully select stimuli that are reinforcers for the individual in a given situation. For example, tickets to a ball game may be reinforcing to some and aversive to others. Recognition is one of the easiest, cheapest, and most universally effective reinforcers.

Shaping

Shaping is a behavior-modification technique used when the response does not meet the criteria. By systematically reinforcing successive approximations, the nurse manager can shape the responses into the desired behavior, and get the nurse to do something new. The manager provides favorable consequences after any attempt at the desired behavior, then withholds consequences until improvement is made. When working with the staff nurse who is chronically absent or late, the manager may acknowledge that the nurse is at work: "I see you were only 30 minutes late today." Later, "I see you were only 15 minutes late today." Still later, "I noticed you were only 5 minutes late today." The manager may initially praise a new employee for attempting a new task and then note improvements in skill as they occur. Once the level of desired performance has been reached, it can be maintained by providing favorable consequences intermittently. Too many positive consequences cause satiation, and they lose their effect on the behavior. Performance that has been intermittently reinforced is most resistant to extinction.

Extinction

Withholding reinforcers will decrease the probability of the occurrence of the behavior and contribute to its extinction. Therefore, if the manager does not mention or otherwise reward undesirable behavior, the lack of action should contribute to extinction. Conversely, any reinforcer that is presented frequently, but not paired with another reinforcer, will lose its effectiveness. Promises of "raises" or "hiring more help and getting some relief" become meaningless if not paired with a pay increase or recruitment and selection of personnel. Managers who praise everyone for everything all of the time will find that their words lose their effectiveness as reinforcers. When the consequences are not worth the effort, the behavior will decrease also.

Punishment

The manager can decrease the probability of a response by pairing the behavior with an aversive stimulus. People who are late to work will not be paid for the time they are absent. There will be no overtime pay for people who did not complete their work on time. Employees who do not meet work standards will be fired. Firing a few workers who were not meeting standards can have an immediate impact on the remaining personnel, who initially work harder to avoid being fired. However, if management does nothing to reinforce the more productive work behavior, avoidance behavior is likely to occur. Employees may cover up for each other, steal from the agency what they rationalize is theirs, or resign. By using aversive stimuli to control behavior, management pairs itself with those stimuli and becomes viewed as aversive.

Once managers have started an aversive stimulus, they should not stop it until the behavior has been corrected or the cessation may act as a positive reinforcer. Absences, tardiness, excuse making, rationalizing, placing blame elsewhere, and other avoidance behaviors will increase if they successfully reduce the aversive stimuli. If the manager gruffly asks a nurse why some work has not been done (aversive stimulus), and the manager backs off when the staff nurse replies that he or she thought someone else was doing it, blaming others is reinforced. Although punishment causes behavior to occur less frequently, it does not teach new behaviors and is likely to increase avoidance behaviors. Most motivation problems are caused by punishment, absence of consequences, or insufficient consequences.

Behavior Modification for the Employee with a Performance Problem

Besides being aware of the subtle ways that one's behavior may reinforce, shape, or reduce behavior of others, the nurse manager may apply behavior modification to personnel with performance problems. First one must identify the performance problem and analyze the antecedent, behavior, and consequence. What happened before the behavior occurred? Each time nurse A was late to work, he had worked the evening shift the night before. Each time nurse B yelled at her staff, an emergency treatment was being performed. Head nurse C was condescending to his staff after a physician had scolded him. What happened after the behavior occurred? Someone had already done part of nurse A's work by the time she got to the ward. Staff nurses responded quickly when nurse *B* yelled at them during an emergency procedure. Nurse *C*'s staff avoided him.

Once the performance problem has been identified, the baseline frequency is determined. The baseline measure is the frequency before any attempts to change it. If nurses are interested in modifying their own behavior, they may collect the baseline data themselves. The behavior must be precisely defined, observable, and consequently countable. Written records should be kept, preferably on a portable recording system that is present when the behavior occurs, so the nurse can record it immediately A tailor-made tally sheet is useful because one can see data in relation to time:

	M	T	W	Th	F	Sat	Sun
7:00	I I I	I I	I I	I I I	I I		
8:00			I				
9:00	I I			I	I		
10:00		I		I			
11:00			I		I		
12:00				I	I		
1:00		I	I		I		
2:00	I I	I	I I	I I	I		
3:00	I I I	I I	I I I	I I	I I I		

If the behavior occurs daily, it should be recorded for 1 week. If there are large variations in the behavior from one day to the next, observations should be recorded for 2 weeks. A time-sampling technique can be used by busy managers by randomly selecting short periods to observe and tally behaviors. This is effective only for high-frequency behavior. The manager must consider if the period of data collection was representative of the normal situation and use a stable baseline rate as a clue to start the intervention.

If one transfers the information from the tally sheet to a graph that depicts frequency over time, it is easy to visualize the effect of the intervention strategy. One can put a wavy vertical line on the graph to depict the point where intervention was started.

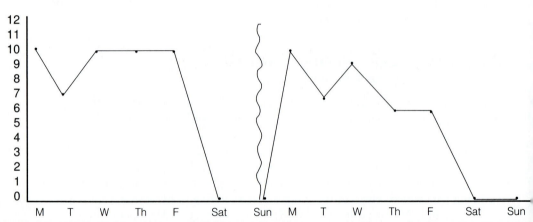

After identifying the relevant variables, the supervisor and nurse select appropriate reinforcement, extinction, punishment, or any combination of intervention strategies to decrease the frequency of the undesirable behavior. If the desired performance is punished, the punishment should be removed. Instead of making fast workers finish everyone else's work, they can be allowed time to do what they choose, such as read in the library or meditate in the chapel, receive a bonus day at a specified frequency, or be given a merit pay increase specifically for doing more than their share of the work. If undesirable behavior is rewarded, the reward should be removed. Instead of having slow employees' work completed by others, the manager should inform the workers that they are responsible for so much work by themselves, must have that work completed before going home, and will receive no overtime pay for completion of the normal workload.

If desired behavior has not been rewarded, the manager should arrange a consequence. This may be as simple as orally acknowledging a nurse's accomplishment occasionally. Nurses' accomplishments can be acknowledged in the agency's newsletter. Awards can be created to recognize desirable behavior.

If obstacles are identified, they should be removed. Nurses can be referred to professional counseling to help them work through situational crises that are interfering with their work performance. The manager can try to get the resources nurses need to do their job. Nurses should also have the necessary education to do what is expected of them. They may need formal education, on-the-job training, practice sessions, or simply feedback. The staff associate is the best source of information for what can serve as a positive reinforcer because what may be desirable for the manager may be aversive to the staff associate.

Once the intervention strategy has been planned, it should be implemented and the response frequency recorded. The strategy should be evaluated for effectiveness. If it is not working, it should be analyzed and revised. Once the desired behavior is obtained, it should be maintained through intermittent reinforcement.

BIBLIOGRAPHY

Marriner A: Discipline of personnel, *Superv Nurse* 7:15-17, November 1976.
Vestal K: Fired! Managing the process, *JONA* 20:14-16, June 1990.

CASE STUDY

A staff member has violated a policy. What principles of disciplinary action will you observe as you give the staff member an oral reprimand? How will you proceed if the violation is repeated?

CRITICAL THINKING AND LEARNING ACTIVITIES

1. Using Worksheet 24-1, identify a behavior that you would like to change. Determine your baseline behavior. Graph the frequency. Plan reinforcement and extinction strategies.

2. Share your behavior modification plan with a classmate and solicit positive reinforcement from that classmate.

3. Offer your support of a classmate's behavior modification plan.

✎ Worksheet 24-1

Behavior Modification

Behavior to change: _____

Baseline behavior:

Times		Sunday	Monday	Tuesday	Wednesday	Thursday	Friday	Saturday
	12 AM							
	1							
	2							
	3							
	4							
	5							
	6							
	7							
	8							
	9							
	10							
	11							
	12 PM							
	1							
	2							
	3							
	4							
	5							
	6							
	7							
	8							
	9							
	10							
	11							

List reinforcement strategies:

List extinction strategies:

Problem Employees

Chapter Objectives

◆ List at least three types of problem employees.

◆ Identify at least three types of employee counseling.

◆ Explain outplacement counseling.

Major Concepts and Definitions	
Substance abuse	misuse of drugs
Angry	furious, raging, tumultuous
Withdrawn	retreated, isolated
Productivity	results
Absenteeism	absence from work
Termination	end of something
Directive counseling	counselor tells one what to do
Nondirective counseling	client decides what to do
Outplacement counseling	helping dismissed person find a new job

PROBLEM EMPLOYEES

Substance abusers, angry or withdrawn workers, personnel with excessive absenteeism, and the terminating employee provide challenges to nurse managers. In each case, the manager must be alert to symptoms of problems, help the employee solve the problem, and evaluate the results.

Substance Abusers

Substance abuse is not uncommon among nurses. It affects all socioeconomic classes, cultures, and races. Only 5% or less of all alcoholics are skid-row bums. Among alcoholic nurses studied, most had been in the top third of their class, held advanced degrees, held responsible and demanding jobs, and had an excellent work history.

Nurses with alcohol or other drug addictions often exhibit psychosocial problems (see Box 25-1). Personality changes may be noted as the nurse becomes more irritable, withdrawn, and moody. Because of a decreased interest in outside activities, isolation increases. Related social changes include eating alone and avoiding social gatherings.

Changes in personal appearance become apparent. Changes in dress, an unkempt appearance, flushed complexion, red eyes, swollen face, and hand tremors are common. Mental status changes include forgetfulness, confusion, and decreased alertness.

General behavior changes too. Inappropriate responses and irritability occur more frequently. Excuses for behavior become more elaborate. Intolerance and suspicion of others and nervousness increase. Avoidance of others is noted. Work efficiency drops, there is a decline in the quality and quantity of work, and the work pace becomes uneven. Some assigned tasks are forgotten. Arriving late and leaving early and extended lunch hours and break times become patterns of behavior. Accidents increase.

When a nurse reports to work in a state of acute intoxication, the manager notes the signs objectively and asks a second person to validate the observations. The odor

Box 25-1   **SIGNS AND SYMPTOMS OF POSSIBLE SUBSTANCE ABUSE**

SIGNS

Psychosocial problems
  Irritability
  Moodiness
  Tendency to isolate self
Social changes
  Eating alone
  Avoiding social gatherings
Changes in personal appearance
  Changes in dress
  Unkempt appearance
  Flushed complexion
  Red eyes
  Swollen face
  Hand tremors
Mental status changes
  Forgetfulness
  Confusion
  Decreased alertness
General behavior changes
  Inappropriate responses
  Elaborate excuses for behavior
  Intolerance of others
  Suspiciousness
  Nervousness

SYMPTOMS

Odor of alcohol
Slurred speech
Unsteady gait
Errors in judgment

of alcohol, slurred speech, unsteady gait, and errors in judgment are symptoms of intoxication. The intoxicated nurse is removed from the situation, confronted briefly and firmly about the behavior, and sent home to rest and recuperate. Then the incident is recorded. The manager describes the observation, states the action taken, indicates future plans, and has the employee sign and date the memo after returning to work. Refusal to sign and date the memo should be noted by the manager and a witness.

Hutchinson has described three stages in the self-annihilation trajectory that nurses experience as they become addicted: the experience, the commitment, and the compulsion. The experience is the nurse's introduction to alcohol or drugs and involves the three phases of initiating, connecting, and experimenting. Initiating is the first experience with drugs and is often experienced as a patient. The use of alcohol or drugs is associated with the relief of pain in the connecting phase. During the experimenting phase the person uses a variety of drugs to find the one of choice.

The commitment stage has three phases, too: dialogue with self, disengaging, and routinizing. Commitment is the decision to use alcohol or drugs in one's lifestyle. It requires finding a source. After finding the chemical of choice, the person dialogues with self to justify the use of the chemical to alleviate psychological or physical pain. Denying, bargaining, and justifying are common dialogues. After the self-diagnosis, a disengaging process occurs. People disengage from their conscience and their usual behavior. They disengage from their family, friends, and colleagues, and the values of nursing and society. They transform themselves into alcohol or drug users. They start using chemicals routinely to relieve their distress. Alcoholism is easier than drug addiction. The alcoholic nurse is more likely to miss work because of hangovers, whereas the drug-addicted nurse is likely to work overtime to have additional access to drugs. Many conning strategies are used to obtain chemicals.

The third stage, compulsion, has two phases—craving and surrendering. It is when the physical addiction becomes dominant. Some people stay in the experience stage for up to a year, but once they become committed the compulsion stage follows.

Chronic performance problems are more common than acute intoxication. Each time performance problems are observed, they should be documented, including date, time, who was observed by whom, and a description of the incident and circumstances. At a prearranged conference, the nurse is confronted with the observations and how they affect job performance and patient care. The nurse is allowed to give an explanation. Alternatives are explored, and a course of action is planned. When substance abuse is identified as the problem, the offender is encouraged to take voluntary action. The manager refers the nurse to a local treatment facility and meets with the nurse periodically to monitor progress. The manager is not to serve the role of therapist.

Hutchinson identified four phases of recovery: premotivation, breakthrough, early recovery, and extended recovery. During the premotivation phase the person may decide to stop using drugs to please someone. The person may hope to use chemicals only occasionally and employ a strong denial system. Denial decreases and the person admits to an addiction problem during the breakthrough phase. The person begins to cope with loss of the chemical, rediscovers values, and gains an image of self as a drug-free person during early recovery. The extended recovery begins after about 6 months in early recovery. People acknowledge their feelings about themselves and their relationships. They gain respect for themselves and their skills. They acquire control of their lives. This is the stage when the nurse can return to work and be productive.

Instead of disciplining and firing personnel whose job performance is impaired, more and more health care organizations are trying to help them regain their health and productivity through employee assistance programs (EAPs). At first EAPs focused on alcohol and drug abuse, but the services have broadened to include financial, legal, and marital problems; gambling; work addiction; and eating disorders. EAPs have increased productivity, reduced absenteeism, and lowered insurance costs. Assessment, diagnosis, and early intervention benefit the employee and the organization.

Many state nurses' associations have started peer assistance programs. Ideally the association intervenes early in the addiction process before legal action is necessary. Often reports of impairment are made through a confidential telephone call or as a referral to the chairperson of the peer assistance program. The chairperson verifies that an impairment exists and may coach the nurse manager about documentation, verification, and intervention. A regional representative or local intervener contacts the person in question and makes an appointment.

The local intervener typically outlines the purpose of the visit with the impaired person, presents information about chemical abuse, and identifies behavior and circumstances in which the impairment has been evident. The fact that the disease is progressive is stressed. Various treatment options are presented. Issues such as hospitalization, insurance coverage, use of sick time and accrued vacation time, and family responsibilities are discussed. If the person denies impairment or refuses treatment, the impaired nurse may be reported to the state board of nursing by the employer.

When an impaired nurse participates in a peer assistance program an advocate is assigned. The advocate maintains contact with the impaired nurse during treatment and until a solid recovery is established. A contract made by the peer review program advocate and the impaired nurse typically identifies employment restrictions, random urine screens, attendance at Alcoholics Anonymous or Narcotics Anonymous meetings, attendance at nurses' support groups, and contacts with the advocate.

When alcoholics or drug abusers refuse counseling or fail to follow the plan of care, they are told treatment is mandatory for continued employment. If they still refuse mandatory participation in the treatment, they are terminated in accordance with the hospital's policies.

Angry or Withdrawn Employees

Nurse managers often deal with angry or withdrawn employees. Anger and withdrawal are the fight and flight responses to anxiety. The angry nurse is more likely to be considered a troublemaker. The withdrawn person may be viewed as nice. However, both need help.

Anxiety occurs from the frustration of unmet expectations or loss of self-respect. The anxiety is transformed into feelings or actions and relief is felt. Angry, hostile, and destructive behavior is a primary response to frustration. It is intended to gain mastery over the situation. The angry employee may become hostile and use critical, sarcastic, and obscene language with others. Consequently, interpersonal relationships suffer, and productive work may be impaired. Anger can also be displaced to patients and others.

Withdrawn persons do not invest emotional energy in others. Fear of self-disclosure or having others become attached to them is frightening. Withdrawal is a protective mechanism to avoid hurt. Withdrawn persons sit through meetings without becoming involved. They are not assertive and do not protect their rights. They may be delegated more than their fair share of the work because they are so cooperative and polite. This leads to more feelings of use, abuse, and helplessness.

Nurse managers need to recognize aggressive and passive behaviors among employees, teach and display assertive behavior, and encourage problem solving. They should help personnel understand themselves and their job responsibilities, develop trust, and promote group harmony. Employees should be encouraged to express themselves without fear of reprisals. Managers should be sincere, firm, and fair. Job expectations need to be clear and personnel rewarded liberally and disciplined justly.

Decreased Productivity

Decreased productivity is a side effect of personnel problems. Managers should make sure that desired performance is not being punished or undesirable behavior rewarded. Expectations are clarified. Employees are taught how to do what they are expected to do. If boredom is a problem, job rotation and special projects are considered.

Absenteeism

Absenteeism is also a side effect of personnel problems. Ineffective management, poor working relationships, boredom, lack of control over decisions affecting one's life, and overwork are contributing factors. Some workers are immature and lack the self-discipline to get themselves to work. Others stay away to avoid an unpleasant or boring job. Some are poorly motivated, do as little as possible to prevent being fired, and do not see their job as a means toward an end. The hypochondriac uses absenteeism to get attention and sympathy from others. Abusive absenteeism may be used to get even with a manager. Some personnel are exhausted from overwork, have lost their enthusiasm for the job, or are burned out.

Managers should make sure that there are attendance policies, that the policies do not reward nonattendance, and that they are enforced consistently. Attendance records should be maintained, and grievance procedures should be established.

Documented attendance policies greatly influence absence rates. Traditional sick leave policies have rewarded employees for absenteeism and have encouraged them to be dishonest to collect sick pay or be punished by losing it. Employees who receive sick pay are absent considerably more than those who do not. Some agencies have required a physician's excuse before an employee can receive sick pay to decrease the dishonest use of sick time. Because most people are only sick 1 or 2 days at a time, some hospitals do not compensate for the first 2 days of any sickness. The third and successive days are compensated. Other agencies have gone to paid time off. Each employee receives a certain amount of paid time off inclusive of holiday, vacation, and sick leave with few restrictions as to its use. It is typically collected at a rate calculated by length of continuous service. It simplifies record keeping but provides incentive to use the days whether sick or not.

Absenteeism data need to be collected and analyzed to determine trends and patterns of individuals and personnel in general. Recording the date of absence, the reason and whether excused or unexcused, day of the week, preceding or following a day off, the employee's job classification, shift, tenure, age, sex, marital status, or any other information thought to be useful provides information to detect trends and pinpoint problems. Absenteeism often occurs more frequently in certain job classifications or departments, on specific days or shifts, or among a group working under a specific manager. Problems need to be identified so managers can develop control measures. Baseline data are also useful to determine the success of the control program.

A progressive discipline policy that imposes increasingly severe penalties is appropriate. Such a policy allows employees to know in advance the consequences of their behavior. Progressive discipline often starts with an oral reprimand that is documented and progresses through a written warning, pay deduction, suspension without pay, and dismissal.

Terminating Employees

Working with a terminating employee (whether voluntary or involuntary) is also challenging for the nurse manager. The manager must help the employee deal with the related feelings. A sense of loss and grief are common. A period of shock or denial that is then followed by disorganization, anger, guilt, and loneliness is normal. This is followed by a deorientation period and a reestablishment phase.

The manager can help terminating employees by providing an opportunity to talk about their feelings. Airing feelings about leaving, self-image, not working anymore or filling another position, and other interests that may be pursued helps relieve the anxiety. Helping the employee plan for the future is also useful.

It is not uncommon for terminating employees to detach themselves from the job and do little for some time before the termination. The manager can assign tasks that are considered important that can either be finished or transferred to someone else at the time of the employee's termination.

Rituals such as best wishes cards and going away parties serve to acknowledge the termination and provide a rite of separation that facilitates the termination process.

EMPLOYEE COUNSELING

Counseling helps improve employees' mental health, thus enhancing understanding, self-control, self-confidence, and consequently their ability to work effectively. Counseling accomplishes several activities on a directive to nondirective scale. It provides an opportunity to give advice, offer reassurance, improve communication, release emotional tension, clarify thinking, and reorient.

When giving advice, a counselor tells the employee what the counselor thinks the employee should do. Unfortunately, it is almost impossible to understand another person's complicated problems, and consequently the advice may not be sound. Advice may foster feelings of inferiority and dependence on the counselor.

Reassurance provides courage to face a problem and confidence that one is handling the situation appropriately. False reassurance is dangerous. It may prevent the employee from getting the professional help needed. It offers little comfort when the counselee knows that the counselor cannot predict the outcome. Even if there is some comfort obtained, it tends to dissipate when the person faces the problem again.

Counseling improves both upward and downward communication. It allows employees to express their feelings to management. Although individual names must be kept confidential, feelings can be grouped into categories and interpreted to higher management. The counseling session allows the counselor to explain company policies and activities to the employee, thus achieving downward communication.

Catharsis or the release of emotional tension often occurs when people have the opportunity to talk about their frustrations. They become more relaxed, and their speech becomes more coherent and rational as they explain their problems to a sympathetic listener. Then, as emotional blocks to clear thinking are eliminated, thinking becomes more rational. People may realize that their emotions are not appropriate for the situation. This may help people recognize and accept their limitations and bring about a reorientation or change in values and goals. The manager should refer an employee to professional help when reorientation is needed.

Directive counseling occurs when the counselor listens to the employee's problems, decides how to solve the problems, and tells the employee what to do. The counselor predominantly gives advice. This type of counseling does give some emotional release, can be reassuring, and fosters communication. Thinking may be clarified in a limited way. Reorientation seldom occurs.

Nondirective counseling is client centered. The counselor listens and encourages employees to explain their problems, identify alternatives, explore the ramifications of each option, and determine the most appropriate solution. Emotional release occurs more frequently in nondirective than in directive counseling. Clear thinking and reorientation are fostered. Reassurance may be used, but advice should be limited. This approach can be very beneficial, but managers must be cautious not to neglect their normal directive leadership responsibilities.

Nondirective counseling is more time-consuming and costly than directive counseling. To be effective, the employee must have the intelligence to identify problems and assess solutions and the emotional stability to deal with them. The nondirective counselor must be cautious not to allow emotionally dependent employees to avoid their work responsibilities.

Cooperative counseling is a compromise between directive and nondirective counseling. It is the cooperative effort by the counselor and employee through an exchange of ideas to help solve the problem. The cooperative counselor starts by listening, as would a nondirective counselor. As the interview progresses, however, the cooperative counselor offers information and insight and is likely to discuss the problems with a broad knowledge of the organization's point of view. This may help change the employee's perspective. Cooperative counseling combines the advantages of both directive and nondirective counseling and avoids most of the disadvantages.

The manager usually provides cooperative counseling when employees have job-related emotional problems. Because of employees' rights to privacy, it is appropriate for the manager to refer an employee to professional help when personal problems are interfering with job performance or when a person needs reorientation.*

OUTPLACEMENT COUNSELING

Although not many registered nurses are fired, during economic recessions there is an increasing incidence in reduction in workforces. Outplacement counseling can be used to minimize the emotional and professional scarring that results from being dismissed from one's position.

Poor job performance, tardiness, absenteeism, substance abuse, inappropriate behavior, and staff reduction are the most common reasons for discharging nurses. A termination of this nature is usually a progressive process. However, for some offenses, nurses can be terminated immediately. These are likely to include abuse of patients and visitors, insubordination, intoxication, possession of drugs, theft, gambling, disorderly conduct, willful destruction of property, sleeping on duty, or falsification of records.

The termination procedures used must be consistent with the agency policies. Termination usually involves several steps, beginning with an oral warning. If the employee does not change the offending behavior in response to the oral warning, written warnings with corrective interviews are used. There need to be well-documented, sufficient grounds for termination. The nurse manager can use anecdotal

---

* Employee counseling is discussed in more detail in Davis K: *Human behavior at work: organizational behavior,* New York, 1981, McGraw-Hill.

notes to record both strong and weak attributes of the worker. They should contain factual information about who was observed by whom, where, and the background of the incident. There should be a sufficient number of observations to establish a pattern of behavior.

Written warnings used with corrective interviews should state the expected level of performance and the consequence if that standard is not met. Suspension is typically used before termination. The counseling note should be signed by both the nurse manager and the worker. If the worker refuses to sign, a witness can validate that the worker has read the counseling notes and refuses to sign them.

Poor job performance should be analyzed. Have employees been taught how to do what is expected of them? If not, they should be taught. Do they practice the skill often enough to keep their talents refined? If not, practice sessions could be made available. Specific, descriptive feedback should be given. Demonstrations and return demonstrations are appropriate. The feedback should be as close to the act as possible. Positive reinforcement for what was done well is as important as identifying weaknesses and making plans to overcome them. Follow-up by noting changes is also important.

A problem-solving approach can be used for tardiness and absenteeism. Why is the person late or absent so often? If a person has difficulty getting children to a babysitter and to work by 7 AM, could that person's hours be changed to 8:00 AM to 4:30 PM? This will allow the employee to fulfill his or her parental responsibilities, and it will also help provide a smooth transition at the change of shift. If the person is a night owl who has difficulty getting up in the morning, could that person be assigned the evening shift? Is the person working two jobs to make ends meet? Are financial assistance and counseling available? Are family problems interfering with attendance? Is the person hung over when reporting to duty? The social services that are available for patients should also be used for staff, for example, self-help groups such as Alcoholics Anonymous, Single Parents, and Shelters for Women. Social services, the chaplain, or family counseling are also useful.

Repeated failure to meet performance standards, lack of compliance with company policies, and staff reductions are just causes for termination. Each should be a progressive process. The employee should know what level of performance is expected to prevent termination and the risk of termination.

Support services are needed by people who are terminated. The agency should have termination policies regarding severance pay, terminal vacation, accrued holidays and sick time, and insurance. The person may need information about unemployment. This is an opportune time for a counselor in personnel to help terminating employees reassess their location and vocation. Where do they want to live? What type of climate do they like? What type of work interests them and provides the most satisfaction? What do their educational background and skills prepare them to do? What can they do to prepare themselves better to reach their goals? How important are salary, fringe benefits, retirement plans, work hours, and opportunities for advancement?

Once terminating employees decide what they want to do and where, they may need assistance to locate job openings. Professional journals, employment agencies, and college placement services are sources of information. Recruiters are often present at professional meetings. Friends, relatives, and acquaintances may help locate positions, and employers can be contacted directly.

Terminating employees are likely to need help preparing résumés, writing marketing letters, and interviewing. They do not need to state the reason that they left the last job on this marketing letter, résumé, or job application. However, they should be prepared to address the issue during an interview. They should be honest about the reason for termination, speak about the treatment they have had, if any, and focus on the knowledge and skills they have learned on the last job that they can transfer to the new one. They should not be critical of the last employer.

The sooner one accepts the fact that one has been fired, the sooner one can put the pieces back together and move on. The boss should be very clear about the reason. The termination should not come as a surprise. With the progressive process, the employee should know the consequences of not meeting the performance standards. Any reduction in workforce should be done with fair warning and target dates. Employees should be informed of the grievance policy and procedure when reflecting if they have been fairly treated. The outplacement counseling can help the person know what questions to ask about pay and benefits, how to tell the family, how to solicit help from friends and acquaintances, and how to budget to protect securities until another job can be obtained. Career counseling and job placement counseling are useful.

Being fired initiates stress and can be quite devastating. Outplacement counseling can help reduce the related personal and professional scarring that inevitably results from being dismissed.

BIBLIOGRAPHY

Bartholomew S: Chemical dependence: recognition and intervention, *Physician Assistant* 14:15-18,21-22,24-26, July 1991.

Beebe GC: Efficacy of a substance abuse primary prevention skills conference for nurses, *Journal of Continuing Education in Nursing* 23:231-234, September-October 1992.

Brennan SJ: Recognizing and assisting the impaired nurse: recommendations for nurse managers, *Nurs Forum* 26:12-16, 1991.

Clark MD: Preventing drug dependency: educating and supporting staff part 2, *JONA* 19:21-26, January 1989.

Compton MA: A Rogerian view of drug abuse: implications for nursing, *Nurs Sci Q* 2:98-105, Summer 1989.

Hughes TL, Fox ML: Patterns of alcohol and drug use among women: focus on special populations, *AWHONN'S Clinical Issues in Perinatal and Women's Health Nursing* 4:203-212, 1993.

Hutchinson S: Chemically dependent nurses: implications for nurse executives, *JONA* 17:23-29, September 1987.

Hutchinson S: Chemically dependent nurses: the trajectory toward self-annihilation, *Nurs Res* 35:196-200, July-August 1986.

Hutchinson S: Toward self integration: the recovery process of chemically dependent nurses, *Nurs Res* 36(6):339-343, November-December 1987.

Kaufman E, McNaul JP: Recent developments in understanding and treating drug abuse and dependence, *Hosp Community Psychiatry* 43:223-236, March 1992.

Lewis-Ford BK: Management techniques: coping with difficult people, *Nurs Manage* 24:36-38, March 1993.

Louie KB: RNs and DAs collaborate to prevent drug abuse, *Nursing Connections* 4:5-11, Winter 1991.

Marriner-Tomey A: Chemical dependency profile and attitudes of Indiana State Nurses' Association Members, *Main Dimensions* 4:1-4, January 1993.

Morrisett WR: Substance abuse: a call for a comprehensive approach, *Physician Assistant* 16:75-76, March 1992.

Murphy SA: An empirically based substance abuse course for graduate students in nursing, *J Nurs Educ* 30:274-277, June 1991.

O'Quinn-Larson J, Pickard MR: The impaired nursing student, *Nurse Educator* 14:36-39, March-April 1989.

Rassool GH: Nursing and substance misuse: responding to the challenge, *J Adv Nurs* 18:1401-1407, September 1993.

Sisney KF: The relationship between social support and depression in recovering chemically dependent nurses, *Image: Journal of Nursing Scholarship* 25:107-112, Summer 1993.

Smith HL, Mangelsdorf KL, Louderbough AW et al: Substance abuse among nurses: types of drugs, *Dimensions of Critical Care Nursing* 8:159-169, May-June 1989.

Spencer-Strachan FL: Attitudes of registered nurses toward perceived substance abusing peers and education specific to substance abuse, *ABNF Journal* 1:27-32, Fall 1990.

Virden J: Impaired nursing: the role of the nurse manager, *Pediatr Nurs* 18:137-138, March-April 1992.

CASE STUDY

One of the nurses with whom you work has developed an unkempt appearance, frequently has red eyes, has increased irritability, and has been late to work several times in the past few weeks. Today you smell alcohol on the nurse's breath when the nurse reports to work. How are you going to handle the situation as the charge nurse?

CRITICAL THINKING AND LEARNING ACTIVITIES

1. Use Worksheets 25-1, 25-2, and 25-3 to help you distinguish among different types of problem employees and types of employee counseling.

2. Discuss in class experiences with substance abusers. What were the symptoms of the abuse? How was the situation handled? How might it have been handled?

3. Have at least one classmate contact the state nurse's association for information about the peer review committee. Have a guest speaker from the state nurse's association peer review committee or the state board of nursing. Discuss the differences in roles between the state nurses association and the state board of nursing regarding chemical dependency.

4. Role-play handling an angry employee.

✍ **Worksheet 25-1**

Problem Employees

List at least three types of problem employees and briefly describe their behavior.

1.

2.

3.

✍ **Worksheet 25-2**

Employee Counseling

Describe at least three types of employee counseling.

1.

2.

3.

✍ **Worksheet 25-3**

Outplacement Counseling

Explain outplacement counseling, using the following questions as guidelines:

1. What is the purpose of outplacement counseling?

2. What are some potential sources of outplacement counseling?

   a.

   b.

   c.

   d.

   e.

3. What services might be useful to the terminating employee as a part of outplacement counseling?

Chapter

26

Stress Management

Chapter Objectives

◆ Identify at least six sources of stress.

◆ List at least twelve symptoms of stress.

◆ Identify and discuss at least twelve stress management techniques.

> **Major Concepts and Definitions**
>
> | | |
> |---|---|
> | Stress | the body's nonspecific response to any demand |
> | Eustress | a positive form of stress that adds excitement and challenge |
> | Distress | a negative form of stress that threatens effectiveness |

STRESS MANAGEMENT

Sources of Stress

Adjustment to change is stressful. Many events in life produce individual stress reactions. Death of a spouse or close family member, divorce, marital separation, marriage or remarriage, and personal injury or illness are highly stressful events. Change in the health of a family member, pregnancy, gain of a new family member, marital reconciliation, increased arguing with spouse, sexual difficulties, changes in financial state, mortgages, trouble with in-laws, a son or daughter leaving home, and the death of a close friend are stressful. Changes in living conditions and personal habits such as changes in work, residence, school, recreation, church activities, social activities, sleeping habits, and eating habits cause stress. Even personal achievements, vacations, and holidays are stressful. These personal stressors can affect one's job performance.

In addition to the personal stressors, there are many sources of stress at work. Dismissal and retirement are highly stressful. Business readjustments such as changing jobs or responsibilities, changes in working hours or conditions, and problems with the boss are stressful. Even outstanding achievement is stressful. Poor physical working conditions; physical danger; work overload; time pressures; responsibility for people; role ambiguity and conflict; conflicts with superiors, peers, and subordinates; restrictions; little participation in decision making; over-promotion or underpromotion; and lack of job security are stressors common to jobs.

Nurses face stress with life-and-death situations; heavy workloads involving physical and mental strain; knowledge of how to use numerous pieces of equipment and the consequences of equipment failure; reporting to numerous bosses; communication problems among staff members, physicians, families, and other departments; and awareness of the serious consequences of mistakes. A hospital is one of the most stressful work environments.

People often needlessly increase their own stress. The difference between demands people place on themselves or perceive from others and the resources they perceive as available to meet the demands is a threat or stress. Individuals are typed by the demands they place on themselves. Type A people set high standards, are competitive, and put themselves under constant time pressure. They are very demanding of themselves even in leisure and recreation activities. Type B people are more easygoing and relaxed. They are less competitive and more likely to accept situations than fight them.

Box 26-1   **THREE STAGES IN STRESS RESPONSE**

Alarm reaction—mobilization of resources to confront threat
Resistance stage—increase in energy consumption
Exhaustion—depletion of the body's energy reserves

Stress Response

Stress is impossible to avoid. It is a nonspecific response of the body to any demand. There are two types of stress: (1) eustress, a positive force that adds excitement and challenge to life and provides a sense of well-being, and (2) distress, a negative force caused by unrelieved tension that threatens effectiveness. Whether one will experience eustress or distress largely depends on the person's perceptions, physical activity or inactivity, mental activity or inactivity, sound nutrition, and meaningful relationships.

A stressor is anything an individual perceives as a threat. Stressors produce a state of stress by disrupting homeostasis. There are three stages in the stress response (see Box 26-1). First, the alarm reaction is the mobilization of resources to confront the threat. Second, in the resistance stage, there is a large increase in energy consumption. Once the reserve energy has been used, the body needs time to recover and to replenish the supply. When stress continues for long periods of time, the energy is used but not replaced and the third stage, exhaustion, results.

Consequently, unrelieved stress interferes with one's physical and mental well-being. After the stress event, the body returns to a state of equilibrium. Stable periods for bodies to restore adaptive energy allow one to meet new stressful situations.

Symptoms of Stress

Numerous symptoms indicate that stress is becoming distress. These include but are not limited to those shown in Box 26-2.

High stress levels accumulated over several months are likely to result in physical and psychological reactions. The amount of stress necessary before one manifests symptoms varies, depending on factors such as heredity, habits, personality, past illnesses, and previous crises and coping mechanisms. Well-educated, intelligent, creative people in management are at high risk for burnout. They may become workaholics but get little accomplished, experience chronic fatigue, feel they do not want to go to work, take increasing amounts of sick time, become negative, blame and criticize others, engage in backbiting, and talk behind others' backs.

Stress Control

Nurse managers can prevent and control burnout by setting personal and professional goals, establishing priorities, practicing good health habits and relaxation techniques,

Box 26-2   **SYMPTOMS OF STRESS**

Fatigue	Nightmares
Depression	Early morning waking
Tearfulness	Feeling of not being able to get anything done
Restlessness	Feeling that everything is too much
Nervousness	Forgetfulness
Withdrawal or sudden gregariousness	Lack of concentration
Irritability	Tendency to be demanding
Anger	Loss of appetite or overeating
Feeling of being unloved	Indigestion
Insecurity	Constipation or diarrhea
Feeling of vague anxiety	Nausea
Pessimism	Coughing
Self-criticism	Headaches
Frequent frustration	High blood pressure
Loss of interest in going out	Rapid pulse
Loss of interest in people and things	Heart palpitation
Decrease in self-care	Perspiration
Disorganization	Aching neck and shoulder muscles
Inability to relax or rest	Low back pain
Accidents	Allergy problems
Arthritis	Dermatitis
Asthma	Influenza
Colds	Hives
Colitis attacks	Menstrual distress
	Ulcers

improving their self-esteem by obtaining the skills they need, and using support systems.

Values clarification.   Values clarification is a useful activity. Values should be chosen freely from alternatives with thoughtful consideration to the consequences of each alternative. They should be cherished and shared with others. The value should be integrated into one's lifestyle, and actions should be consistent with the values. To help clarify one's values, one may assign priorities to a list of values as the following:

Affection	Pleasure
Duty	Power
Expertise	Prestige
Health	Security
Independence	Self-realization
Leadership	Service
Parenthood	Wealth

One can also list in order of priority characteristics such as the following:

Ambitiousness	Honesty
Broadmindedness	Imagination
Cheerfulness	Independence
Cleanliness	Logic
Courage	Lovingness
Forgiveness	Responsibility
Helpfulness	

Goal setting.   Goals should be consistent with one's values, and one should consider goal alternatives. To do this, one considers why a goal is desired. One may want a promotion for recognition or for economic reasons. If the promotion is not forthcoming, one may receive recognition through community service. Money might be generated through wise investments or fees for community services. The achievement of desired outcomes through different approaches increases flexibility and decreases stress caused by unmet goals.

Stress avoidance and regulation.   When reappraising situations, one should avoid troublesome transactions. The frequency of stress-inducing situations should be minimized. Every change takes energy. Therefore during periods of high stress, routines and habits should be maintained as much as possible. One should be cautious about moving and starting a new job at the same time one is getting a divorce. That also would be a particularly poor time to try to stop smoking or lose weight. Unnecessary changes should be prevented during periods of high stress. Deliberately postponing some changes helps one deal with unavoidable change constructively and reduces the need for multiple adjustments at one time. However, increasing positive sources of tension that foster growth, such as learning a sport, can help offset the deleterious effect of negative tension.

Time blocking.   Time blocking is the setting aside of specific time for adaptation to a stressor. To reduce the stress from having been promoted to a management position, one could set aside time for reading about management or for observing a manager. This helps ensure that concerns are addressed and tasks accomplished. It decreases anxiety, time urgency, and feelings of frustration.

Time management.   Time management helps control stress. Much time can be conserved when one knows one's value system and acts consistently with it, sets goals, and plans strategies for accomplishment of those goals. One can also use organizers such as to-do lists and calendars to plan good use of one's time.

Assertiveness.   When one asserts oneself, one increases self-esteem and reduces anxiety, thus reducing stress. As with time management, assertiveness involves thinking through goals and acting consistently with one's values through the use of effective work habits and by setting limits on others' attempts to block one's goals. It involves stating what one wants and how one feels, making requests, taking compliments, handling put-downs, and setting limits. An assertive person makes eye contact with others, stands straight, sits in an open, listening posture, and speaks in a clear voice. Assertive people choose for themselves and achieve desired goals through self-enhancing behavior that reduces stress.

Feeling pauses.   Feeling pauses are useful. One should take time to identify a feeling, label it, distinguish between thinking and feeling, and accept the feeling for what it is rather than talking oneself into what it should be. One should be aware if one is feeling the following:

Amusement	Hope
Calmness	Joy
Care	Love
Compassion	Passion
Elation	Relaxation
Excitement	Satisfaction
Forgiveness	Thrill
Happiness	

One should also acknowledge negative feelings:

Anger	Fear
Anxiousness	Frustration
Confusion	Hurt
Depression	Jealousy
Embarrassment	Restlessness
Envy	Terror

Then one should determine whether the feeling is appropriate for the situation and decide how to express the feeling in a safe and appropriate way. Feelings can be expressed in "I feel" messages rather than "You" messages that blame or attack others. Feelings can be talked about with an uninvolved person. One can fantasize about how one would like to handle the situation better the next time. Negative feelings may be acted out symbolically by punching a pillow, drawing a picture, or writing a poem. One may set aside negative feelings by getting involved in something pleasant such as exercise, hobbies, music, television, or talking to a friend. Feelings can also be experienced vicariously by getting involved in another's experience through reading a book, watching a movie, or listening to someone.

Inner shouting.   Inner shouting is the process of shouting "I feel . . ." inside one's head; the person blurts the feeling out spontaneously rather than saying it quietly. Anger should be viewed as a symptom. Pains should be focused on to help one take responsibility for feelings of hurt and humiliation.

Anchoring.   Anchors are associated feelings that are initiated either by an event or by the memory of that event. Anchors may be sounds, sights, smells, tastes, or touches that stimulate positive or negative feelings. Birds chirping may remind one of happy lazy mornings with the family. One may recall an awful accident at the sight of blood.

One might remember fall walks through the woods with a lover at the smell of dry leaves. A taste may revive memories of grandma's home cooking. A light touch to the face may remind one of earlier loving moments and cause one to experience a sense of well-being. Our lives are filled with anchors that cause associations. We can use anchoring in a useful way to experience desired feelings. Because touch can be inconspicuous and easy to replicate, one can associate a positive feeling with a familiar touch to the body. This may be so simple as clasping one's hands and being reminded of soft music, beautiful colored glass, and the peaceful sanctuary of church. Exact pressure at a very specific spot makes the anchor work most accurately and should be done when one desires to bring back a pleasurable feeling.

Sorting. Sorting is choosing the interpretation of an event. One can have an optimistic or pessimistic interpretation of events. Is the glass half full or half empty? We become what we think and therefore can make ourselves happy or miserable. To be more happy and fun loving, one should focus on the positive aspects of situations.

Thought stopping. Thought stopping helps get rid of negative thinking. Excessive rehearsals in our minds of negative past events are unhelpful thoughts that waste time, reduce our self-esteem, and encourage maladaptive behavior patterns. To prepare for thought stopping, one should think of beautiful pleasant experiences: a sunrise, a waterfall, a flower, a pet, favorite music, baking bread, holding hands. One should also identify not-so-helpful thoughts: I'm stupid; I'm fat; Nobody likes me. One should identify the negative thoughts that are most bothersome. In private, one can think about a negative thought momentarily and suddenly yell, "Stop!" while clasping one's hands or hitting one's head or leg. One startles oneself, and the thought escapes. Immediately one should insert a pleasant thought. If the negative thought returns, the procedure can be repeated. It is reinforced when the negative thoughts are stopped. Thoughts lead to feelings that can lead to behaviors, so by changing the way one thinks, one can change the way one behaves. Thought stopping should not be used, however, when physical or emotional safety and grieving are involved.

Compartmentalization. Compartmentalization of thought is the deliberate decision to think negative thoughts at specified times of the day. During the alloted time, one thinks about worry, guilt, or jealousy. One does not allow oneself to think these thoughts at other times of the day.

Environmental changes. Environmental changes can be designed to reduce stress. This may be as extreme as changing jobs or residence or as minor as painting a room a favorite color or adding a picture, candle, or basket. The short time inconvenience of remodeling may be worth the long-term stress reduction. Temporary changes in jobs can add variety and stimulation.

Humor. Humor related to an attitude toward life is most likely to reduce stress. There is a cluster of qualities that characterize this frame of mind, including flexibility, spontaneity, unconventionality, shrewdness, playfulness, humility, and irony. These are qualities that can be developed. Flexibility is the ability to examine all sides of the issues. One should try to look at a situation from several different viewpoints: the boss's, the subordinate's, the client's. Spontaneity is the ability to swing from one mood to another quickly. One might practice the body language of several emotions, including fear, anger, sadness, and love. One can free oneself from current values, places, and occupations through unconventionality and imagine living a day as a favorite animal, a famous historical person, an Eskimo, a Native American, or an astronaut. Shrewdness is refusal to believe that people or things are what they appear to be. One can think of a list of people and things and give an example of how each is not what it seems to be. Playfulness is the ability to see life as an amusing game. One can visualize life as a game and give the game a name. One should identify times of various emotions—fun, enjoyment, fear, anger, sadness—and chart wins and losses. Humility is a willingness to question the importance of one's values, ideas, achievements, and existence. One must consider the meaning of one's life and consider how difficult situations have brought happiness and how happy relationships have included suffering. Irony is the ability to see that situations are not black or white.

Centering.   Centering helps reduce stress by bringing the mind and body back into balance. With left-sided dominance, intuitive, aesthetic, and creative functions are reduced under stress. To center oneself, one is to put one's tongue on the centering button, which is about a quarter of an inch behind the upper front teeth. This spot apparently stimulates the thymus gland, weakens the effect of stress, and balances the cerebral hemispheres. Other activities that seem to balance the two hemispheres of the brain include reading a poem in a rhythmic fashion; listening to a person with a soothing voice; listening to classical music; listening to natural sounds, such as cats purring, birds chirping, or brooks or waterfalls babbling; looking at pictures of pleasant landscapes or smiling people making caring gestures; swinging one's arms during a vigorous walk; and taking a shower. Good posture is also beneficial.

Nutrition.   Good nutrition helps maintain the body for full functioning. Eating a balanced diet, taking vitamin supplements, and drinking plenty of water are important. In general, Americans need to reduce fat and cholesterol, sugar, salt, and food additives consumption. American diets contain high levels of fat and cholesterol, which are abundant in red meats, eggs, cheese, and prepared foods. Excessive consumption of fat is associated with cardiovascular diseases. Americans are obtaining an increasing proportion of their calories from sugar, which is associated with obesity, tooth decay, diabetes, and heart disease. There is a growing concern that additives and pollutants are related to cancer. These food additives include preservatives, coloring, flavoring, and stabilizers that extend shelf life and make processed food taste better. In addition, pesticides and other chemical pollutants are health hazards.

The increasing consumption of saturated fats and sugar coupled with a decrease in activity levels contributes to a widespread occurrence of obesity. In general, Americans need to increase exercise while decreasing caloric intake, particularly from fats and sugars. At the same time, the percentage of calories from foods containing fiber, such as fresh fruits, vegetables, and whole grains, should be increased. Canned, frozen, and prepared foods are usually devoid of their original fiber content and often have sugar and salt added. The grains we eat have often been refined to white flour and rice, thereby losing much of the roughage. Although improving eating habits may not prevent stress, it is one way to maintain the level of fitness needed to fight stress.

Exercise.   Regular, vigorous exercise can also help one withstand chronic stress. Aerobic exercise elevates the heart rate during and for a period after the exercise. The range of elevation necessary to produce an aerobic effect is from 60% to 80% of the maximal heart rate the person can achieve, which is calculated at 220 minus the person's age in years. Jogging, cycling, and swimming are particularly good aerobic exercises. Dance allows one to stretch and strengthen muscles and to reduce tension.

Regular exercise develops greater capacities in several areas of function. It increases the strength of cardiac contractions, the size of the coronary arteries, the blood supply to the heart, the size of the heart muscle, and the blood volume per heartbeat. It decreases the heart rate at rest and with exertion and reduces vulnerability to cardiac arrhythmias. It increases the blood oxygen content, blood volume, and efficiency of peripheral blood distribution and return. Exercise increases the blood supply to the lungs and the functional capacity during exercise. It increases lean muscle mass and functional capacity during exercise. Exercise also reduces strain and nervous tension resulting from psychological stress and reduces the tendency for depression.

Sleep.   Sleep is also important for dealing with stress. Sleep needs decrease with age, and people may awaken several times during the night as they grow older. This should not be confused with insomnia, which is a prolonged inability to sleep. There are three types of insomnia: (1) initial, when it takes more than 15 minutes to fall asleep; (2) intermittent, with awakening during the night and difficulty returning to sleep; and (3) terminal, with early morning awakening and inability to go back to sleep.

Physical, emotional, and nutritional factors may contribute to insomnia. A lack of physical exercise, digestive problems, heart trouble, and high blood pressure interfere with sleep. Disturbing emotional states such as anger, fear, guilt, depression, and anxiety create tension that interferes with sleep. An unbalanced diet, alcohol, caffeine consumption, and a large meal shortly before bedtime can interfere with sleep.

To foster a good night's sleep, the day's activities should be tapered off before getting ready for bed. Regular exercise promotes deep sleep but should not be done for a couple of hours before bedtime. Likewise, biofeedback and meditation have stress-reducing properties that foster sleep but should not be done before bedtime because they can boost energy and alertness. Chocolate, cola, coffee, tea, and other foods and beverages containing caffeine should be restricted, particularly in the evening. Overeating, particularly heavy foods, should also be avoided at night. The bed should be associated with sleep, and the room should be dark and quiet.

Relaxation

Abdominal breathing.   There are numerous techniques that can be used to foster relaxation. Abdominal breathing is a quick method. When stressed, people tend to breathe in short, shallow breaths. Consequently, the lungs do not fill up completely. The remaining air is stale, and oxidation of tissues is incomplete. Muscle tension results. Without being conspicuous, one can take a few abdominal breaths almost anywhere at any time. It is best to do abdominal breathing for 5 to 10 minutes once or twice a day while sitting upright. It may be done during normally low times or to reverse the stress response when it has been triggered. To do abdominal breathing, one should inhale slowly through the nose while keeping the back straight. First the abdomen expands, then the chest, and finally the shoulders. Then one should exhale slowly and hold the breath for a second or two before starting another inhalation.

Massage.   Massage can relieve tension, provide a passive form of exercise, and foster tactile communication. It stimulates relaxation and flexibility. Self-massage can be done from a chair. It can be done as a full-body massage or to a part of the body that is particularly tense. To do a full-body massage, one may start by placing both hands on the top of the head and moving them in slow circular motions down the back of the head, neck, and shoulder area. The neck and shoulder are common sites for tension. They may be most easily massaged by crossing hands over so that the right hand massages the left shoulder and the left hand massages the right shoulder. Then the hands are returned to the top of the head and moved forward in circular motions over the forehead, face, neck, and chest. To relax the right arm, one grasps the fingertips of the right hand with the left hand and moves up the hand and arm to the shoulder in circular motions with the fingers on top and the thumb on the underside. Then one massages down the right side of the chest. The procedure is repeated up the left arm and down the left side. Then hands are placed on the lower abdomen with fingertips touching. Circular motions are used up to the chest.

The low back is another area that is commonly tense, particularly from sedentary work. One places the hands on the lower back with fingertips touching at the coccyx. The fingertips then massage up as high as one can reach. A foot should be massaged with the massage continuing up the foot, over the ankle, and up the calf and thigh. Then the massage should be repeated on the other foot and leg. This full-body massage can be done after a warm bath at bedtime to foster sleep.

Progressive relaxation.   Progressive relaxation may also be used to foster sleep. It is the conscious contraction and relaxation of muscles. By deliberately tensing muscles, one can learn to identify what muscles are tight and learn to relax them. It can be used before, during, or after an anxious situation. If done routinely once or twice a day, it can help keep one's level of anxiety down.

Progressive relaxation can be done in a standing, sitting, or lying position. There is greater likelihood of falling asleep in a lying position. In a sitting position, one should keep the head squarely on the shoulders, back against the chair, feet on the floor, legs uncrossed, and hands on the lap in a relaxed position. During progressive relaxation, one tenses specific muscles to a maximal degree and notices how the tight muscles feel for about 5 seconds. Then the muscle is relaxed, and the pleasant feeling of relaxation is enjoyed for about 10 seconds. For a head-to-toe progression, one starts by wrinkling up the forehead and noticing where it feels particularly tense. Then one relaxes that part slowly, identifies the muscles that are relaxing, notices the difference between tension and relaxation, and enjoys the relaxed feeling. Box 26-3 contains abbreviated instructions for other body parts.

With experience in progressive relaxation, one can also learn to relax without tension. One first concentrates on relaxing each body part and then on generalized relaxation with deep breathing. One takes a deep breath, holds it, and then exhales slowly while relaxing the entire body from head to toe, saying "relax" so that the "x" is said as the focus reaches the toes.

Box 26-3 **PROGRESSIVE MUSCLE RELAXATION**

Close eyes tightly
Wrinkle nose
Place teeth together and press lips against teeth into a forced smile
Press tongue hard against the roof of the mouth
Clench teeth
Pucker lips
Pull chin toward chest
Put head back as far as it will go
Press head to right shoulder
Press head to left shoulder
Hold arm out straight, make a fist, and tighten the whole arm or pull elbow tightly into side
Repeat with the other arm
Push shoulder blades toward each other
Pull chest in
Pull stomach in
Tighten muscles in lower abdomen, buttocks, and thighs and raise self in the chair
Push foot against the floor, then point toes toward the head and repeat with the other leg and foot

Biofeedback. Biofeedback uses mechanical devices to gain self-regulation to control autonomic responses. The galvanic skin response uses electrodes attatched to the fingertips to measure skin resistance, which is moisture of the skin that indicates nervousness. Arteries contract under stress and dilate with relaxation. A thermistor on the finger detects changes in peripheral skin temperature that are associated with activity of the smooth muscles in peripheral arteries. This skin temperature is particularly useful for control of migraine headaches. The electroencephalograph uses electrodes attached to the scalp to detect electrical activity on the brain's cortex. Different brain wave patterns are associated with different states of mind. The electromyograph uses electrodes attached to the forehead or forearm to measure muscle tension from electrical impulses generated by muscles. People with migraine and tension headaches, hypertension, and gastrointestinal problems have responded well to biofeedback. Because the instruments convert skin resistance, skin temperature, brain waves, and muscle tension into readily observable signs, people can tell if they are controlling their body responses or not. They can also learn to read and interpret body signals without the use of instruments to modify their responses.

Autogenic training: self-hypnosis. Autogenic training produces deep relaxation through self-hypnosis. These regular but brief sessions of passive concentration on physiologically adapted stimuli reduce other extraneous stimuli and have helped people with asthma, arthritis, constipation, hypertension, migraine headaches, and sleep disturbances.

To do self-hypnosis, one should lie down with eyes closed in a quiet room and take a few deep breaths. Each autogenic training session should last 2 to 20 minutes, preferably 20 minutes two or three times a day. There are six phrases. When learning autogenic training, only one phrase should be added at a time once a week.

The first phrase focuses on heaviness, the next on warmth, then on heartbeat, breath, the solar plexus, and the forehead. Supporting phrases such as "I am relaxing" or "I am at peace" are interspersed between induction phrases. For the heaviness induction, one systematically concentrates on thinking that each part of the body feels heavy: "My face is heavy. I am relaxing. My neck is heavy. I am at peace. My shoulders are heavy. I am resting. My chest is heavy. I am quiet." For the warmth induction phrase, one substitutes "warm" for "heavy" in the previous phrases. The heart induction phrase is, "My heartbeat is calm and regular." Then one concentrates on, "My breathing is relaxed and comfortable." Next one puts one's hands on one's abdomen to create warmth and repeats, "My solar plexus is warm." Finally, one thinks, "My forehead is cool." To return to an alert state, one takes a few deep breaths and thinks, "I will arise refreshed and alert," then moves one's arms and legs, opens one's eyes, and slowly gets up.

Meditation.   Meditation focuses attention on an experience, helps one become aware of one's response, and facilitates the integration of the physical, mental, emotional, and spiritual aspects of one's life. There are many methods for meditating. One may focus on an object such as a candle, chant, listen to music, or meditate on one's own breath. To meditate on one's breath, one can count while breathing: one on inhalation, two on exhalation, three on inhalation, and four on exhalation. That process can be repeated until the allotted time for meditation is over. Usually people experience an inner calm and sense of well-being from meditation.

Visualization and mental imagery.   Visualization and mental imagery can be used to relax. One starts in a relaxed position and visualizes pleasant thoughts. One can meditate on a visualized colored object, such as a blue sky, white cloud, green tree, red apple, or pink flower. One can imagine being in a favorite place, such as a sandy beach, in the mountains, or in front of a fireplace in a favorite room listening to music. One can concentrate on the sights, sounds, smells, tastes, and feelings of the pleasant thoughts.

Poetry.   Poetry reading or writing is useful for reducing tension, particularly if one is depressed and movement and verbalizing have not worked sufficiently. Poems are chosen for their rhythm, their mood, and the feelings expressed. Poems can be read in a one-to-one or group meeting. Discussions about the meaning can help verbalize feelings.

Music.   Soft classical music can help release feelings and emotions and bring about relaxation.

Baths.   Water is a relaxant. One should fill the bathtub with water that is body temperature and immerse oneself up to one's neck for about 15 minutes.

Enhancing Self-Esteem

Positive affirmations can be used to enhance one's self-esteem. One can become more comfortable with positive thoughts about oneself and decrease the amount of self-devaluation. Several methods can be used. One might imagine positive scenes and see oneself as one wants to be. One can repeat positive affirmations such as, "I am happy," "I am healthy," or "I am beautiful." One can also write positive affirmations on cards, put them in conspicuous places, and read them often. People may take turns making positive comments about each other.

Support Groups

Support systems are synergistic. One can accomplish more through support groups than alone. Support groups provide a feeling of being accepted, valued, loved, and esteemed, and a sense of belonging. In addition to providing emotional support, support systems help provide a social identity and are a source of information, services, and material aid.

There are several types of support systems. Usually, the family is the natural support system that constitutes the primary support group. Peer support groups are also important. They are composed of people who have had similar experiences, have adjusted, and want to share their insight. A head nurse may receive support from other head nurses or a jogger from other joggers. Religious organizations provide a congregation that sets guidelines for living, shares values, and provides traditions. Voluntary service groups and self-help groups provide support for specific purposes such as to lose weight, to stop drinking alcohol, to quit smoking, or to adjust to a mastectomy or a stoma. Family, friends, and peers are usually sought out before professional support systems, but the helping professions are available when support from others is inadequate.

It is extremely important that managers take excellent care of their own well-being. They can function at their best if they are healthy. They need considerable energy to be supportive of others and will not have strength to share if they are hurting. Likewise, staff nurses need a sense of health and well-being to provide the best nursing care. Managers are responsible for providing care to the caregivers.

The manager should help protect personnel from undue stress. Personnel may be taught identification of stress symptoms and stress management. Annual physical examinations could be required. Vacations are provided and encouraged. Counseling and referral services can be provided as support systems. Nutrition, educational, and health promotional programs are presented, and nutritious food is served in the cafeteria. Exercise programs can be provided and encouraged. Managers should monitor stress levels and intervene when necessary.

BIBLIOGRAPHY

Benson H, McKee MG: Relaxation and other alternative therapies, *Patient Care* 27:75-78, Dec 15, 1993.

Burns C, Harm NJ: Emergency nurses' perceptions of critical incidents and stress debriefing, *J Emerg Nurs* 19:431-436, October 1993.

Detert RA, Schindler JV: Stress-management education in schools: a factor analysis of content elements, *Health Values: Achieving High Level Wellness* 14:3-13, November-December 1990.

Francis ME, Pennebaker JW: Putting stress into words: the impact of writing on physiological, absentee, and self-reported emotional well-being measures, *Am J Health Promotion* 6:280-287, March-April 1992.

Frisch SR, Dembeck P, Shannon V: The head nurse: perceptions of stress and ways of coping, *Can J Nurs Adm* 4:6-7,9-13, November-December 1991.

Grant CA: Stress management: self-appraisal and intervention, *Dermatology Nursing* 1:22-26, Oct 1989.

Harbert K, Hunsinger M: The impact of traumatic stress reactions on caregivers, *Journal of the American Academy of Physician Assistants* 4:384-394, July-August 1991.

Hinds PS, Quargnenti AG, Hickey SS, Mangum GH: A comparison of the stress-response sequence in new and experienced pediatric oncology nurses, *Cancer Nurs* 17(1):61-71, February 1994.

Hiscox C: Stress and its management, *Nursing Standard* 5(21):36-40, February 13-19, 1991.

Jung FD, Hartsell M, Tranbarger R: Evaluation of peer support program for staff nurses, *Nurs Econ* 9:419-425, November-December 1991.

Kellet J: Facilitating support groups: a pilot study, *Nursing Standard* 6:34-36, February 26-March 3, 1992.

Kunkler J, Whittick J: Stress-management groups for nurses: practical problems and possible solutions, *J Adv Nurs* 16:172-176, February 1991.

Lees S, Ellis N: The design of a stress-management programme for nursing personnel, *J Adv Nurs* 15:946-961, August 1990.

Madela EN, Poggenpoel M: The experience of a community characterized by violence: implications for nursing, *J Adv Nurs* 18:691-700, May 1993.

Narasi B: A tool for living through stress, *Nurs Manage* 25:73-75, September 1994.

Peddicord K: Strategies for promoting stress reduction and relaxation, *Nurs Clin North Am* 26:867-874, December 1991.

Stachnik T, Brown B, Hinds W et al: Goal setting, social support, and financial incentives in stress management programs: a pilot study of their impact on adherence, *Am J Health Promotion* 5:24-29, September-October 1990.

CASE STUDY

A number of nurses on your staff are married, raising small children, taking classes toward a degree, and feeling stressed. They are starting to develop some negativism. How will you approach this problem?

CRITICAL THINKING AND LEARNING ACTIVITIES

1. Using Worksheets 26-1 and 26-2, list your major stresses and the symptoms that indicate that you are stressed. Reflect on your major stresses and consider ways to prevent stress, such as leaving the house a few minutes earlier to avoid heavy traffic or getting a credit card so you don't have to worry about having enough cash with you to buy gas for the car.

2. Look at the list of values in Worksheet 26-3 and indicate whether each one is of high, medium, or low value to you.

3. Write three of your goals. Evaluate each one for its consistency with your values.

4. Pause for a moment and think about how you are feeling: calm, excited, happy, hopeful, or satisfied; or angry, anxious, confused, depressed, embarrassed, or frustrated.

5. Look at the jokes in the newspaper. Start a file of jokes and review it periodically. Watch a situation comedy on TV. Go to a funny movie or read a funny book.

✍ Worksheet 26-1

Stressors

List your major stressors:

School/work:	Personal:
1.	1.
2.	2.
3.	3.
4.	4.
5.	5.

✍ Worksheet 26-2

Symptoms of Stress

List the symptoms that indicate you are stressed:

1.

2.

3.

4.

5.

Now list strategies you might employ to help you manage your stress. Describe why each strategy might work well for you.

1.

2.

3.

4.

5.

✍ Worksheet 26-3

Values

Rate the values listed below as high, medium, or low value to you.

Value	High	Medium	Low
Affection			
Duty			
Expertise			
Health			
Independence			
Leadership			
Parenthood			
Pleasure			
Power			
Prestige			
Security			
Self-realization			
Service			
Wealth			

Chapter

27

Program Evaluation

Chapter Objectives

◆ Itemize activities that could be on a calendar of events for program evaluation.

◆ Identify and discuss at least six internal and external sources of invalidity.

◆ Identify and discuss at least six research designs. In the discussion identify which sources of invalidity the design controls for and which could still be a problem.

◆ Describe issues related to inventory control.

◆ Explain fixed, variable, direct, and indirect costs as they relate to break-even calculations.

Major Concepts and Definitions	
Program	outline of work to be done, plan of procedure
Evaluation	valuation
Validity	measurement of what is to be measured
Internal invalidity	extraneous variables that confound the effects of the experimental variable
External invalidity	factors that reduce the findings' generalizability
Statistics	facts or data of a numerical kind, assembled, classified, and tabulated so as to present significant information about a given subject
Audit	to examine and check
Inventory control	consideration of the purchasing, order, storage, and costs of long and short stock in order to determine the most economical level of goods in stock
Break-even calculations	direct and indirect costs equal income
Direct costs	specific costs of program
Indirect costs	generalized costs such as maintenance, and administration allocated to the program
Variable costs	costs that vary in direct proportion to volume
Fixed costs	costs unrelated to volume
Semifixed costs	costs that are fixed within a range of activity
Semivariable costs	costs that are fixed at zero output and increase with volume

PROGRAM EVALUATION

Program evaluation is an essential part of effective administration. It is the evaluation of a set of activities designed to determine the value of the program or of the program elements. Evaluative research is the use of scientific research methods to make an evaluation. Program evaluation may be formative or summative. Formative evaluations provide information about the program during the developmental stages. Summative evaluations provide information for judging a developed program. Evaluation may be descriptive or comparative.

Programs are evaluated for any number of reasons. Federal, state, or local agencies may require program evaluation. Program evaluation can be used to improve programs systematically or to determine the state of the programs. It can be used to evaluate the effect of new technologies on programs and help determine if parts responsible for success in one program can be used in other parts of the system.

Once the program to be evaluated and the purpose for its evaluation have been decided, someone should be made accountable for the evaluation. Credibility is the major argument in favor of an external evaluator. A person who is part of the program may have difficulty in being objective about the program's strengths and weaknesses because of pride, loyalty, or job security. On the other hand, an internal evaluator may be as objective as an external one and has knowledge about the program, its history, and circumstances; such knowledge facilitates the evaluation.

Calendar of Events

One of the first things the evaluator should do is develop a calendar of events that depicts the tasks to be done, the schedule, and organization of the project. A calendar of events for program evaluation itemizes activities to be done down the left-hand margin and projected dates across the top.

	Jan.– Feb.	March– April	May– June	July– Aug.	Sept.– Oct.	Nov.– Dec.
Inform personnel of purpose of the evaluation and who is responsible	X					
Define goals	X					
Determine criteria	X					
Develop instrument		X				
Train data collectors		X				
Pilot test			X			
Collect data			X			
Analyze data				X		
Report findings				X		
Correct deficiencies					X	
Reassess (follow up)						X

The projected date for each activity is estimated. This is a valuable tool for planning and judging the progress of the program evaluation.

Program Evaluation Model

The formulation of program goals is essential for program evaluation. The goals should be clear, specific, and measurable. The evaluator will need to develop indicators to measure the extent to which the goals are achieved. These program-outcome indicators are the dependent variables of the study. The standards set by accrediting agencies such as the American Nurses' Association, the National League for Nursing, and the Joint Commission on Accreditation for Hospitals can be used to determine goals and criteria.

Methods of data collection should be decided next. There are numerous sources for the collection of data, including questionnaires, interviews, observations, ratings, government statistics, instructional records, policy and procedure manuals, financial records, documents such as minutes of meetings or transcripts of trials, and tests.

Box 27-1   MODEL FOR PROGRAM EVALUATION

Goal	Standard	Observation
Nursing service has a current written organizational plan.	Organizational plan delineates the functional structure and the mechanism for cooperative planning and decision making.	Content analysis of the organizational plan.
Nursing service has goals.	Goals are written and made known to all personnel.	Locate written goals; interview management regarding how personnel are informed of goals; questionnaire to personnel.
Nursing committees are formally organized.	Purpose and function of each standing committee are defined; nursing is represented on committees concerned with nursing service.	Content analysis of documents for purpose and function of standing committees; content analysis of committee composition; interviews; questionnaires.

A model that depicts the program goals, the indicators to determine the extent to which the goals are achieved, and sources of the data helps direct the evaluation project. Box 27-1 is an example.

Sources of Internal and External Invalidity

When designing research, the evaluator gives careful consideration to sources of internal and external invalidity. Validity is the measurement of what is to be measured. Extraneous variables can confound the effects of the experimental variable and are therefore sources of internal invalidity. Factors that reduce the generalizability are sources of external invalidity.

There are several sources of internal invalidity. History is a problem when an event extraneous to the purpose of the study occurs between the pretest and posttest and confounds the effect of the experimental variable. It is a hidden treatment or a change-producing event that occurred in addition to the treatment. The problem of history is a more plausible explanation of the change the longer the time lapse between pretests and posttests. It can be controlled with experimental isolation, which can almost never be used when human subjects are involved. For example, a group-training technique to reduce racial prejudice against African Americans has been developed. A group of prejudiced individuals is convened, pretested, trained, and posttested. If an African American political leader is assassinated during that time, one would suspect that history confounded the experimental effect. The reduced prejudice can probably be attributed to sympathy for the assassinated African American politician rather than to the therapy.

Maturation is another internal invalidity problem. It is a systematic change over time in a person's biological or psychological condition, including growing older or becoming tired or hungry. Prescribed plan activities to promote walking for 12- to 15-month-olds or bladder control for 2- to 3-year-olds would be questionable because children normally learn those skills during those times.

Testing is a practice effect or the effect on the scores of the posttest of taking the pretest. The practice effect is larger for the same test than for an alternative form of the test. A form of test wiseness, the practice effect lasts about 3 months. People taking an achievement, intelligence, or personality test for a second time within a 3-month period will usually do better than people taking them for the first time, although it is unlikely that they have become brighter or better adjusted.

Instrumentation becomes a problem when there are changes in the measuring instrument over time. Changes in tests, judges, measuring devices, or calibrations cause instrumentation problems. Results from one test cannot usually be compared with results of a different test. Instrument decay or the fatiguing of spring scales causes invalidity problems. Observations produce instrumentation problems. There are intrahuman differences of the observer through fatiguing, the process of learning, the process of increased skill with practice, and learning to establish rapport. There are differences in observations by the same person at different times. One may be more lenient at one time than at another. One becomes more skillful with experience. There are also interhuman differences, such as knowledge and skill. Researchers observing disruptive behavior in psychiatric patients before and after a treatment may become more aware of disruptive behavior by the second observation and record more behaviors, or they may record fewer minor disruptions the second time because of the high level of disruptive behavior they had observed. In either case, the treatment effect is difficult to determine.

Statistical regression becomes a problem when groups have been selected because of their extreme scores. The phenomenon of regression toward the mean is the inevitable tendency of persons whose scores are extreme (far above or below the norm) on the first test to be less extreme on the second test. Patients chosen for a therapy group because of their high anxiety would show less anxiety on a second test regardless of the treatment.

Selection is a problem when the experimental group differs from the control group. For example, we may have a selection problem if we try to compare a control ward with an experimental ward because patients were assigned as a function of systematic characteristics, such as presenting symptoms or histories. Randomization is a control for selection. This problem often occurs when the subjects are already formed into groups for reasons other than the study.

Experimental mortality is a differential loss of subjects from comparison groups. It includes lost cases, cases on which only partial data are available, and cases who refuse to participate. The experimental group may appear stronger or more intelligent only because the weak and stupid dropped out of it. Heavy smokers and drinkers are likely to be the first to drop out of therapy groups to reduce smoking and drinking, leaving the clients who appear most successful with the therapy.

Researchers must also be aware of external invalidity problems that complicate the generalizability of the findings. Subjects who are available to the experimenter may not represent the population, and consequently the results of the research are not generalizable. Random sampling solves this problem. The independent variable needs to be operationally defined so that replication of the research is possible. Multiple-treatment interference, Hawthorne effect, novelty effect, and experimenter effect are considered. When two or more treatments are given consecutively to the same subjects, it is difficult, if not impossible, to know the cause of the results, and multiple-treatment interference occurs. When one knows one is a subject, one may change one's behavior, not because of the treatment, but because one knows one is being observed. This is the Hawthorne effect. The subject may react either positively or negatively because of the newness of the treatment, thus producing the novelty effect. The experimenter effect occurs when the subject is influenced by the experimenter. Such subtle behavior as smiling and nodding one's head during an interview may unintentionally influence the subject.

Pretest sensitization is the same as the testing internal validity problem except as it relates to generalizability of the results, which makes it an external validity problem. Identification of the dependent variables and selection of instruments to measure those variables are necessary for external validity. One must also consider if the effect will be lasting or if one is likely to get different results at different times. In the situation where the African American political leader was assassinated, thereby reducing prejudice against African Americans among those in group therapy, we had a history internal validity problem. Now we have an interaction-of-treatment-with-time external validity problem. The racial prejudice may have been temporarily reduced as a result of the assassination but will probably not be maintained for long. Treatments to reduce smoking may appear most successful right after a cancer scare but not as successful later. One must have internal validity to obtain external validity, which is the ability to generalize the research results. With program evaluation there may be little intent to generalize the results.

Research Designs

Next, the evaluator should design the evaluation. Will the evaluation be one shot only or a continuous process? Will a program be assessed, or will programs be compared? Will an experimental or a quasi-experimental design be used? The pretest-posttest control group, posttest-only control group, Solomon four group, and factoral are experimental designs.

Experimental designs. In the *pretest-posttest control group,* experimental subjects are randomly divided into two comparison groups as follows:

R O X O

R O   O

R = Randomly assigned individuals

O = Observation

X = Experimental treatment

The control and experimental groups are randomly assigned. The two groups are considered equivalent during initial observation. During final observation, the difference between groups should be the result of a variable being applied to one group but not to the other. The pretest-posttest control group true experimental design controls for history, maturation, testing, instrumentation, regression, selection, and mortality. One should consider the Hawthorne and novelty effects because the interaction of the testing and the experiment are not controlled.

In the *posttest-only control group,* experimental subjects are randomly divided into two groups to be compared as follows:

R X O

R   O

The control and experimental groups are randomly assigned. A pretest is not administered. A treatment is applied to one group only. Because of the random selection, it is assumed that the groups are equivalent before the treatment is administered to one group and that the difference noted on the posttest is due to the treatment. This design controls for history, maturation, testing, instrumentation, regression, selection, mortality, and the interaction of the testing and the experiment. It is superior to the pretest-posttest control design unless there is a question about the randomness. This design is appropriate when a pretest is awkward and is convenient for maintaining anonymity. The Solomon four group design is a better design but may not be worth more than double the effort.

The *Solomon four group* design uses four randomly selected groups. It combines the pretest-posttest control group and the posttest-only control group designs as follows:

R O X O

R O   O

R   X O

R   O

It is considered the most desirable of the experimental designs because it allows the investigator to examine the effects of the treatment in four independent comparisons. The Solomon four group design controls for history, maturation, testing, instrumentation, regression, selection, mortality, and the interaction of testing and the experiment. However, it may not be worth the effort.

Factoral design allows for observation of some subjects at all levels of all experimental variables and can be used when the situation is under the complete control of the experimenter, which is rarely the situation.

Quasi-experimental designs.   The evaluator usually cannot control the time and subjects to whom experimental variables are applied. However, the evaluator may be able to select the time and persons on whom observations will be made and can consequently gain some control through the use of quasi-experimental designs.

A *time series* involves a series of measurements over a period of time with an experimental variable introduced at some point in the sequence as follows:

$$O \; O \; O \; O \; X \; O \; O \; O \; O$$

Maturation is controlled because it is not likely to cause the difference between each of the observations. Testing, regression, and selection are controlled. History is the most probable problem, and the longer the time over which the observations are made, the more probable the problem. Instrumentation is also a potential problem. It is important not to change the instruments or their calibration. It is best if this design is repeated by several researchers in separate situations.

When the *equivalent-time-samples design* is used, the time available for making the observations is divided into equal time periods as follows:

$$XO \; XO \; XO \; XO \; XO$$

The times to make observations are randomly selected. This design controls for history, maturation, testing, instrumentation, regression, selection, and mortality. The multiple-treatment effect is a problem, and generalization of the findings is limited to similar populations.

In the *nonequivalent control group*, the broken line (- - - -) means the groups are not equivalent samples:

$$O \; X \; O$$
$$\text{-------}$$
$$O \qquad O$$

For this design, a control and an experimental group are both given a pretest and posttest. However, the groups are not randomly selected and do not have sampling equivalence. It is better than a one-group pretest-posttest design because it controls for history, maturation, testing, and instrumentation. Regression, mortality, and interaction between selection and maturation need to be considered as potential problems.

The *counterbalanced designs* are sometimes called Latin square, switchover designs, crossover designs, and rotation experiments. The following is an example:

$$X_1O \; X_2O \; X_3O \; X_4O$$

$$X_2O \; X_4O \; X_1O \; X_3O$$

$$X_3O \; X_1O \; X_4O \; X_2O$$

$$X_4O \; X_3O \; X_2O \; X_1O$$

Four experimental treatments are applied in a random manner in turn to four individuals or groups. Counterbalanced designs control for history, maturation, testing, instrumentation, regression, selection, and mortality. Multiple treatment interference is a problem. Strength can be obtained through replication.

For *separate-sample pretest-posttest design,* a pretest is given on one group and a posttest on another as follows:

R O (X)

R   X O

This simulated before-and-after design is weak, but it is better than a single-group pretest-posttest design because it controls for testing, regression, and selection. History, maturation, and mortality are not controlled, and the instrumentation needs to be questioned.

For the *separate-sample pretest-posttest control group,* two groups are pretested, one receives the experiment, the two are posttested. This excellent design controls for history, maturation, testing, instrumentation, regression, selection, and mortality. Because it is an expensive design, it has probably never been used.

R O (X)

R   X O

R O

R   O

For the *multiple time-series design,* a series of measurements is taken over a period of time on two separate groups with an experimental variable introduced at some point in the sequence of one of the groups as follows:

O O O X O O O
- - - - - - - - - - - - - - -
O O O   O O O

This excellent design can be used to compare one agency with a similar one. Controlling for history, maturation, testing, instrumentation, regression, selection, and mortality, it is the best of the more feasible designs. Power is increased through repeated measures.

The *recurrent institutional cycle design* is a patched-up design that starts with an inadequate design and adds features to control for sources of invalidity. It becomes an accumulation of precautionary checks that approaches experimentation.

X O
- - - - - - - - -
O X O

In *regression-discontinuity analysis design,* the solid line (—) means the groups are not equivalent. They differ by known amounts along a variable. The treatment is applied to individuals or groups that exceed a certain level of a variable rather than randomly. This design controls for history, maturation, testing, regression, and selection. Instrumentation and mortality would need to be questioned.

$$
\begin{array}{c}
\underline{X\ O} \\
\underline{X\ O} \\
\underline{X\ O} \\
\underline{O} \\
\underline{O} \\
O
\end{array}
$$

As with other research, data must be collected and analyzed. It is particularly important to communicate the results to appropriate people so that corrective actions can be taken, to do follow-up reassessments to make sure the corrections were made, and to check the results.

TOOLS FOR CONTROL

Statistics, Reports, and Observations

Statistical analysis of data may be of a historical or forecast nature and may be presented in tabular or chart form. The use of charts makes it easier for the manager to visualize trends and relationships and to make predictions. Special reports with analysis in addition to the statistical analysis are helpful in problem areas. Recommendations for corrective actions may be included in the report. A manager can also collect considerable data by walking through the institution, doing site visits, and visiting with personnel.

Audits

External audits are usually done by a public accounting firm to determine whether the agency's records of financial transactions accurately represent the agency's financial condition. The external audit verifies the accuracy of records by spot checking financial transactions, thus encouraging honesty from employees. If the internal control system is considered effective, the auditor's sample will be smaller and less expensive than if the internal control is deemed weak.

Internal audits are done by agency staff to determine the effectiveness of other controls. Internal audits may check accounting controls to safeguard assets and to ensure reliability of information generated by the accounting process. They may also be used to check administrative controls for efficiency and for compliance with policies. Internal audits protect the interests of the agency by assessing the accuracy of accounting and statistical data; the safety of the agency's assets; and compliance with policies, procedures, and plans. They further the interest of the organization by assessing the organizational structure, lines of authority, policies, procedures, practices, and performance. Internal auditing should be continuous and constructive.

Inventory Control

The manager needs to determine the most economical level of inventory because supplies represent a significant cost factor. The purchasing, order, storage, and costs of long and short stock must all be considered to determine the most economical level of inventory. The purchasing cost is the price paid per item. Cost may be related to the size of the order with cost per item decreasing as the size of the order increases. Purchasing cost equals PD, with P being the cost or price per unit and D being the number of units purchased.

The order costs involve writing specifications, soliciting and analyzing bids, writing orders, receiving the supplies, accounting for the materials, and paying the bills. The order cost may be relatively large the first time an item is purchased or relatively small for routine purchasing processes. The order cost varies with the number of orders placed. The more orders per year, the greater the annual costs will be. Annual order cost equals $(D/Q)O$ when D is the number of units purchased, Q is the order size, and O is the average cost of placing a single order.

The carrying cost is the expense involved with holding inventories. It involves expenses such as storage, insurance, and security. To keep carrying costs down, small orders should be placed frequently; this approach is in direct conflict with keeping the purchasing and order costs low. Carrying cost equals $HQ + IPQ/2$ when H is the cost of storage per item and Q is the order size. $IPQ/2$ is the opportunity cost element, in which I represents the highest obtainable rate of return at the current interest rate, P is price per unit, and Q is the order size.

The short or stock-out costs involved with holding an insufficient amount of inventory must be considered. The manager considers the consequences of running out of stock. Not only is a sale lost, but client satisfaction may suffer. Although this expense is difficult to measure, it is a real cost.

Total cost is expressed as follows:

$$TC = PD + \frac{DO}{Q} + \left(HQ + \frac{IPQ}{2} \right) + L + S$$

TC = Total cost $HQ + \dfrac{IPQ}{2}$ = Carrying cost

PD = Purchase cost L = Overstocked cost

$\dfrac{DO}{Q}$ = Order cost S = Stock-out cost

The economical order quantity is expressed as follows:

$$EOQ = \sqrt{\frac{2DP}{C}}$$

EOQ = Economical order quantity
D = Usage in units or demand
P = Order cost
C = Annual cost of carrying one unit in inventory

A large order size is merited when there is a large demand, high order cost, and low carrying cost. However, a smaller order size is desired when there is little demand for the item, the order cost is small, and the carrying cost is high.

A high inventory turnover is desired. Low inventory turnover may be caused by poor purchasing policies, overstocking, and a decrease in demand for the item. The inventory turnover can be calculated as follows:

$$\text{Inventory turnover} = \frac{\text{Total cost of supplies}}{\text{Inventories}}$$

To determine when to reorder, the manager needs to know the average daily usage and the lead time required to receive the supplies. A manager needs to keep the average daily usage multiplied by the number of days it takes to receive the goods in order not to run out of stock.

Some managers use the *ABC* method for maintaining inventories. *A* refers to a small number of items that account for a large percentage of the budget and are carefully monitored; *B* refers to moderate cost items that receive some monitoring; and *C* refers to a bulk of inexpensive, expendable items, such as rubber bands, that receive little monitoring.

Break-Even Calculations

Full costs equal all direct costs that can be traced to a source plus indirect costs such as maintenance, administration, and the building that are allocated to the source. Cost finding is an attempt to find the full cost and to allocate indirect costs. Indirect costs allocated may include housekeeping calculated by square feet, utilities by square feet, laboratory by number of tests, and dietary services by number of meals served.

The cost-volume-profit relationships can be visualized on a break-even chart. The manager considers variable, fixed, semifixed, and semivariable costs when doing a break-even analysis. Variable costs vary in direct proportion to volume (Figure 27-2). Two disposable syringes probably cost twice as much as one. Fixed costs are relatively fixed in total regardless of changes in volume (Figure 27-3). A nurse receives a certain salary regardless of the number of injections the nurse gives. Semifixed costs are fixed within a range of activity (Figure 27-4). One nurse can give just so many injections per shift, and beyond that a second nurse will need to be hired. Semivariable costs are fixed at zero output and increase with volume (Figure 27-5). The break-even point is

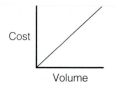

Figure 27-2 Variable costs.

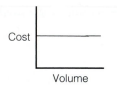

Figure 27-3 Fixed costs.

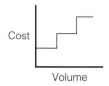

Figure 27-4 Semifixed costs.

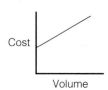

Figure 27-5 Semivariable costs.

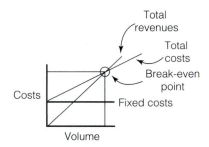

Figure 27-6 Break-even costs.

depicted on a break-even chart where revenues equal expenditures (Figure 27-6). The formula for break-even analysis is

$$R = FC + VC + P$$
$$R = \text{Total revenue}$$
$$FC = \text{Fixed cost}$$
$$VC = \text{Variable cost}$$
$$P = \text{Profit}$$

Average cost is the full cost divided by the volume of service units. The average cost decreases as the volume of patients increases because more patients share the fixed costs.

Mixed costs contain both the variable and fixed costs elements.

Marginal costs are the extra costs created by providing care to one more service unit. It is the difference in the total costs before and after adding one more service unit. Decisions about changes should be decided on the basis of marginal costs versus average or full costs.

Cost estimation is the prediction of costs. It is a complicated process involving dividing historical costs into fixed and variable components and by adjusting historical costs for inflation to predict future costs.

To adjust cost for inflation, the historical cost is multiplied by the current value of the appropriate price index divided by the value of that index when the cost was incurred.

Regression analysis considers costs as the dependent variable and service units as the independent variable. The coefficient of the independent variable represents the variable costs, and the constant term of the regression represents fixed costs.

Contribution margin is the price minus the variable costs per service unit and represents the additional financial benefit for each additional service unit.*

BIBLIOGRAPHY

Barrett-Barrick C: Promoting the use of program evaluation findings, *Nurse Educ* 18:10-12, January-February 1993.

Bray ML, Edwards LH: A primary health care approach using Hispanic outreach workers as nurse extenders, *Public Health Nurs* 11:7-11, February 1994.

Broughton W: Qualitative methods in program evaluation, *Am J Health Promotion* 5:461-465, July-August 1991.

Broughton W: Reporting evaluation results, *Am J Health Promotion* 6:138-143, November-December 1991.

Buccini R, Ridings LE: Using licensed vocational nurses to provide telephone patient instructions in a health maintenance organization, *JONA* 21:27-33, January 1994.

Ecklund S: Increasing nurse satisfaction: providing home visit opportunities, *Recruitment and Retention Report* 6:3-7, December 1993.

Fitzgerald E, Illback RJ: Program planning and evaluation: principles and procedures for nurse managers, *Orthop Nurs* 12:39-44, September-October 1993.

Fries JF, Fries ST, Parcell CL, Harrington H: Health risk changes with a low-cost individualized health promotion program: effects at up to 30 months, *Am J Health Promotion* 6:364-371, May-June 1992.

Grant P: Formative evaluation of a nursing orientation program: self-paced vs. lecture-discussion, *Journal of Continuing Education in Nursing* 24:245-248, November-December 1993.

Hixon AK, Padios E, Schmucker S, Shank F: Improving continuity of care by evaluation of post-discharge outcomes, *SCI Nurs* 9:42-45, June 1992.

Jung FD, Hartsell M, Tranbarger R: Evaluation of a peer support program for staff nurses, *Nurs Econ* 9:419-425, November-December 1991.

Jung FD, Pearcey LG, Phillips JL: Evaluation of a program to improve nursing assistant use, *J Nurs Adm* 24:42-47, March 1994.

Lengacher CA, Mabe PR, Bowling CD et al: Redesigning nursing practice: the partners in patient care model, *JONA* 23:31-37, December 1993.

Lishner K, Puetz B: Program evaluation: as the program director sees it; as the evaluator sees it, *Journal of Continuing Education in Nursing* 17:125-130, July-August 1986.

Patrick DL, Beery WL: Measurement issues: reliability and validity, *Am J Health Promotion* 5:305-310, March-April 1991.

---

*Finkler SA, Kovner CT: *Financial management for nurse managers and executives,* Philadelphia, 1993, WB Saunders, pp 143-178.

Pevny V: Outcome of a quality assurance review: development of a documentation tool for chemotherapy administration, *Oncol Nurs Forum* 20:535-541, April 1993.

Rogers J, Grower R, Supino P: Participant evaluation and cost of a community-based health promotion program for elders, *Public Health Rep* 107:417-426, July-August 1992.

Sarnecky MT: Program evaluation: a responsive model proposal part 2, *Nurs Educ* 15:7-10, November-December 1990.

Thompson JC: Program evaluation within a health promotion framework, *Can J Public Health* 83(suppl 1):S57-71, March-April 1992.

Tibbles LR, Smith AE, Manzi SC: Train the trainer for hospital-wide safety training, *Journal of Nursing Staff Development* 9:266-269, November-December 1993.

Williams S: Evaluating a continuing education program, *Aust J Adv Nurs* 9:21-28, December 1991-February 1992.

Woodhouse LD, Livingood WC: Exploring the versatility of qualitative design for evaluating community substance abuse prevention projects, *Qualitative Health Research* 1:434-445, November 1991.

CASE STUDY

Services are changing from having physicians to having nurse practitioners do physical examinations. Consequently there is less use of large gloves and an increased use of smaller gloves. What factors should you consider when determining how many gloves to order how often?

CRITICAL THINKING AND LEARNING ACTIVITIES

1. Evaluate the research design of a research report related to management.

2. Form small groups. Identify research designs and discuss the invalidity problems that are controlled and those that are not.

3. Form small groups. Using Worksheet 27-1, identify a situation in a health care agency with which you are familiar and list all the costs you can think of that are associated with it. Identify whether each cost is variable, semivariable, fixed, or semifixed.

✍ **Worksheet 27-1**

Costs

1. Briefly describe the situation in the space below:

2. In the chart below, list each separate cost that is associated with the situation described above and identify whether it is variable, semivariable, fixed, or semifixed.

Cost	Variable	Semivariable	Fixed	Semifixed

Chapter

28

Risk Management and Quality Management

Chapter Objectives

◆ List the five steps in the risk management process.

◆ Identify at least three sources for identifying potential risks.

◆ Describe the importance of patient relations in relationship to risk management.

◆ Identify the three conceptual frameworks most commonly used for quality assurance.

◆ Describe the research process as applied to quality improvement.

◆ List rules to remember for testifying.

◆ Discuss the relationship of torts, negligence, and malpractice.

Major Concepts and Definitions	
Risk management	development and implementation of strategies to prevent patient injury, minimize financial loss, and preserve agency assets.
Patient relations	public relations striving for patient satisfaction
Quality assurance	A retrospective view of quality of care
Total quality management	a philosophy of management that uses a problem-solving approach to improve quality of care while reducing costs
Continuous quality improvement	preventive problem solving that results in exemplary service
Torts	legal wrongs
Negligence	unintentional tort where harm results by not behaving in a reasonable and prudent manner
Malpractice	negligent acts of people with professional education
Legally liable	legally responsible
Plaintiff	complaining party
Defendant	answering party

RISK MANAGEMENT

Risk management involves the development and implementation of strategies to prevent patient injury, minimize financial loss, and preserve agency assets. Risk management focuses on liability control. It assesses areas in which claims can be prevented. By reducing the frequency and severity of injuries to patients, the likelihood of litigation can be decreased and litigation costs lessened. The risk management process includes risk identification, analysis, treatment, evaluation, and follow-up (Stull and Pinkerton, 1988).

The first step in risk management is identifying potential risks for accidents, injury, and financial loss. Energy should be put into preventive activities such as providing a safe physical environment, fostering good personnel relations, satisfying patient desires, and providing high-quality service. The present institutionwide monitoring system should be reviewed. Evaluate the completeness of the monitoring system, including audits, committee minutes, incidence reports, patient questionnaires, and oral complaints. Determine whether additional systems need to be implemented to provide data for risk management control.

After data have been collected, they should be analyzed to determine the frequency and severity of problems in general categories. Then a plan to reduce the risks as much as possible should be developed and implemented. Safety procedures should be reviewed, and laws and codes related to patient care, consent, and safety should be monitored. Needs for personnel, patient, and family education should be identified and education implemented. The results of the risk management program should be evaluated and reported to appropriate groups (Sullivan and Decker, 1988).

Risk management programs should include patient relations, safety and security, quality assurance, quality management, and liability control.

NATIONAL SAFETY COUNCIL

The safety movement began in ancient times with the Egyptians, Greeks, and Romans, and in the Middle Ages guidelines were established regarding working conditions. The safety movement became a major force in industry during the Industrial Revolution. In 1913, the National Council for Industrial Safety (later renamed the National Safety Council) was founded. It developed a forum to develop national standards. Other groups also formed and started keeping statistics on accident and injury rates in industry.

Occupational diseases and safety issues were identified, and methods to control hazardous and toxic materials and to protect the people who handle them were developed. On-the-job safety issues received serious attention. Since World War II, the safety movement has not only reduced injuries and deaths but has shown administrators that money spent on safety measures returns a profit of up to several hundred percent.

The National Safety Council encourages cooperation among labor, management, and government to develop legislation and upgrade safety standards. The National Safety Council seeks to improve investigative methods and supports special research projects. Changes in the workforce, new technologies and their hazards, environmental hazards, blood-borne diseases, and drug and alcohol abuse are challenges for the future.

The mission of the National Safety Council is to promote health and protect life by providing assistance, knowledge, and expertise to safety professionals in all areas. Moral responsibility exists in a philosophy of accident prevention. The employer is responsible for ensuring a safe, healthful work environment, and employees are accountable for following safety guidelines and standards.*

OCCUPATIONAL SAFETY AND HEALTH ACT

The purposes of the Occupational Safety and Health Act of 1970 and the Mine Safety and Health Act of 1977 are to ensure safe and healthful working conditions and to preserve the nation's human resources. They established nationwide guidelines and standards for the first time. The Secretary of Labor and the Occupational Review Committee are responsible for administration and enforcement of the acts. Research and education activities are the responsibility of the Secretary of Health and Human Services and are implemented by the National Institute for Occupational Safety and

---

* National Safety Council: *Accident prevention manual for business and industry,* Chicago, 1992, National Safety Council.

Health (NIOSH). The Assistant Secretary of Labor for Occupational Safety and Health acts as the chief of the Occupational Safety and Health Administration (OSHA).

OSHA's primary responsibilities are (1) to promulgate, modify, and revoke health and safety standards; (2) to approve or reject state plans for programs; (3) to require employers to keep records of safety and health data; (4) to conduct investigations and inspections and to issue citations and propose penalties; (5) to petition the courts to restrain imminent danger situations; and (6) to provide educational programs, consulting, funding for state plans, and statistical records of illnesses, injuries, and accidents.

The Occupational Safety and Health Review Commission (OSHRC) is a three-member quasi-judicial board that hears cases when OSHA actions are contested by employees and employers. The committee decisions can be reviewed by state and federal courts.

NIOSH is the federal agency responsible for research, education, and training. The representatives can inspect agencies and ensure compliance but are not authorized to enforce OSHA regulations. The main functions of NIOSH are (1) to develop educational programs, (2) to develop occupational health and safety standards, and (3) to conduct research. The responsibility to establish research methods and conduct statistics surveys is with the Bureau of Labor Statistics.

With few exceptions, OSHA applies to every employer in all 50 states and all U.S. possessions who has one or more employees and who engages in business affecting commerce. All local, state, and federal government employees and mine operators and their employees are exempt from coverage.

Under OSHA, the employer is responsible for providing a safe, healthful work environment and for complying with the applicable standards. The employees must comply with applicable standards. The employer is liable for the state and federal sanctions for violating standards. Employees are subject to their employer's sanctions.

All standards promulgated by OSHA are published in the Federal Register. OSHA requires employers to keep records of all occupational illnesses and accidents and to report either to OSHA or to the state plan within 48 hours. OSHA can grant two types of variances from the standards: temporary and permanent. Employers must show just cause for either variance and inform the employees of the application.

Workplace inspections are usually conducted without prior notice. Investigations of imminent dangers are top priority, followed by catastrophic and fatal accidents, followed by employee complaints regarding hazards and reinspections. General inspection procedures include an opening conference, a walk-through documenting alleged violations, interviews with workers, and a closing session. Citations and penalties vary according to the seriousness of the violation. Violation citations are to be posted near where the violation occurred. If an employer wants to contest a case, the area office that initiated the action should be contacted. OSHA encourages states to assume responsibility for administering and enforcing occupational safety and health laws. Areas needing regulations include but are not limited to blood-borne pathogens, lifting guidelines, confined-space regulations, ergonomic guidelines, respiratory guidelines, and egress.

Administrators need to identify the tasks to be performed, identify the tools necessary, evaluate the environment in which the tasks will be performed, assess the organization in which this takes place, and make necessary changes to provide a safe work environment for the employee.*

PATIENT RELATIONS

The dissatisfied customer is the one most likely to pursue litigation. Therefore it is important to identify incidents that might lead to claims, educate patients and their families about the care, and handle patient complaints. To handle complaints, listen and let the patients express themselves before speaking. Don't become defensive. Avoid reacting emotionally. Negotiate. Ask for the patient's expectations and explain what you can or cannot do. Agree on actions to be taken and a time frame. Follow through. A caring attitude can be very effective. It is also important to teach personnel about customer relations and how to prevent and handle complaints.

SAFETY AND SECURITY

A safety and security program should provide safety for patients, their families and other visitors, and personnel. Risks from custodial negligence should be controlled. There should be plans for natural disasters, fire, electrical shock, and power loss. There should be an equipment maintenance program (Stull and Pinkerton, 1988).

QUALITY ASSURANCE TO CONTINUOUS QUALITY IMPROVEMENT

In the late 1950s, planning, organizing, and evaluating health care services became a public concern. In 1952, the Joint Commission on Accreditation of Hospitals—now the Joint Commission on Accreditation of Healthcare Organizations (JCAHO)—was formed. The American Nurses' Association (ANA) and the National League for Nursing (NLN) both published manuals in 1959 to help establish standards for health care.

During the 1960s, the ANA started a division of nursing practice to develop standards for nursing practice, which became the basis for quality assurance programs. The ANA also developed a process to evaluate the quality of patient care.

In October 1972, the Ninety-second Congress passed Public Health Law 92-603, an amendment to the Social Security Act that mandated the establishment of Professional Standards Review Organizations (PSRO) to review the quality and cost of care received by clients of Medicare, Medicaid, and Maternal Child Health programs. Health facilities were to develop quality control programs by 1976 or the government would do it for them. Consequently, quality assurance has received considerable attention. The ANA developed guidelines for standards of nursing practice under the PSRO system; the American Hospital Association and the JCAHO developed a retrospective review of care. Individuals and agencies developed criteria and processes for the measurement of quality of care.

---

* National Safety Council: *Accident prevention manual for business and industry,* Chicago, 1992, National Safety Council.

JCAHO required audits of care delivered in its initial quality assurance standards and increased the number of multidisciplinary audits required in 1975. Nursing then became a major contributor for evaluation of documentation. More recently, JCAHO has had nursing examine a nursing care problem quarterly, document assessment of the problem, develop and implement the plan for correction, and evaluate the effectiveness of the implemented actions.

Instruments for measuring nursing care were developed during the 1970s, but limited data were generated or published in quality assurance studies. The quality assurance program recommended by the Joint Commission on Accreditation of Hospitals was a retrospective review of patient care through a closed-chart audit that focused on patient-care outcomes.

Committee Selection and Functions

Each agency needs a quality assurance committee to establish criteria and a process for quality assurance and to evaluate care, make recommendations, and do follow-up work. A chairperson with enthusiasm and attention to detail helps ensure a successful program. Members also need to be interested in quality assurance and knowledgeable about channels of communication, hospital resources, patient population, and nursing needs. Representation of staff nurses, head nurses, clinical specialists, and in-service instructors from various nursing units helps produce a wide variety of ideas. Preset meeting times allow for staffing to accommodate attendance, and large committee membership supplies personnel to do the work.

Conceptual Framework

Structure, process, and outcome or any combination of these are the common approaches to evaluation. The structure approach focuses on the delivery system by which nursing care is implemented. Committee members evaluate policies, procedures, job descriptions, orientation schedules, in-service schedules, and charting. The process approach measures what the nurse does while delivering patient care. Both nurse and patient may be interviewed to collect evidence of professional judgment and functions. The outcome approach measures the results of the care administered to the patient and evaluates whether the goals were reached, by considering clinical manifestations, patient knowledge, and the client's self-care.

Audits may be concurrent or retrospective. Concurrent audits evaluate care as it is being administered and may include observation of staff; inspection of patient; open-chart auditing; staff and patient interviews; and group conferences including participation from the client, family, and staff. Retrospective audits judge care after it has been delivered through the study of patient charts or care plans after the patient has been discharged, postcare questionnaires, patient interviews, or all of these.

Review of the Literature

A review of the literature locates instruments, criteria, and standards that have been developed and allows committee members to benefit from others' accomplishments and mistakes.

Maria C. Phaneuf also recommends a retrospective review of the records of discharged patients. She developed 50 components and descriptive statements for the 7 dependent and independent nursing functions identified by M.J. Lesnik and Bernice E. Anderson in *Nursing Practice and the Law*. These functions are (1) application and execution of the physician's orders, (2) observation of symptoms and reactions, (3) supervision of the patient, (4) supervision of caregivers, (5) reporting and recording, (6) execution of nursing procedures and techniques, and (7) promotion of health by direction and teaching. Phaneuf's instrument focuses on the patient and patient care rather than on the nurse and the nurse's activities for appraising the content and process of the care. Care is rated on a graded scale as excellent, good, incomplete, poor, or unsafe.

The Slater scale, originally constructed by Doris Slater Stewart, contains 84 items: 18 actions directed toward meeting individual psychosocial needs, 13 actions related to group psychosocial needs, 13 activities to satisfy physical needs, 16 operations to meet general needs, 7 communication items, and 17 behaviors reflecting professional expectations. A cue sheet listing several examples to illustrate each of the items is also included. The nurse is rated for each action as best, average, or poor. The cue sheet contains additional columns for not applicable and not observed. The quality of care expected from first-level staff nurses is the standard of measurement. Unlike Phaneuf's work, the Slater scale focuses on the nurse instead of the patient and measures the nurse's competencies as care is being provided. It yields both numerical and descriptive information of the nurse's strengths and weaknesses. The Slater scale can be used to improve the nurse's performance.

Qualpacs, the Quality Patient Care Scale, is a revision of the Slater Nursing Performance Rating Scale. It lists 68 items under the same subsections used in the Slater scale: individual psychosocial, group psychosocial, physical, general, communication, and professional implications. A cue sheet lists examples to illustrate each item. The care is rated according to best, average, or poorest care, with not applicable and not observed options. The care expected of a first-level staff nurse is the standard of measurement. This is a concurrent process-oriented approach.

Sharon Van Sell Davidson and peers have identified concurrent and retrospective review criteria for numerous health conditions in *Nursing Care Evaluation* (1977). Susan Martin Tucker and others (1975) outline observations, immediate care, ongoing care, patient teaching, and discharge planning for numerous medical-surgical, obstetric, and pediatric conditions. Other books and articles about quality assurance are plentiful and contain material that can be adopted or modified.

Instrument Development

An operational definition of quality of care gives direction to instrument development. Instruments may be general and appropriate for all patients or structures or applicable only to a specific process or to a homogeneous group in which differences in scores are due to variations in the concept being evaluated rather than to other factors. Medical diagnosis, symptom, acuity, age, and health care settings often are used to determine homogeneity. A taxonomy of nursing diagnoses is being developed. Identification of homogeneous patient groups for the development and application of instruments necessitates the development of numerous tools.

Once the patient group or specific process has been identified, selection of goals, criteria, and items is the priority. The goal is a statement of the end that one strives to attain. Criteria are the standards or scales against which judgments are made. Criteria describe what is implied in the goal in concise, measurable statements of desired structure, process, or outcome. They are written for a specific condition and are understandable, clinically sound, and achievable.

Brainstorming is a common approach for identifying items. Actual problems—those that patients generally experience—and potential problems—those with a high risk of occurring—are identified, and the structure, process, or outcome to resolve or prevent them is determined. The generation of as many ideas as possible without immediate evaluation is recommended initially. Later, items can be eliminated, checked for comprehensiveness, put into a uniform format, precisely defined, and quantified. A pilot study to collect data with the instrument can clarify which items should be retained, discarded, or rewritten.

Scales and measurements must be developed. A checklist to determine whether a characteristic is present; ratings to give each item a measure of worth such as good, average, or poor; and ranking by comparison, such as more or less than the standard, are common measurements. Scales are either nominal, ordinal, interval, or ratio. The simplest type is the nominal. Its categories are collectively exhaustive, and each is mutually exclusive, meaning that there is a category for all the observations and that each observation can fit only one category. Sex, marital status, and the presence or absence of a condition are examples. Ordinal scales classify observations into a specific order of more or less, such as good, average, or poor. Interval scales are ordered with equal measurement between each class, but the unit of measurement is determined arbitrarily. Examples are the thermometer and sphygmomanometer. Ratio scales contain the properties of the other scales plus an absolute-zero point. Multiplication and division are possible because each number has a relationship to any other number. Currency systems are examples.

Validity and Reliability

Establishment of validity and reliability is important. Validity is the measurement of what is supposed to be measured and is difficult to establish. Face validity is an analysis of the instrument's appearance as valid. Someone simply looks at an instrument and decides if it has face validity. It is the easiest assessment of validity but is a questionable criterion because of its high degree of subjectivity. Content validity is a judgment that the content of the instrument is appropriate and closely related to what is to be measured. It is best determined by a jury of experts. Construct validity is particularly important when phenomena or concepts that are not directly observable, such as intellectual skills, human characteristics, and personal adjustment, are involved. The construct is a hypothetical definition that clearly defines observable phenomena. Construct validity is theory oriented. An instrument contains predictive validity to the extent that it predicts future behavior. It can be determined by checking the prediction after a period of time. Concurrent validity reveals the behavior that is being demonstrated presently and is particularly important for concurrent audits.

Reliability is repeatability and is easier to determine than validity. Scores obtained by different raters' observations of the same event at the same time or by the same rater at different times can be compared. The test-retest method involves administration of the same test again after a period of time with the hope that the results will be consistent. The fact that people may remember items from the first administration or that people change over time are problems. This method is appropriate for stable characteristics but is problematic for unstable traits. The split-half method compares halves of the test to determine internal consistency. Reliability is suggested when the results of both halves are similar. To use the split-half method, both halves need to contain enough items to be reliable. Statistical methods to check reliability include the Kuder-Richardson test for internal consistency and the Spearman-Brown formula for a coefficient for the total test.

Methods of Data Collection

Observation, interviews, questionnaires, and content analysis of charts and care plans are the most common methods for data collection. When observation is used, the quality assurance committee determines what to observe, develops observational procedures, and trains observers. Observations should be planned and recorded systematically and subjected to controls. Observation is suitable for concurrent audits. Behavior is observed and recorded as it occurs, and the process can be noted. Because observation does not demand participation of the observed, it is relatively independent of the subject's willingness to cooperate and therefore makes subjects readily available. Observation is a comparatively inexpensive method that lends itself to simple data-gathering instruments and recording equipment. Although it can be stopped at any time, it is limited to the length of the occurrence. The timing of an event may be difficult to predict, and consequently the observer may waste time waiting for something to happen. The presence of an observer also may influence the subject's behavior. Observations may be difficult to record, are subject to observer bias, and may vary between observers. Consequently, observers need training. Specifications of observer tasks; detailed instructions; sharp, measurable categories; immediate, detailed recording; observation averaging; and the use of recording equipment such as cameras and tape recorders help overcome observer bias and variability.

Interviews of both clients and staff may be used to evaluate care. Interviews may be (1) nondirective—subjects talk about whatever they desire; (2) focused—the subject speaks to a list of topics; (3) nonstandardized—the interviewer makes up the questions; (4) semistandardized—the interviewer asks a specific number of questions and probes; and (5) standardized—the interviewer conducts each interview in exactly the same manner using the same wording without probing. The interviewer can minimize misunderstanding by probing, clarifying, pursuing topics in depth, and observing nonverbal communication. Subjects do not need to be literate. Interviewing provides more flexibility and a greater response rate than questionnaires. However, it is an expensive method because it requires so much time. The subject may be nervous or may attempt to please the interviewer, and the recording of answers is problematic.

Questionnaires are less time-consuming and consequently less expensive than interviews. They are particularly useful when subjects are dispersed over a large geographical area. Less skill is needed to administer a questionnaire than to conduct an interview. Questionnaires put less pressure on the subject for immediate response, standardize instructions and questions, and offer anonymity. The participants, however, must be literate. Unfortunately, often only a small percentage of questionnaires are returned, and the effect of nonrespondents is difficult to evaluate. Items may be omitted or misunderstood. A forced choice may not be an actual choice, and probing is not possible.

When preparing a questionnaire, the subjects' frame of reference and information level and the social acceptability of the item need to be considered. Language should be gauged to the level of the subjects. Lengthy or leading questions and double negatives are to be avoided, and each question should contain only a single idea. Questions are arranged from general to specific. A pretest is helpful for identifying problems with the instrument. A high proportion of omissions, "other," "don't know," or all-or-none responses suggests poor questions. Added qualifications and comments and variation in answers when questions are reordered also suggest problems.

The percentage of returns of the questionnaires is influenced by a personal cover letter requesting cooperation, sponsorship by the health agency, attractive format, short length, ease of filling out and returning, and inducements for replying. The best response is from people interested in the topic.

Content analysis of charts and care plans is a common method of data collection. It is a method of observation and measurement that is systematic, objective, and quantitative. Frequency of occurrences usually is noted on a checkoff list. Descriptive statements can then be given about frequency of occurrences and changes in conditions. Unfortunately, it can take a long time to review records; classification systems may be too ambiguous for a phenomenon to fit a category; the chart chosen may not represent the phenomenon; and prejudices in the scoring method can bias the results.

Sampling

Sampling is a technique of selecting a sample from the whole population being studied. Evaluators want to be able to generalize their conclusions concerning the quality of care given the total population. Adequacy of sample size is important, especially with small samples, if the quality assurance committee members are to have confidence in their inferences. The more homogeneous the population, the smaller the sample size necessary to be representative. Budgetary and time restrictions greatly influence sample size.

The best sampling technique is random sampling, which allows each patient an equal chance to be included in the sample. A table of random numbers that can be located at the back of most statistics books is frequently used. To use this method, patient records are numbered. Evaluators close their eyes and point to a number on the table to start the selection. They then systematically progress by row or column until the appropriate number of records is selected. A roulette wheel can be used. The wheel is spun, and the patients' charts whose numbers are chosen by the pointer are selected for review. The wheel is repeatedly spun until the desired sample size has been reached. A third possibility is to put pieces of paper with a chart number or patient name on each into a large container. The evaluator draws a piece of paper, rotates the papers, and draws another until the desired sample size is reached.

Systematic sampling consists of selecting every-nth patient. Selection can be according to admission, discharge, or an alphabetical listing. The evaluator makes a random start and then selects systematically. The size of the interval is determined by the percentage of the population desired in the sample size. For example, if one wants the sample to be 10% of the population, the evaluator chooses every tenth patient.

Stratified sampling divides the population into sections and then takes a random sample from each section to ensure that important variables are represented. For instance, patients may be classified according to body systems by the major diagnosis. If 30% of hospital admissions are classified as cardiovascular cases, 30% of the sample would be drawn from those cases.

Cluster sampling uses small samples from various sections of the population. A certain number of audits may be selected from each hospital unit. Instead of randomly selecting 100 patient charts, 10 charts may be randomly selected from each of 10 hospital units.

Multistage sampling randomly selects some percentage of the population and then randomly samples smaller subunits. For instance, in a large hospital system, the evaluator would randomly select which hospitals are to be audited. Next, the specialty area to audit within the selected hospitals is randomly selected. Finally, the specific units within those specialty areas and the specific patients on those units are randomly chosen.

Incidental or convenience sampling uses readily available subjects. The families of patients who happen to be in the coffee shop at a particular time or patients who happen to be in their rooms at a particular time may be interviewed.

The sample mean is not truly representative of the total population average. It is an attempt to approximate it. The difference between the mean or average of the sample and the total population is the sampling error.

Analysis of Data

Simple scoring is preferred and can be subjected to descriptive measures. Frequency distribution indicates how many times observations were assigned to specific categories. Measures of central tendency can be calculated from the frequencies. The mean is the average. It is calculated by adding all the scores and dividing that sum by the total number of scores. The mode is the most frequently occurring score, and the median is the score in the middle with half the number values above it and half below it.

Expected Level of Performance

The quality assurance committee must determine the level of expected performance below which they will take corrective action. Staff should know what criteria are being used to evaluate the quality of care and should have an opportunity to review reports of audits. The committee identifies performance discrepancy and completes problem analysis. Once they identify the problem, they can recommend corrective measures. The corrective action recommended, time schedule for completion, and responsible person are documented and shared with appropriate people. A reaudit determines if the corrective action was implemented successfully.

Sharing favorable audits and evidence of improvement in care provides recognition for good work and increases morale. Research regarding the cost and effects of audits is still needed.

JCAHO'S 10-STEP MONITORING AND EVALUATION PROCESS

Box 28-1

1. Assign responsibility

2. Delineate scope of care

3. Identify important aspects of care

4. Identify indicators

5. Establish thresholds for evaluation

6. Collect and organize data

7. Evaluate care

8. Take action to improve care

9. Assess actions and document improvement

10. Communicate information

From JCAHO: *Transitions: from QA to CQI*, Chicago, 1991, JCAHO.

Quality Management Focus in Accreditation

In 1988, JCAHO revised the nursing quality assurance standards for nursing care to be evaluated objectively against preestablished standards and criteria. The results need to be analyzed to determine problem areas and a plan developed to correct practice deficiencies. A method to reevaluate the effectiveness of the corrective action is expected.

The JCAHO developed a 10-step model as a basis for an effective quality assessment and improvement process (see Box 28-1). It focuses on monitoring, evaluating, and problem solving to facilitate effective use of resources to manage quality of care. It broadens the scope of quality assurance to continuous quality improvement.

The 10-step model has been modified with a framework for improving performance. Expansions include (1) focusing on process of care and services rather than on outliers and individual performance; (2) extension of activities into all areas, not just clinical nursing; (3) identification of customer and supplier relationships; and (4) the role of leadership in the process.

The quality management focus of the 1990s is on organizationwide programs and total organizational quality. It encourages innovative methods to improve patient care delivery, teamwork, control of costs related to delivery of care, and development of multidisciplinary standards.

The dimensions of performance include doing the right thing through efficacy and appropriateness and doing the right thing well through availability, timeliness, effectiveness, continuity, safety, efficiency, and respect and caring (see Box 28-2).

Box 28-2   DEFINITIONS OF DIMENSIONS OF PERFORMANCE*

I. Doing the Right Thing

The **efficacy** of the procedure or treatment in relation to the patient's condition

> The degree to which the care/intervention for the patient has been shown to accomplish the desired/projected outcome(s)

The **appropriateness** of a specific test, procedure, or service to meet the patient's needs

> The degree to which the care/intervention provided is relevant to the patient's clinical needs, given the current state of knowledge

II. Doing the Right Thing Well

The **availability** of a needed test, procedure, treatment, or service to the patient who needs it

> The degree to which appropriate care/intervention is available to meet the patient's needs

The **timeliness** with which a needed test, procedure, treatment, or service is provided to the patient

> The degree to which the care/intervention is provided to the patient at the most beneficial or necessary time

The **effectiveness** with which tests, procedures, treatments, and services are provided

> The degree to which the care/intervention is provided in the correct manner, given the current state of knowledge, in order to achieve the desired/projected outcome for the patient

The **continuity** of the services provided to the patient with respect to other services, practitioners, and providers and over time

> The degree to which the care/intervention for the patient is coordinated among practitioners, among organizations, and over time

The **safety** of the patient (and others) to whom the services are provided

> The degree to which the risk of an intervention and the risk in the care environment are reduced for the patient and others, including the health care provider

The **efficiency** with which services are provided

> The relationship between the outcomes (results of care) and the resources used to deliver patient care

The **respect and caring** with which services are provided

> The degree to which the patient or a designee is involved in his/her own care decisions and to which those providing services do so with sensitivity and respect for the patient's needs, expectations, and individual differences

*Used with permission from JCAHO: *1994 accreditation manual for hospitals,* vol 1, Standards, Oakbrook Terrace, Ill, 1993, JCAHO.

An unscheduled, unannounced, or random unannounced survey can be done at any time during an organization's 3-year accreditation cycle. JCAHO can do an unscheduled or unannounced survey when there is a potentially serious standards compliance problem. An organization usually receives notice 24 to 48 hours before an unscheduled survey, but no advance notice is given for an unannounced visit. Unannounced visits may be made when there is substantial deterioration in clinical care, an immediate threat to patient health or safety, or credible allegations of falsified accreditation information. Effective July 1, 1993, 5% of a random sample of accredited organizations will receive an unannounced survey.

To prepare for surveys, nurses should familiarize themselves with the JCAHO standards, the accreditation manual, and scoring guidelines. Review policies and procedures mentally and discuss them. Have workshops about standards and processes. Think about how you make decisions. Be direct and honest, but do not ventilate complaints. Focus on being confident by smiling and acting relaxed.

The accreditation review begins even before the survey team arrives at the agency with staff reviewing hospital documentation. The on-site visit is scheduled ahead of time and lasts from 2 to 5 days depending on the type and size of the agency. The first day the team holds a brief opening conference with the administrators and other staff. The surveyors then review important documents such as policies, procedures, bylaws, and rules and regulations. During the rest of the survey, the team members spend much time on patient care units and do interviews with patients. The site visitors typically do an in-depth review of at least one of several charts the nurse manager has selected for review. The reviewer is looking for competency and collaboration and may ask nurses or doctors how they are implementing the others' plan of care. Patients are likely to be asked questions to validate the doctors' and nurses' responses.

Site visits are likely to include ambulatory sites, anesthesia sites, clinical lab, dietary, emergency service, endoscopy suite, imaging, laundry, physical rehabilitation, social work, supply, and respiratory care. Interdisciplinary interviews may include discussions of competency, ethics, infection control, information management, leadership, medication usage, operative invasion, patient care conference, patient family education, performance improvement, and strategic planning. Structural interviews include nursing as well as the chief operating officer and medical staff.

The surveyor discusses the problems uncovered with fellow team members. The team scores each of the JCAHO standards. The agency passes or fails each standard. JCAHO staff determine or recommend to the Accreditation Committee of the Board of Commissioners one of several accreditation statuses: accreditation with commendation, accreditation with or without type 1 recommendations, conditional accreditation, deny accreditation, defer consideration while additional information about the agency's compliance status is reviewed by JCAHO staff, and provisional accreditation.

Accreditation decision is the conclusion reached regarding the agency's status after evaluation of the results of the on-site survey, recommendations of the surveyors, and other information such as documentation of compliance, plans to correct deficiencies, and evidence of improvements.

Accreditation with commendation is the highest accreditation decision.

Conditional accreditation is a determination that substantial standards compliance deficiencies exist in an agency. Correction must be demonstrated through a follow-up survey to get full accreditation.

Not accredited is a decision that results when an agency has been denied accreditation, has had its accreditation withdrawn by the JCAHO, withdrew from the accreditation process, or did not apply for accreditation.

Accreditation survey is an evaluation of an agency to assess its level of compliance with applicable JCAHO standards and to make determinations about its accreditation status.

Focused survey is a survey conducted during the accreditation cycle to assess the degree to which an agency has improved its level of compliance regarding specific recommendations.

Survey team is the group of health care professionals (usually a nurse, physician, and administrator) who perform the accreditation survey.

Scoring guideline is a descriptive tool that is used to assist agencies in complying with JCAHO standards and to determine the degree of compliance. It is described in the *Accreditation Manual for Hospitals,* volume II.*

QUALITY MANAGEMENT: THE HEROES

W. Edwards Deming is the genius who revitalized Japanese industry with his focus on total quality management and continuous quality improvement. The Deming Chain Reaction is as follows: (1) Improve quality. (2) Decrease costs with fewer mistakes, less rework, fewer delays, and better use of time and materials. (3) Improve productivity. (4) Capture the market with better quality at lower prices. (5) Stay in business. (6) Provide jobs. Box 28-3 outlines the 14 key points of the Deming Management Method.

Joseph M. Juran is an advocate for total quality management (TQM). His quality trilogy includes three activities: quality planning, control, and improvement (see Box 28-4).

Philip B. Crosby defines quality as conformance to requirements. He believes that the system for creating quality is prevention of errors instead of appraisal. He has identified 14 steps to quality improvement, some of which are parallel (see Box 28-5).

Quality improvement differs from quality assurance (see Table 28-1). The process of quality improvement includes the following steps:
1. Identify the customers and their expectations and the outputs using brainstorming, focus groups, and interviews.
2. Describe the current process using flowcharts and focus groups.
3. Measure and analyze the discrepancy between desired expectations and reality using check sheets, logs, time charts, trend charts, histograms, and surveys.
4. Focus on an improvement opportunity using decision matrix, Pareto charts, and voting.
5. Identify root causes of inefficiencies through brainstorming, affinity charts, cause-and-effect diagrams, tree diagrams, relationship diagrams, force field analysis, and focus groups.

---

* From JCAHO: *1994 accreditation manual for hospitals,* vol 1, Standards, Oakbrook Terrace, Ill, 1993, JCAHO.

1. Create constancy of purpose for improvement of products and services. Dr. Deming suggests that the purpose is to stay in business and provide jobs through maintenance, research, innovation, and constant improvement.

2. Adopt the new philosophy. Mistakes and negativism should be unacceptable.

3. Cease dependence on mass inspection. Dr. Deming maintains that quality arises from improvement in the process rather than from inspection and that workers should participate in improvement in the process. When quality is addressed at the inspection phase, workers are paid to make the mistake and then paid to correct it, which is very expensive.

4. End the practice of awarding business on the price tag alone. Buyers should get the best quality in a long-term relationship with a single supplier for any specific item rather than purchasing the lowest-priced and often poor-quality items from the cheapest vendor.

5. Constantly improve the system of production and service. Management must always look for ways to reduce waste and improve quality.

6. Institute training. Workers cannot be expected to do their jobs well if no one tells them how to do so.

7. Institute leadership. Dr. Deming believes that people who do not do well are just misplaced. It is the leader's responsibility to identify workers who need individual attention, find an appropriate place for them in the organization, and help them do a better job.

8. Drive out fear. Many workers are afraid to ask questions or point out problems for fear of being blamed for the problem. They may continue to do something wrong or not at all. For the best quality and productivity, people need to feel secure.

9. Break down barriers between staff areas. Often departments compete with each other or have goals that conflict. It is better to have teamwork to solve problems.

10. Eliminate slogans, exhortations, and targets for the workforce. It is better for workers to develop their own slogans.

11. Eliminate numerical quotas because they deal with numbers, not quality. They often contribute to inefficiency and high cost because workers meet quotas at any cost to keep their jobs.

12. Remove barriers to pride of workmanship. People are eager to do a good job. Barriers such as faulty equipment, defective materials, and misguided managers should be removed.

13. Institute a vigorous program of education and retraining. Both managers and staff need to be educated about new methods and teamwork.

14. Take action to accomplish the transformation. Managers and staff need a plan of action to carry out the quality mission. A critical mass of people must understand the 14 points about continuous quality improvement.

*These 14 points are discussed in Walton M: *The Deming management method,* New York, 1986, Putnam; and Walton M: *Deming management at work,* New York, 1990, Putnam's Sons.

Box 28-4 **JURAN'S QUALITY TRILOGY***

QUALITY PLANNING

1. Determine who the customers are.

2. Determine the needs of the customers.

3. Develop product features that respond to the customers' needs.

4. Develop the processes that produce those product features.

5. Transfer the resulting plans to the operating forces.

QUALITY CONTROL

1. Evaluate actual quality performance.

2. Compare actual performance to quality goals.

3. Act on the difference.

QUALITY IMPROVEMENT

1. Establish the infrastructure needed to secure annual quality improvement.

2. Identify the specific needs for improvement, which become the improvement projects.

3. Establish a project team with responsibilities for bringing the project to successful closure.

4. Provide the resource and training needed by teams to diagnose the problems, develop a remedy, and establish controls to maintain the gains.

*Modified from Juran JM: *Juran on leadership for quality,* New York, 1989, The Free Press.

6. Generate and select solutions to the problem by brainstorming and using decision matrices and tree diagrams.
7. Map out a trial run through brainstorming, force field analysis, action planning, tree diagrams, and flowcharting.
8. Implement the trial run using check sheets, logs, and histograms.
9. Evaluate the results using check sheets, logs, surveys, focus groups, histograms, and trend charts.
10. Draw conclusions using Pareto diagrams, focus groups, and force field analysis.
11. Standardize the change using force field analysis, brainstorming, action planning, tree diagrams, and flowcharting.
12. Monitor holding the gains through check sheets, trend charts, surveys, histograms, and control charts.

Box 28-5

CROSBY'S 14 STEPS TO QUALITY IMPROVEMENT*

1. Commitment from management

2. Use of quality improvement teams composed of people with process knowledge and commitment to actions

3. Quality measurement to identify areas that need improvement and change

4. Measuring the cost of quality and nonquality

5. Quality awareness by all personnel

6. Corrective actions through opportunities for improvement

7. Zero defects planning—do it right the first time

8. Employee education for quality improvement

9. Zero defect day as demonstration of commitment to quality

10. Goal setting toward zero defects

11. Error-causal removal by removing barriers

12. Recognition for meeting goals

13. Quality councils to assist people in quality improvement

14. Do it all over again

*From Crosby PB: *Quality is free,* New York, 1979, McGraw-Hill; Crosby PB: *Quality without tears,* New York, 1984, McGraw-Hill; Crosby PB: *Let's talk quality,* New York, 1989, McGraw-Hill.

HEALTH CARE REFORM

For nearly a century, various groups have recommended proposals for health care reform. In 1915, a group recommended a focus on prevention and sharing of health care costs by employers, employees, and the government. In 1932, a commission encouraged doctors to form group practices to share responsibility for cost-effective, high-quality health care. In 1933, President Franklin Roosevelt initiated the Social Security Act, which he intended to include national health insurance. In 1946, President Harry Truman introduced a plan for national health reform, declaring that health is a right, not just a privilege. In 1972, President Richard Nixon advocated that employers take responsibility and contribute to their workers' health care. In 1993, President Bill Clinton advocated a bold health care reform.

President Clinton outlined six principles basic to the Health Security Act: (1) security—guaranteeing comprehensive benefits to all Americans; (2) simplicity—cutting red tape and consequently simplifying the system; (3) savings—controlling the costs of health care; (4) quality—making health care better; (6) choice—preserving and increasing the options available; and (7) responsibility—making everyone responsible for health care.

Table 28-1   Comparison of Quality Assurance and Quality Improvement

Quality Assurance	Quality Improvement
Detection oriented	Prevention oriented
Reactive	Proactive
Narrow focus	Cross-functional
Getting by	Raising standards
Tradition and safety	Experimentation and risk
Busyness	Productivity
Leadership not vested	Leadership leading
Leader as director	Leader as empowerer
Employee as expendable	Employee as customer
Responsibility of few	Responsibility of all
Problem solving by authority	Problem solving by all
We-they thinking	Organizational perspective
Cynicism	New optimism

Security is accomplished by providing every American with a comprehensive health benefits package that cannot be taken away. Simplicity is achieved by reducing paperwork, that wastes time and costs billions of dollars. Savings can be achieved through group purchasing. Quality involves emphasizing keeping well and giving consumers information to judge quality themselves. Choice means the right to choose one's health care provider to protect the doctor-patient relationship. Responsibility means that every employee and every employer contributes to the cost of health care.*

The Clinton health care reform plan was complex and coherent, with interlocking parts that fit together logically. There was an emphasis of universal health care coverage and broad comprehensive coverage that includes preventive care, prescriptive medications, mental health services, home health benefits, and long-term care. It was designed to slow the current rate of increase in health care costs until they are comparable to the rate of inflation while providing access to economical, high-quality health care.

LIABILITY CONTROL

Policies and procedures for handling incidents and claims should be developed and implemented. Some incidents may relate to medication errors, falls, procedures (particularly invasive procedures), patient or family refusal of treatment, and patient or family dissatisfaction with care. Because of the negative connotation of the word

* The White House Domestic Policy Council: *Health security: the president's report to the American people,* Washington, DC, 1993, The White House Domestic Policy Council.

incident, some agencies use the terms *event, occurrence,* or *situation* instead. Filing an incident report is not admitting guilt. It is reporting something that is not a part of routine care.

It is preferable that incident report forms contain questions that can be answered yes or no or by multiple choice. Narrative should be limited. The observer should give a factual, nonjudgmental account of what was seen, heard, felt, or smelled. No impressions, interpretations, or opinions should be stated. All of the information needed should be in one place.

Documentation is critically important. The quality of the documentation often determines the outcome of lawsuits. Medical records are legal documents that can be introduced in court. Nurses and other personnel must be well versed in accurate and comprehensive documentation. Nurses should also know how to testify in court and how to serve as expert witnesses (Stull and Pinkerton, 1988).

Tort law is the branch of civil law that concerns legal wrongs committed by one person against the person or property of another. Torts may be intentional or unintentional.

Negligence is an unintentional tort that involves harm resulting from the failure of people conducting themselves in reasonable and prudent ways. Careless is not thinking before one acts or not paying attention. One can be careful and still be negligent for not acting as prudently as others would in the same circumstances.

Malpractice is negligent acts of people with specialized education. Malpractice reflects negligence, but not all negligence is malpractice. When people are held legally responsible for their negligent acts they are legally liable and may be required to pay for damages. Medical malpractice refers to the negligent acts of any health professional when conducting patient care responsibilities. Nursing malpractice refers specifically to nurses conducting their patient care responsibilities. Common causes of malpractice claims against nurses are medication errors from misreading the medication order or not clarifying an incomplete or ambiguous order and technique in giving injections.

Negligent conduct depends on the act itself and the surrounding circumstances, including (1) the nature of the nursing function, (2) the nurse's qualifications to perform the function, (3) the urgency of the situation, and (4) the foreseeable harm if the care is not implemented. The emergency room nurse is not held to the same standards of care expected under more normal circumstances. Being a minor does not exempt a nurse from liability for acts of malpractice, and the nurse's state of mind and physical condition are not considered relevant.

The rule of personal liability means that people are responsible for their own tortious conduct even when someone else may share that liability under some other law. Supervisors will not usually be held liable for the negligent acts of those they supervise because all professional persons are held liable for their own negligent behavior. However, a supervisor may be found guilty of negligence for making an assignment beyond a worker's capabilities without giving adequate supervision in carrying out the delegated functions. If a supervisor believes that certain staffing will jeopardize patient safety and potentially precipitate litigation, the position should be documented and the hospital administrator informed.

The doctrine of *respondeat superior* applies to the United States government because the government has agreed to be sued for negligent acts of its employees under the Federal Tort Claims Act (FTCA). By virtue of special statutory enactments, nurses employed by the Veterans Administration and the United States Public Health Service have complete immunity from personal liability for acts of negligence in the implementation of their government responsibilities. However, the aggrieved patients may sue the government for injuries they have sustained. Occupational health nurses are potentially exposed to a greater risk of being sued for negligent conduct than other nurses because of the joint effect of the doctrine of respondent superior and workers' compensation laws. Workers' compensation laws usually prevent an employee from suing an employer, so the aggrieved employee can sue only the nurse.

A nurse is legally required to implement medical procedures ordered by a licensed physician or a physician's assistant acting on behalf of the physician employer unless the nurse has reason to believe harm would result from doing so. Failure to carry out the physician's order will subject the nurse to liability for subsequent harm to the patient if there is not reason to question the order. Consequently nurses must know how to implement the procedure and the effect of the procedure on the patient. When nurses question physician's orders, they should tactfully question the physician. If the physician is insistent, the nurse should take the matter to the supervisor or responsible hospital official. Patient safety is of utmost concern. The nurse has a legal responsibility not to follow the order when there are reasonable grounds to believe that the action would harm the patient.

Consent is not legally required when immediate care is necessary to save the life and consent cannot be obtained either from the patient or an authorized legal representative. Constructive consent or consent implied by law is effective. Minors are not legally capable of giving valid consent to medical treatment, but minors who live apart from their parents and are married are considered emancipated and are capable of giving consent. The law presumes every adult is mentally competent until adjudicated otherwise. After people have been declared mentally incompetent in a judicial proceeding they cannot give valid consents. When patients have been deemed clinically incompetent but not legally incompetent, nurses should seek the participation of the patient's next of kin in making decisions. When family members cannot agree, treatment should be postponed until a legal guardian is appointed with the authority to make the necessary medical decisions.

Informed consent is given by the patient who fully understands what is being consented to. Consent may be given orally or in writing. Both are legally effective, but it is advisable to get the consent in writing. The patient must be told the nature of the proposed treatment, alternative treatments possible, and the risks involved to be able to give an informed consent. Liability or negligence can result if the dangers of a procedure are minimized to obtain the patient's consent.

Most false-imprisonment cases in health care involve locking mentally ill patients in their rooms. An agency can be held liable for the conduct of a nurse-employee who unlawfully confines or detains a patient against the patient's will because of the doctrine of respondeat superior.

The plaintiff is the complaining party in a malpractice suit. The defendant is the answering party. All nursing malpractice suits consist of the following elements: (1) a claim that the nurse owed the plaintiff a special duty of care; (2) a claim that the nurse was expected to meet a specific standard of care; (3) a claim that the nurse's failure to meet that standard of care resulted in harm to the patient; and (4) a claim for money damages to compensate the plaintiff for the harm sustained.*

Battery is an intentional tort involving unpermitted and intentional contacts with one's person or extension of the body to clothing, object in the hand, car, and so forth. A hostile intent of the defendant is not necessary. It is the absence of the plaintiff's consent to the defendant's contact that is the issue. Direct contact with the plaintiff is not necessary, and the personal integrity exists even when the plaintiff is under anesthesia or asleep. The defendant is liable for all harm, including unforseeable consequences from the conduct.

Assault involves mental disturbance of personal integrity, including fright and humiliation. It does not include actual contact.

Grounds for civil actions regarding assault and battery include forcefully handling an unconscious patient, forcing a patient out of bed to walk, forcing a patient to submit to treatment even if a consent had been signed because resistance implies withdrawal of consent, lifting a protesting patient from bed to a stretcher or chair, threatening to strike or striking a child or adult unless in self-defense, and in some states performing alcohol, blood, urine, or other health tests for presumed drunken driving without consent. Some states have implied consent statutes in motor vehicle codes for the privilege of driving. Intentional torts such as assault and battery often are not covered in malpractice insurance.

TESTIFYING

Testifying under oath can be a terrifying experience, but understanding procedures and a few rules can make the experience less stressful. Appearance is important. One should dress neatly and conventionally. A business suit is usually appropriate. If one is testifying just before, after, or during a shift, a uniform is appropriate.

A pleasant demeanor is also important. One should project a polite, sincere, and cooperative image. One should know the facts before testifying. It is appropriate to review the record, particularly the part one is responsible for. The health care agency record should never be falsified. It may be helpful to make a sketch or diagram if placement of persons and objects is important.

The court recorder records everything said, so one should enunciate clearly. Questions must be answered orally because nodding the head and other nonverbal responses are difficult to record and subject to interpretation. One is likely to be asked for personal and professional information such as residence, age, marital status, educational background, grades received, and employment history. One should be sure the question is understood before answering it. Making an inaccurate response because the question was not understood can adversely affect the outcomes. Pausing before answering the question is appropriate to formulate an answer and to allow time for an attorney to raise objections. If the attorney objects to a question, refrain from responding until the issue is resolved. The lawyer will direct you if an answer is required. One should keep answers brief, tell the truth, and answer only the question asked. One should try to give favorable facts and avoid such questionable words as *think, guess,* and *maybe.* Sometimes matters of amount, distance, and time are crucial.

---

* Bernzweig EP: *The nurse's liability for malpractice: a programmed course,* St Louis, 1990, Mosby.

Do not be forced into guessing. If unable to make a reliable judgment, "I don't know" is an appropriate response. When asked to identify an exhibit such as a medical record, one should scrutinize it carefully and indicate whether it is recognized or not. Whoever calls one as a witness has the first opportunity to ask questions. Afterward, the opposing party's attorney has the opportunity to ask questions (Kilmon, 1985).

EXPERT WITNESSES

Because malpractice litigation has increased and physicians are serving as expert witnesses for nursing less than they did before the 1970s, nurses are increasingly acting as expert witnesses. Some state nurses associations are developing resource banks of nurse expert witnesses. Nurses may need to submit a letter of intent describing their qualifications as a nurse expert, résumé, and letters of reference. Some state nurses associations provide continuing education regarding legal issues and being an expert witness to ensure a pool of adequately prepared expert witnesses.

Attorneys often want to meet experts before selecting them. They also need résumés and letters of reference. Attorneys often contact experts by telephone and provide brief case summaries. Then the nurse must decide which cases to accept. The case must match the expert's area of expertise. Experts should review only records that are within their specialty. The expert compares the facts of the case with standards of care and offers a professional opinion. The expert should understand clearly whether the attorney wants the expert to defend the nurse or dispute the nurse's credibility. The cases selected should not involve matters concerning places where the expert has worked or people with whom the expert has worked because the issue of bias could be raised. Fees negotiated should include time required to review the records, write a report, and provide testimony (Salmond, 1986).

BIBLIOGRAPHY

Bohnet NL, Ilcyn J, Milanovich PS et al: Continuous quality improvement: improving quality in your home care organization, *JONA* 23:42-48, February 1993.

Brooms L: The goal is quality improvement, *Nurs Manage* 24:51-52, January 1993.

Buss HE: Continuous quality improvement: adaptation of the 10-step model with postanesthesia care unit application, *Journal of Post Anesthesia Nursing* 8:238-248, August 1993.

Cesta TG: The link between continuous quality improvement and case management, *JONA* 23:55-61, June 1993.

Churchill M: Employees are also our customers, *ANNA J* 19:152, April 1992.

De Laune S: Risk reduction through testing, screening and infection control precautions—with special emphasis on needlestick injuries, *Infect Control Hosp Epidemiol* 11(suppl):563-565, October 1990.

Dixon IL: Continuous quality improvement in shared leadership, *Nurs Manage* 24:40-45, January 1993.

English JFB: Reported hospital needlestick injuries in relation to knowledge/skill, design, and management problems, *Infect Control Hosp Epidemiol* 13:259-264, May 1992.

Foreman JT: Continuous quality improvement in home care: do it right the first time, *Caring* 12:32-37, October 1993.

Goldman TA: Risk management concepts and strategies, *J Intravenous Nurs* 14:199-204, May-June 1991.

Haiduven DJ, DeMaio TM, Stevens DA: A five-year study of needlestick injuries: significant reduction associated with communication, education, and convenient placement of sharps containers, *Infect Control Hosp Epidemiol* 13:265-271, May 1992.

Hollander SF, Smith M, Barron J: Cost reductions part 1: an operations improvement process, *Nurs Econ* 10(5):325-330, Sept-Oct, 1992.

Jones KR: Outcomes analysis: methods and issues, *Nurs Econ* 11:145-152, May-June 1993.

Kilmon EL: Do you swear to tell the truth? *Nurs Econ* 3:98-102, March-April 1985.

Leimnetzer MJ, Ryan DA, Niemann VG: The hospital Visiting Nurse Association partnership: a continuous quality improvement program 23:20-23, November 1993.

Marriner A: The research process in quality assurance, *Am J Nurs* 79:2158-2161, December 1979.

Masters ML, Masters RJ: Building TQM into nursing management, *Nurs Econ* 11:274-278, 291, September-October 1993.

Murray JA, Murray MH: Benchmarking: a tool for excellence in palliative care, *J Palliat Care* 8:41-45, Winter 1992.

Phaneuf MC: A nursing audit method, *Nurs Outlook* 12:42-45, May 1964.

Phaneuf MC: The nursing audit for evaluation of patient care, *Nurs Outlook* 14:51-54, June 1966.

Phaneuf MC: Analysis of nursing audit, *Nurs Outlook,* 16:57-60, January 1968.

Phaneuf MC: Quality of care: problems of measurement. I. How one public health nursing agency is using the nursing audit, *Am J Public Health* 59:1827-1832, October 1969.

Phaneuf MC, Wandelt MM: Quality assurance in nursing, *Nurs Forum* 13:328-345, 1974.

Salmond SW: Serving as an expert witness, *Nurs Econ* 4:236-239, September-October 1986.

Sherman JJ, Malkmus MA: Integrating quality assurance and total quality management/quality improvement, *JONA* 24:37-41, March 1994.

Ventura NR, Rizzo J, Lenz S: Quality indicators: control maintains—propriety improves, *Nurs Manage* 24:46-50, January 1993.

CASE STUDY

You are the evening charge nurse caring for 20 critically ill patients with the help of one LPN and two aides. There are many medications and treatments to give. You don't think it is possible for you and the LPN to do all of the medications and treatments and don't believe the aides are qualified to do most of the work that needs to be done. What are you going to do?

CRITICAL THINKING AND LEARNING ACTIVITIES

1. Fill out Worksheets 28-1 and 28-2 to help reinforce your knowledge of risk and risk management.

2. Inquire about the patient relation program at a local health care facility.

3. Interview someone who serves on a quality assurance committee about the business conducted by that committee.

4. Watch a movie or television program involving a court case to become more familiar with the proceedings.

5. Interview a nurse expert witness about experiences as a witness. After completing Worksheet 28-3, determine whether the witness followed the "rules" you have identified as guidelines for testifying.

✍ **Worksheet 28-1**

Risk Management Process

Briefly describe the five steps in the risk management process.

1.

2.

3.

4.

5.

✍ **Worksheet 28-2**

Potential Risks

Identify at least three sources for identifying potential risks.

1.

2.

3.

✍ **Worksheet 28-3**

Testifying

List rules to remember for testifying.

1.

2.

3.

4.

5.

6.

Chapter

29

Labor Relations

Chapter Objectives

◆ Describe the four phases of unionization.

◆ Explain the decertification process.

◆ Identify advantages and disadvantages of collective bargaining.

Major Concepts and Definitions	
Labor relations	relations between the workers and management
Unionization	organization of workers
Collective bargaining	organization of workers to bargain for working conditions

LABOR RELATIONS

Why Employees Join Unions

Employees essentially join a union to increase their power to get certain responses from management. Management's actions or inactions have probably caused the employees to reach their limit of tolerance. Poor working conditions and job inequities in wage increments, promotion, and benefits cause distress. Poor quality of immediate supervision, arbitrary treatment from management, and poor communications between employer and employee are major reasons for unionization. Instead of quitting their jobs and giving up their seniority, security, and friends to move to another job, they form a union.

Labor Law

In 1935 the National Labor Relations Act (NLRA), or the Wagner Act, was passed in an effort to end the depression. It prevented some employers from cutting wages in the hopes that higher worker incomes and increased spending would lessen the severity of the economic depression. Unfortunately, some employers went bankrupt because they could not reduce wages. Employers could not legally fire employees who sought unionization. The NLRA created the National Labor Relations Board to investigate and initiate administrative proceedings against employers who violated a law that listed employer violations only.

Because the NLRA was biased toward unions, it was amended in 1947 by the Taft-Hartley Act, or Labor Management Relations Act. It listed union restrictions to restore equality between employers and employees. Nonprofit health care institutions, however, were exempted from the law. The unions developed public relations problems when some of them went on strike during the war and when unions were blamed for the postwar inflation.

In 1959 the laws were further modified by the Landrum-Griffin Act, or Labor-Management Reporting and Disclosure Act, to safeguard against corrupt financial and election procedures used by some unions. The Union Members' Bill of Rights resulted.

In 1974, Public Law 93-360, the Nonprofit Health Care Amendments to the Taft-Hartley Act, extended federal collective bargaining rights to private sector employees. It created notification procedures that must precede a strike and ensured employees of the right to join, or refrain from joining, a union.

Unfair labor practices by management. The NLRA's section 8(a) prohibitions on management are known as the unfair labor practices. They include interference, 8(a)(1); domination, 8(a)(2); discrimination, 8(a)(3); discrimination, 8(a)(4); and refusal to bargain, 8(a)(5). Restraining or coercing or otherwise interfering with employees during the exercise of their right to organize is an unfair labor practice. Management may not contribute financial or other support or otherwise dominate or interfere during the development or administration of a labor organization. The employer may not discriminate in hiring or tenure or other terms of employment to encourage or discourage membership in a labor organization. Nor can the employer discriminate against an employee for filing charges or giving testimony. The employer is also forbidden to refuse to bargain with representatives of the employees.

Unfair labor practices by unions. Before 1935, management's power had few limitations. From 1935 to 1947 managers had to contend with unfair labor practice limitations, but no such unfair labor practices were defined for labor organizations. In 1947, the Labor Management Relations Act amended the NLRA and added restrictions for labor organizations. These include interference, 8(b)(1); induced discrimination, 8(b)(2); refusal to bargain, 8(b)(3); strikes and boycotts, 8(b)(4); initiation fee, 8(b)(5); featherbedding, 8(b)(6); and recognition picketing, 8(b)(7). Labor organizations may not restrain or coerce an employer in the selection of a representative for collective bargaining. The union may not cause an employer to discriminate against an employee who is not a member of the union. Nor can a union representative of the employees refuse to bargain with the employer. With adherence to required notification procedures, an employee organization may strike against the employer when negotiations have failed. A primary boycott is a strike action taken by union members against their employer. The illegal or protected status of strikes or boycotts depends on the union objectives and the tactics used. Labor unions may not force an employer to join any organization or cease using specific products or doing business with someone, thus making "hot cargo" clauses illegal. Hot cargo agreements are stipulations on the employer's use of products that give the union power over other organizations. A secondary boycott that is directed at a customer or supplier of the employer is also illegal. An employee group may not force an employer to bargain with them if the employees are represented by another bargaining agent. Labor organizations may not force "any employer to assign particular work to employees in a particular labor organization . . . rather than to employees in another labor organization," and they may not honor strike lines against other employers by refusing to cross the picket lines. Informational picketing is not barred because it does not disrupt the employer's operation. Recognition picketing to get an employer to recognize an employee group is lawful except when the employer has recognized another labor organization, when it is within 12 months preceding a valid election, and when picketing has been conducted without a petition. The union may not charge discriminatory or excessive initiation fees or cause an employer to pay for services not performed, a practice called featherbedding.

UNIONIZATION

Organizing Phase

To form a union, an organizer must establish internal contacts. In a hospital or other health agency the organizer needs at least one nurse on each shift to assist with unionization. The organizer should be known by a majority of the nurses, be knowledgeable about related laws, and be able to use free time for organizing. The organizers ascertain the level of interest informally by listening, asking questions, and supplying information. After an assessment period, the organizers meet, discuss the prevailing climate, identify the frustration level, enumerate the kinds and extent of employment problems, and assess the nurses' interest in unionization. If interest is minimal, further organizing efforts should be postponed. If nurses show interest in organizing, the campaign is planned.

There must be commitment from the nurses before a formal organization can be established. To achieve this, the organizers hold informational meetings. Coordination of efforts, development of unity, identification of problems and concerns, education about collective bargaining, and active participation of nurses are the tasks to be accomplished in the organizing meetings. The organizers should work in nonwork areas on their own time. The organizers contact the labor organization that they want to represent them for information and authorization cards. The labor organization can send a letter to the employer informing management that the nurses within that agency are organizing and that the activity is protected by law. Box 29-1 contains a list of questions that the manager can ask to help determine whether staff members are in the organizing phase.

Recognition Phase

The organizers must get at least 30% of the nurses to be represented to sign individual authorization cards before the labor organization can act on behalf of the group. Handing out authorization cards is solicitation and cannot be prohibited by management anywhere in the agency during nonworking time. Recognition of the labor organization by the employer is necessary before collective bargaining can begin. Some employers will recognize the labor organization on a voluntary basis when given proof of the majority representative status. However, employers often refuse to recognize the labor organization voluntarily on the basis of a good faith doubt of majority representation. Thus it becomes necessary to obtain certification from the National Labor Relations Board (NLRB).

The NLRB does not start an election until requested to do so by an employee organization. A petition for an election must be accompanied by designation cards signed by 30% of the employees in the bargaining group to indicate a substantial show of interest. Labor organizations usually obtain signatures from at least 50% of the potential members before they file a petition.

A preliminary hearing is held before an election is scheduled. This provides participants an opportunity to express their opinions. The regional director of the NLRB assesses that the employer is under the board's jurisdiction; determines that other criteria are met; determines the bargaining unit and voter eligibility; and sets the

Box 29-1

QUESTIONS TO HELP DETERMINE WHETHER STAFF ARE IN THE ORGANIZING PHASE

A "Yes" answer to the following questions may indicate that personnel are in the organizing phase:

- Have you seen union authorization cards anywhere on the agency premises?
- Have you heard of any union-sponsored meetings outside the organization?
- Have you heard of any employee meetings being held at an employee's home?
- Has there been an increase in the number of peer work social activities?
- Have you noticed a repeated presence of strangers or ex-employees mingling with employees outside the agency as employees are coming to and going from work?
- Have you seen employees talking together in small groups and either breaking up their conversation and walking away or becoming silent as you or other members of management approach?
- Has there been any significant increase in the number of employee complaints about wages or conditions of employment?
- Has there been an increase in employee complaints regarding schedules, staffing levels, content or frequency of in-service education programs, unclear and overlapping job classifications?
- Has there been a change in the rate of turnover?
- Are you aware of any other factors that appear to be out of the ordinary and seem to be separating administration from employees?

date, hours, and place for the election. The election usually takes place during working hours on the employer's premises about a month after the hearing. All employees in the bargaining unit who were on the employer's payroll during a given payroll period in the recent past are allowed to vote. This rule prevents hiring people to vote in the election.

The number of bargaining units within an agency is held to a minimum. Appropriate bargaining units include (1) technical employees, such as x-ray technicians, surgical technicians, and licensed practical nurses; (2) service and maintenance employees, such as employees doing kitchen work, laundry, and housekeeping; (3) business office clerical employees, such as receptionists, clerks, and switchboard operators; and (4) professional employees, such as nurses.

Spouses and children of the employers, temporary employees, and managerial employees are not eligible to vote. People who have the authority to hire, fire, and direct others are considered managers. This may include nurse managers, head nurses, and charge nurses. As a member of management, the director of nursing is ineligible to vote.

During the preelection period, the employer is required to post NLRB election notices stating the time, date, and place of the election. On election day the field examiner from the regional board sets up the election machinery and does not allow electioneering around the polling place. Eligible employees cast secret ballots. Ballots are counted in the regional office. The tabulation of votes is forwarded to the office of the General Counsel in Washington, D.C., and the General Counsel decides the election. If employees no longer want to be represented by the labor organization, they can initiate a decertification election with a requisite 30% show of interest. If a bargaining unit is denied because of the vote tabulation, the labor organization is not permitted to seek certification among the same people until after a 12-month moratorium, and the management group should rectify the problems identified during the organization. If a union wins the election, both parties prepare to negotiate.

Contract Negotiation Phase

The piecemeal, total, and combination approaches are used for contract negotiations. The piecemeal is a step-by-step approach that tries to settle the issues one by one. The total approach considers nothing settled until everything is settled. This allows for calculation of the effects of the interdependent variables on each other. The combination method uses both approaches. The step-by-step method is used to progress from the easy to the hard issues. The decisions are not irrevocable, trading takes place, and decisions are reworked until negotiations are acceptable to both parties. The union representatives present the solutions to the members for a ratification vote to accept or reject the offer. If the solutions are accepted, the employee and management representatives sign the agreement, and it becomes binding. If they are rejected, the representatives reassemble to continue negotiating the contract.

During contract negotiations, the union is on the offensive and management is on the defensive. The union makes most of the demands, while management defends itself against them and prepares for a strike. The threat of a strike strengthens the union negotiator's position.

Strikes in the health care field require more special and elaborate notification procedures than in other industries. This allows for the delay of new admissions or referral to other facilities. Alternative health care plans are made for ambulatory patients. Some hospitalized patients may be transferred to other agencies, and supervisory personnel are scheduled to care for the remaining patients.

The NLRB categorizes collective bargaining into three groups: illegal, voluntary, and mandatory. Illegal topics violate the NLRB and other laws. Voluntary subjects need not be negotiated unless both sides consent to do so. Voluntary issues include size of the bargaining team, union dues, management salaries, and patient charges. Mandatory subjects are related to conditions of employment, work hours, and remuneration.

Contracts often start with a preamble that states both parties' objectives and a pledge of cooperation. Near the beginning there is a statement of the employer's recognition of the union as the bargaining representative for specific employees with specification of employees who are excluded.

A union security clause requires new workers to join the union. Union security is protected by establishing a closed shop, union shop, agency shop, or maintenance-of-membership arrangement in the contract. The closed shop requires the employer to hire and retain only union members in good standing. However, this is prohibited by the Labor Management Relations Act of 1947 for employers and employees in industries affecting interstate commerce. A union shop requires all employees to become members of the union within a specific time after hiring (usually 30 to 60 days) and to maintain membership as a condition of employment. An agency shop requires all employees in the negotiating unit who do not join the union to pay a fixed amount equivalent to organization dues on a regular basis as a condition of employment. The money may go to the organization's welfare fund or to a charity. The maintenance-of-membership clause requires union members to maintain their membership during a specific period, such as the duration of the contract.

Financial remuneration—including wages and salaries, shift differentials, over-time rates, holiday pay, cost-of-living adjustment, longevity, and merit increases—receives considerable attention. Nonfinancial remuneration—including insurance, retirement plans, employee services such as free lunches and parking, vacations, holidays, leaves, and educational assistance—also receives considerable attention. The union usually strives to have rewards made on the basis of seniority. Guidelines for discipline, grievance procedures, and professional standards are also negotiated. After acceptance of the contract by the union members through a ratification vote, the contract is signed by employee and employer representatives and becomes binding.

Contract Administration

Implementation of the agreement, the final phase of the unionization process, interprets and enforces the agreement developed during negotiations. When one of the parties involved does not abide by the terms of the contract, a grievance may result. Grievances are most commonly filed against management because management has a more active role than the union in the administration of the contract. The grievance procedure is usually addressed in the contract.

Underlying causes of grievances should be identified and corrected so that future grievances will be prevented. Different types of grievances require different reactions from managers and union leaders. A legitimate grievance results when one party violates the agreement between parties. Managers' ignorance of the agreement and lack of commitment are the major causes. It is not uncommon for first-line managers to function without having read the contract and with the attitude that labor relations are a chore. On the other hand, union stewards are more motivated to understand the agreement and must have an interest in labor relations to obtain their positions. Consequently, most legitimate grievances are against management. It is advisable to develop training programs to familiarize managers with the contract and to set labor relations objectives as priorities for managers.

Imagined grievances occur when a party incorrectly believes that there has been a violation. Employees sometimes imagine a grievance because they do not understand their rights. The steward should correct the misunderstanding before it becomes a formal grievance.

Political grievances occur for reasons other than the concern itself. Management may want to appear supportive to subordinate managers and stewards to union members, so they do not adequately advise the complainant. A cooperative atmo-sphere between labor and management is the best way to avoid political grievances.

Harassment grievances are fabricated to distress the other side. They are most commonly used by unions in connection with negotiations. Management usually denies the grievances, forcing the union to drop the grievance or request arbitration.

If the contract indicates that both sides share arbitration expenses, harassment grievances are usually dropped.

Organizations should have a grievance procedure even if they are not unionized. This allows employees access to management regarding issues of concern to them and conveys management's intent to be fair. Grievances should be handled quickly through the use of a grievance procedure. Grievances may be handled in a centralized or decentralized manner. In a decentralized process, the immediate supervisor tries to resolve as many problems as possible, and grievances rarely progress further. This encourages a close working relationship between manager and staff associates. Unfortunately, there may be inconsistent decisions because of the number of different people involved in the process. In a centralized grievance procedure, the immediate manager denies the validity of the grievance, and it is handled by the next level of management or by a personnel department. Thus, decisions are made consistently among units because of the few people involved in the decision making. Unfortunately, cooperation between the manager and staff associate is not fostered.

Arbitration.   Most contracts allow either side to seek arbitration when a grievance is not satisfactorily resolved, but both parties must agree on the arbitrator. The American Arbitration Association and the Federal Mediation and Conciliation Service are primary sources for professional arbitrators. The payment of costs involved is specified in the contract. Commonly, both parties share the costs, but some contracts specify that the loser must pay.

In any case, arbitration is not automatic and must be requested by the dissatisfied party. Both sides select a representative, the grievance is reviewed, fact finding is done, and witnesses are interviewed. Preparation of one's case from the opponent's view encourages one to consider both sides and develop a stronger case. Presenting one's case to a friend who will act as an advocate helps further identify weaknesses in one's presentation and further strengthens the case. Documents should be prepared in triplicate for the hearing so that the arbitrator, opponent, and presenter can each have a copy. Witnesses may be used for the hearing. Their availability should be confirmed. Witnesses should be informed of where and when to attend the hearing and what will be expected of them.

A hearing is similar to courtroom proceedings. The arbitrator makes opening remarks, and the initiating party comments on the purpose of the hearing and outcomes desired. The responding side may respond then or wait until later. Witnesses are presented and cross-examined in an alternating pattern. First a witness testifies for the initiator, and then one for the responding party testifies and is cross-examined. The initiating party makes closing remarks followed by the responding party's closing statement, each pointing out evidence to support that side. The arbitrator studies the evidence and makes a decision. The arbitrator may issue a summary judgment shortly after the proceedings or a written decision to both parties within a month. The decision of the arbitrator is enforceable in court.

Decertification

When employees no longer want to be represented by their present union, they can request a decertification election. Management may also request an election if it is in good faith doubt that the union is representing the majority of employees. The decertification election is similar to the certification process. First a decertification petition must be signed by at least 30% of the bargaining unit to file a show of interest. In reality, more than 50% and probably closer to 75% need to show interest to guarantee a successful election. The petition is filed with the NLRB by the employer. It can be filed on the expiration date of a contract or ideally during the 30-day period before the 90-day period preceding expiration of the contract.

After receiving the decertification petition, the NLRB distributes a notice about it to the union, the petitioners, and the employer. The employer is asked to submit to the NLRB (1) names and addresses of other interested unions, (2) copies of current and recent contracts covering the employees petitioning for decertification, and (3) names and job classifications of all employees in the bargaining unit.

A preelection hearing may be scheduled if there are questions regarding representation. If neither the union nor the employer requests a hearing, an election date and time are set. The selection of the date is extremely important to the success of the election. Campaigning is limited to 24 hours before the election so that the decertification process momentum is not disrupted by a weekend. Wednesday, Thursday, or Friday are preferable days for the election. A day that will ensure maximal turnout, such as payday, is desirable. The election should be held within 3 weeks of confirmation of the election by the NLRB.

Decertification campaigns are similar to certification efforts. Managers should have various meetings, including individual meetings, small group meetings, and entire unit meetings to assure personnel that they are in good hands with management and that they will be better off without a union. However, decertification cannot be accomplished just by holding meetings during the campaign. Management needs to have earned the confidence of the employees over time through the use of good management techniques.

The NLRB conducts the election on the specified date. If the union loses the election, management stops negotiating with the union. If not, the next contract is negotiated.

Key terms used in collective bargaining are defined in Box 29-2.

NURSE MANAGERS' ROLE IN COLLECTIVE BARGAINING

Nurse managers should evaluate their management skills and take continuing education courses to improve them. Motivational techniques are particularly important for nurse administrators to possess because they work through others. They must listen carefully to staff concerns and represent staff associates' wishes to top management. Nurse administrators need to know about labor relations.

The director of nursing should not serve as the chief negotiator during collective bargaining because it would put the director in an adversary role. The agency legal representative is usually the negotiator. During negotiations, the director of nursing defines what is best for the nursing care of patients. Once the contract has been negotiated, nurse managers must learn the terms of the contract and have copies of the contract available to them. Problems should be solved through problem-solving techniques as they arise.

Box 29-2   KEY TERMS USED IN COLLECTIVE BARGAINING

Agency shop: A business where nonmembers are required to join the union as a condition of employment.

Arbitration: Procedures for using the services of a third party to settle labor disputes.

Arbitrator: The person chosen by agreement of both parties to decide the dispute between them.

Authorization cards: Cards the employees sign to authorize representation by a specific union.

Bargaining agent: A person or group accepted by an employer and chosen by members of the bargaining unit to represent them in collective bargaining.

Bargaining unit: An employee group that the state or National Labor Relations Board recognizes as an appropriate division for collective bargaining.

Certification: The official recognition by a labor organization as the exclusive bargaining agent for employees of a specific bargaining unit.

Contract violations: Acts that break the terms of a contract.

Collective bargaining: A legal process used by organized employees to negotiate with an employer about wages and related concerns resulting in an employment contract.

Deadlock: A stall in negotiations when neither party is willing to compromise about an issue.

Decertification: The withdrawal of official recognition of a union as the exclusive bargaining agent for a bargaining unit.

Grievance: Any complaint by an employer or union concerning an aspect of employment.

Grievance procedures: Steps both sides have agreed to follow to settle disputes.

Mediation: A process for settling labor disputes where a mediator helps the parties to reach their own agreements.

Open shop: A business where employees are not required to belong to the bargaining unit.*

*From Mary Foley, RN, and the Center for Labor Relations, ANA.

ADVANTAGES AND DISADVANTAGES OF COLLECTIVE BARGAINING

There are advantages and disadvantages to collective bargaining. Some equalization of power between administrators and staff associates can be obtained because of the staff associates' strength in numbers. Grievance procedures become viable, and staffing for systematic and equitable distribution of work can be established. The quality of services can be influenced. Unfortunately, an adversary relationship may develop between administration and staff associates, and strikes may not be prevented. Unionization is considered unprofessional by many nurses. Leadership for unions may be difficult to obtain, because many professional nurses have little experience in positions of authority. Women tend to view employment as a job instead of a career, minimizing interest in leadership positions, and if the bargaining unit and the professional association are the same, top administrators may have to drop membership in the professional organization, further depleting the leadership.

BIBLIOGRAPHY

Boston C: Breaking down the walls without tearing down the house . . . patient focused care, *JONA* 24:5-6, March 1994.

Flarey DL, Yoder SK, Barabas MC: Collaboration in labor relations: a model for success, *JONA* 22:15-22, September 1992.

Flarey DL: Quality circles and labor relation issues, *Nurs Econ* 7:266-269, September-October 1989.

Wilson CN, Hamilton CL, Murphy E: Union dynamics in nursing, *JONA* 20:35-39, February 1990.

CASE STUDY

In the hospital where you work, patients' length of stay is greatly reduced and the patient census is down. Nurses' time has been cut back. Nurses are increasingly dissatisfied and there is some talk of unionizing. As a manager, what can you do to reduce the felt need to unionize?

CRITICAL THINKING AND LEARNING ACTIVITIES

1. Form small groups and discuss the manager's role in the four phases of unionization. Use Worksheet 29-1 to help you identify the characteristics of the four phases.

2. Outline the decertification process, using Worksheet 29-2.

3. Interview a union member about the pros and cons of unions. Use Worksheet 29-3 to help you identify the pros and cons of the collective bargaining process in general.

✍ **Worksheet 29-1**

Phases of Unionization

Describe four phases of unionization.

Phase 1:

Phase 2:

Phase 3:

Phase 4:

✍ **Worksheet 29-2**

Decertification Process

Outline the steps in the decertification process.

Step 1:

Step 2:

Advantages and Disadvantages of Collective Bargaining

Identify advantages and disadvantages of collective bargaining:

Advantages

1.

2.

3.

4.

5.

6.

7.

8.

Disadvantages

1.

2.

3.

4.

5.

6.

7.

8.

Bibliography
Part Five

Anderson RA: *Stress power!* New York, 1981, Human Sciences Press.

Anderson RP, Fox I, Twomey D: *Business law: principles, cases, legal environment,* ed 11, Cincinnati, 1991, South Western.

Beal EF, Wickersham ED, Kienast P: *The practice of collective bargaining,* Homewood, Ill, 1972, Irwin.

Bean JJ, Laliberty R: *Understanding hospital labor relations,* Reading, Mass, 1977, Addison-Wesley.

Bennis WG, Benne K, Chin R, editors: *The planning of change,* ed 4, New York, 1985, Harcourt Brace College Publishers.

Benson H: The relaxation response, New York, 1992, Random House.

Berger MS et al, editors: *Management for nurses,* ed 2, St Louis, 1980, Mosby.

Berman HJ, Kukla SF, Weeks LE: *The financial management of hospitals,* ed 8, Ann Arbor, Mich, 1993, Health Administration Press.

Bernzweig EP: *The nurse's liability for malpractice: a programmed course,* ed 5, St Louis, 1990, Mosby.

Boyer JM, Westerhaus CL, Coggeshall JH: *Employee relations and collective bargaining in health care facilities,* St Louis, 1975, Mosby.

Brook RH: *Quality of care assessment: a comparison of five methods of peer review,* Washington, DC, 1973, United States Department of Health, Education and Welfare.

Brooten DA, Hayman LL, Naylor MD: *Leadership for change: an action guide for nurses,* Philadelphia, 1988, Lippincott.

Campbell DT, Stanley JC: *Experimental and quasi-experimental designs for research,* Chicago, 1966, Houghton Mifflin.

Carter JH et al: *Standards of nursing care: a guide for evaluation,* New York, 1976, Springer.

Cautela JR, Groden J: *Relaxation,* Champaign, Ill, 1978, Research Press.

Christian WP, Hannah GT: *Effective management in human services,* Englewood Cliffs, NJ, 1983, Prentice-Hall.

Clark CC: *Enhancing wellness: a guide for self-care,* New York, 1981, Springer.

Creighton H: *Law every nurse should know,* ed 5, Philadelphia, 1986, Saunders.

Crosby PB: *Completeness: quality for the 21st century,* New York, 1992, Dutton.

Crosby PB: *Quality without tear: the art of hassle-free management,* New York, 1984, Plume.

Davidson SVS: *PSRO: utilization and audit in patient care,* St Louis, 1976, Mosby.

Davidson SVS et al: *Nursing care evaluation,* St Louis, 1977, Mosby.

Davis K: *Human behavior at work: organizational behavior,* ed 7, New York, 1985, McGraw-Hill.

Deegan AX: *Management by objectives for hospitals,* Germantown, Md, 1982, Aspen Systems.

Duke University Hospital Nursing Services: *Guidelines for nursing care: process and outcomes,* Philadelphia, 1983, Lippincott.

Epstein C: *The nurse leader: philosophy and practice,* Norwalk, Conn, 1982, Appleton & Lange.

The Federal Mediation and Conciliation Service: *Its role in the health care industry:* ℞ *for labor peace,* Washington, DC, 1975, US Government Printing Office.

Flanagan L: *Braving new frontiers: ANA's economic and general welfare 1946–1986,* Kansas City, 1986, American Nurses' Association.

Franklin JL, Thrasher JH: *An introduction to program evaluation,* New York, 1976, Krieger.

French WL: *The personnel management process,* ed 5, Boston, 1982, Houghton Mifflin.

Ganong JM, Ganong WL: *Cases in nursing management,* Germantown, Md, 1979, Aspen Systems.

Ganong JM, Ganong WL: *Performance appraisal for productivity,* Rockville, Md, 1983, Aspen Systems.

Girdano D, Everly G: *Controlling stress and tension,* ed 4, Englewood Cliffs, NJ, 1992, Prentice-Hall.

Goldberg P: *Executive health,* New York, 1979, McGraw-Hill.

Goodman PS, Pennings M, et al: *New perspectives on organizational effectiveness,* San Francisco, 1977, Jossey-Bass.

Haack MR, Hughes TL: *Addiction in the nursing profession,* New York, 1989, Springer.

Hamrie AB, Spross J: *The clinical nurse specialist in theory and practice,* Orlando, Fla, 1989, Saunders.

Health Law Center: *Problems in hospital law,* Rockville, Md, 1974, Aspen Systems.

Hemelt MD, Mackut ME: *Dynamics of law in nursing and health care,* Reston, Va, 1978, Reston.

Hill L, Smith N: *Self-care nursing: promotion of health,* Norwalk, Conn, 1985, Appleton & Lange.

The Joint Commission on Accreditation of Healthcare Organizations: *1994 accreditation manual for hospitals,* Oakbrook Terrace, Ill, 1993, Joint Commission on Accreditation of Healthcare Organizations.

Jablonski JR: *Implementing TQM: competing in the nineties through total quality management,* ed 2, San Diego, 1992, Pfeiffer & Company.

Juran JM: *Juran on planning for quality,* New York, 1988, The Free Press.

Juran JM: *Juran on quality by design: the new steps for planning quality into goods and services,* New York, 1992, The Free Press.

Jernigan DK, Young AP: *Standards, job descriptions, and performance evaluations for nursing practice,* Norwalk, Conn, 1983, Appleton-Century-Crofts.

Johanson BC, Wells SJ, Dungca CU et al: *Standards for critical care,* St Louis, 1988, Mosby.

Kalisch BJ, Kalisch PA: *Politics of nursing,* Philadelphia, 1982, Lippincott.

Kanter RM: *The change masters,* New York, 1985, Simon & Schuster.

Katz J, Green E: *Managing quality: a guide to monitoring and evaluating nursing services,* St Louis, 1992, Mosby.

Koch MW, Fairly TM: *Integrated quality management: the key to improving nursing care quality,* St Louis, 1993, Mosby.

Kilmann RH: *Managing beyond the quick fix,* San Francisco, 1989, Jossey-Bass.

Kjervik DK, Martinson IM: *Women in stress: a nursing perspective,* New York, 1986, Saunders.

Knowles RD: *A guide to self-management strategies for nurses,* New York, 1984, Springer.

Lachman VD: *Stress management: a manual for nurses,* New York, 1983, Saunders.

Lefton RE, et al: *Effective motivation through performance appraisal,* Cambridge, Mass, 1980, Harper Business.

Lippitt G: *Visualizing change: model building and the change process,* La Jolla, Calif, 1973, University Associates.

Lippitt R, Watson J, Westley B: *The dynamics of planned change,* New York, 1958, Harcourt, Brace & World.

Luthans F, Kreitner R: *Organizational behavior modification,* ed 6, Glenview, Ill, 1992, McGraw-Hill.

Mager RF, Pipe P: *Analyzing performance problems of "you really oughta wanna,"* ed 2, Belmont, Calif, 1984, Lake.

Maier NRF: *The appraisal interview: three basic approaches,* La Jolla, Calif, 1976, University Associates.

Martel L: *Mastering change,* New York, 1986, Simon & Schuster.

Mason EJ: *How to write meaningful nursing standards,* New York, 1984, Delmar.

Mayers MG, Norby RB, Watson AB: *Quality assurance for patient care: nursing perspectives,* New York, 1977, Appleton-Century-Crofts.

McConnell EA: *Burnout: in the nursing profession,* St Louis, 1982, Mosby.

Meisenheimer CC: *Quality assurance: a programming guide to effective programs,* Rockville, Md, 1985, Aspen Systems.

Murchison IA, Nichols TS: *Legal foundations of nursing practice,* Canada, 1970, Macmillan.

Murchison I, Nichols TS, Hanson R: *Legal accountability in the nursing process,* St Louis, 1978, Mosby.

National Safety Council: *Accident prevention manual for business and industry,* ed 10, Chicago, 1992, National Safety Council.

Neale JM, Liebert RM: *Science and behavior: an introduction to methods of research,* ed 3, Englewood Cliffs, NJ, 1986, Prentice-Hall.

Nicholls ME, Wessells VG, editors: *Nursing standards and nursing process,* Rockville, Md, 1977, Aspen.

Northrop CE, Kelly ME: *Legal issues in nursing,* St Louis, 1987, Mosby.

Odiorne GS: *Management by objectives: a system of managerial leadership,* Belmont, Calif, 1965, Pitman.

Peale NV: *The power of positive thinking,* New York, 1987, Fawcett.

Pender N: *Health promotion in nursing practice,* Norwalk, Conn, 1987, Appleton & Lange.

Phaneuf MC: *The nursing audit: profile for excellence,* New York, 1972, Appleton-Century-Crofts.

Pinkerton S, Schroeder P: *Commitment to excellence,* Rockville, Md, 1988, Aspen.

Quinn JB: *Strategies for change: logical incrementation,* Homewood, Ill, 1980, Irwin.

Robert M, Weiss A: *The innovation formula,* Cambridge, Mass, 1988, Harper Business.

Rossi PH, Freeman HE: *Evaluation: a systematic approach,* ed 5, Beverly Hills, Calif, 1993, Sage.

Rutkowski B: *Managing for productivity in nursing,* Rockville, Md, 1987, Aspen.

Schaef AW: *When society becomes an addict,* San Francisco, 1988, Harper & Row.

Schein EH: *Organizational culture and leadership,* ed 2, San Francisco, 1992, Jossey-Bass.

Schroeder P: *Improving quality and performance: concepts, programs, and techniques,* St Louis, 1994, Mosby.

Selye H: *The stress of life,* ed 2, New York, 1978, McGraw-Hill.

Selye H: *Stress without distress,* New York, 1978, McGraw-Hill.

Sheridan RS, Bronstein JE, Walker DD: *The new nurse manager: a guide to management development,* Rockville, Md, 1984, Aspen.

Shortell SM, Richardson WC: *Health program evaluation,* St Louis, 1978, Mosby.

Silber MB, Marlborough JL, McLachlan EM: *Dynamic nurse management,* San Diego, Calif, 1988, Cabashon.

Smith HP, Brouwer PJ: *Performance appraisal and human development,* Reading, Mass, 1977, Addison-Wesley.

Stewart CJ, Cash WB: *Interviewing: principles and practice,* ed 7, Dubuque, Iowa, 1994, Brown & Benchmark.

Strauss G, Sayles LR: *Personnel: the human problems of management,* Englewood Cliffs, NJ, 1980, Prentice-Hall.

Sutterley DC, Donnelly GF: *Coping with stress: a nursing perspective,* Rockville, Md, 1982, Aspen Systems.

Tasto DL, Skjei EW: *Spare the couch: self-change for self-improvement,* Englewood Cliffs, NJ, 1979, Prentice-Hall.

Tucker SM: *Patient care standards,* ed 5, St Louis, 1991, Mosby.

Vash CL: *The burnt-out administrator,* ed 3, New York, 1983, Springer.

Wandelt MA, Ager JW, Walton M: *Quality patient care scale,* New York, 1974, Appleton-Century-Crofts.

Wandelt MA, Stewart D: *Slater Nursing Competencies Rating Scale,* New York, 1975, Appleton-Century-Crofts.

Warner-Reitz A: *Healthy lifestyle for seniors,* New York, 1981, Meals for Millions Freedom from Hunger Foundation.

Watson DL, Tharp RG: *Self-directed behavior,* ed 6, Monterey, Calif, 1993, Brooks/Cole.

Weiss CH: *Evaluation research,* Englewood Cliffs, NJ, 1972, Prentice-Hall.

Werther WB: *Unions do not happen, they are caused,* New York, 1978, National League for Nursing.

Werther WB, Lockhart CA: *Labor relations in the health professions,* Boston, 1976, Little, Brown.

Wilkins AL: *Developing corporate character,* San Francisco, 1989, Jossey-Bass.

Willig SH: *The nurse's guide to the law,* New York, 1970, McGraw-Hill.

Wilson CKM: *Hospital wide quality assurance: models for implementation and development,* Philadelphia, 1987, Saunders.

Appendix

Lake View Hospital

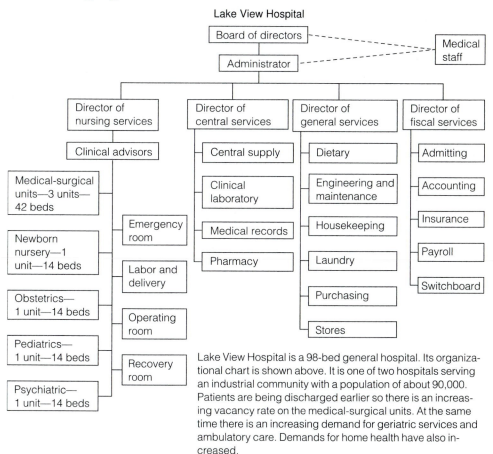

Lake View Hospital is a 98-bed general hospital. Its organizational chart is shown above. It is one of two hospitals serving an industrial community with a population of about 90,000. Patients are being discharged earlier so there is an increasing vacancy rate on the medical-surgical units. At the same time there is an increasing demand for geriatric services and ambulatory care. Demands for home health have also increased.

Organizational chart for Lake View Hospital

Appendix

General Bibliography

Bernhard L, Walsh M: *Leadership: the key to the professionalization of nursing,* St Louis, 1990, Mosby.

Brooten DA: *Managerial leadership in nursing,* Philadelphia, 1984, Lippincott.

Connor PE: *Dimensions in modern management,* ed. 3, Boston, 1982, Houghton Mifflin.

Decker PJ, Sullivan EJ: *Nursing administration: a micro/macro approach for effective nurse executives,* Norwalk, Conn, 1992, Appleton & Lange.

Dienemann J: *Nursing administration: strategic perspectives and application,* Norwalk, Conn, 1990, Appleton & Lange.

Di Vincenti M: *Administering nursing service,* ed 2, Boston, 1977, Little, Brown.

Donnelly JH Jr, Gibson JL, Ivancevich JM: *Fundamentals of management: functions, behavior, models,* Austin, Tex, 1987, Irwin.

Douglas LM: *The effective nurse,* St Louis, ed 4, 1992, Mosby.

Feldman DC, Arnold HJ: *Managing individual and group behavior in organizations,* New York, 1983, McGraw-Hill.

Ganong JM, Ganong WL: *Nursing management,* ed 2, Germantown, Md, 1980, Aspen Systems.

Gibson JL, Ivancevich JM, Donnelly JH: *Organizations: behavior, structure, processes,* Plano, Tex, 1985, Business Publications.

Gillies DA: *Nursing management: a systems approach,* ed 2, Philadelphia, 1989, Saunders.

Hampton DR, Summer CE, Webber RA: *Organizational behavior and the practice of management,* ed 5, Glenview, Ill, 1987, Scott, Foresman & Co.

Hein EC, Nicholson MJ, editors: *Contemporary leadership behavior: selected readings,* Boston, 1990, Little, Brown.

Holle ML, Blatchley ME: *Introduction to leadership and management in nursing,* ed 2, Boston, 1987, Jones & Bartlett.

Kaluzny AD, et al: *Management of health services,* Englewood Cliffs, NJ, 1982, Prentice-Hall.

Kast FE, Rosenzweig JE: *Organization and management: a systems and contingency approach,* ed 4, New York, 1985, McGraw-Hill.

Kazmier LJ: *Management: a programmed approach, with cases and applications,* ed 4, New York, 1980, McGraw-Hill.

Keane CB: *Management essentials in nursing,* Reston, Va, 1980, Appleton & Lange.

Kirk RK: *Nursing management tools,* Boston, 1981, Little, Brown.

Kreitner R, Kinicki A: *Organizational behavior,* Homewood, Ill, 1989, Irwin.

Longest BB: *Management practices for health professionals,* ed 3, Reston, Va, 1984, Appleton & Lange.

Marriner A, editor: *Contemporary nursing management: issues and practice,* St Louis, 1982, Mosby.

Marriner-Tomey A, editor: *Case studies in nursing management,* St Louis, 1990, Mosby.

McConnel CR: *The effective health care supervisor,* Rockville, Md, 1982, Aspen Systems.

Pugh DS, Hickson DJ, Heirings CR: *Writers on organizations,* Beverly Hills, Calif, 1985, Sage Publications.

Rakich JS, Longest BB, Darr K: *Managing health services organizations,* Philadelphia, 1985, Saunders.

Robbins SP: *Organizational behavior: concepts, controversies, and applications,* ed 3, Englewood Cliffs, NJ, 1983, Prentice-Hall.

Rowland HS, Rowland BL: *Nursing administration handbook,* ed 2, Germantown, Md, 1985, Aspen Systems.

Rubin IM, Fry RE, Plomick MS: *Managing human resources in health care organizations: an applied approach,* Reston, Va, 1978, Reston.

Schweiger JL: *The nurse as manager,* New York, 1986, John Wiley & Sons.

Sheridan RS, Bronstein JE, Walker DD: *The new nurse manager: a guide to management development,* Rockville, Md, 1984, Aspen Systems.

Simms LM, Price SA, Ervin NE: *The professional practice of nursing administration,* New York, 1985, John Wiley & Sons.

Stevens BJ: *The nurse as executive,* Rockville, Md, 1985, Aspen Publishers.

Stull MK, Pinkerton SE: *Current strategies for nurse administrators,* Rockville, Md, 1988, Aspen Publishers.

Sullivan EJ, Decker PJ: *Effective management in nursing,* ed 2, Reading, Mass, 1988, Addison-Wesley.

Swansburg RC: *Management and leadership for nurse managers,* Boston, 1990, Jones & Bartlett.

Veninga RL: *The human side of health administration,* Englewood Cliffs, NJ, 1982, Prentice-Hall.

Vestal KW: *Management concepts for the new nurse,* New York, 1987, Lippincott.

Young LC, Hayne AN: *Nursing administration: from concepts to practice,* Philadelphia, 1988, Saunders.

Index

Page numbers followed by *f* indicate boxes, figures or worksheets;
those followed by *t* indicate tables.